Practical Ambulatory Anesthesia

Practical Ambulatory Anesthesia

Edited by

Johan Raeder, MD, PhD
Director of Ambulatory Anesthesia, Oslo University Hospital
Professor of Anesthesiology, University of Oslo, Norway

Richard D. Urman, MD, MBA, CPE
Director of Anesthesia Services – Ambulatory Care Center (Chestnut Hill)
Associate Professor of Anesthesia, Harvard Medical School
Brigham and Women's Hospital, Boston, Massachusetts, USA

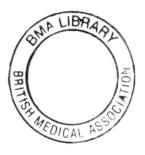

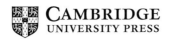

CAMBRIDGE
UNIVERSITY PRESS

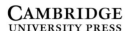

University Printing House, Cambridge CB2 8BS, United Kingdom

Cambridge University Press is part of the University of Cambridge.

It furthers the University's mission by disseminating knowledge in the pursuit of education, learning and research at the highest international levels of excellence.

www.cambridge.org
Information on this title: www.cambridge.org/9781107065345

First published 2015

Printed in the United Kingdom by TJ International Ltd. Padstow Cornwall

A catalog record for this publication is available from the British Library

Library of Congress Cataloging in Publication data
Practical ambulatory anesthesia / edited by Johan Raeder, MD, PhD,
Director of Ambulatory Anesthesia, Oslo University Hospital and
Professor of Anesthesiology, University of Oslo, Norway Richard
D. Urman, MD, MBA, CPE, Director of Anesthesia Services – Ambulatory Care Center
(Chestnut Hill), Assistant Professor of Anesthesia, Harvard Medical School,
Brigham and Women's Hospital, Boston, Massachusetts, USA.
    pages   cm
ISBN 978-1-107-06534-5 (hardback)
1. Anesthesia.   2. Ambulatory surgery.   I. Raeder, Johan.   II. Urman, Richard D.
RD82.P73   2015
617.9′6–dc23
                                                                      2015021118

ISBN 978-1-107-06534-5 Hardback

....

Contents

Contributors

Claude Abdallah, MD, MSc
Pediatric Anesthesiologist, Children's National, George Washington University, Washington, DC, USA

Fatima Ahmad, MD
Associate Professor of Anesthesiology, Director of Loyola Ambulatory Surgery Centre at Oakbrook Terrace, Loyola University Medical Center, Maywood, IL, USA

Jennifer M. Banayan, MD
Assistant Professor of Anesthesia and Critical Care, University of Chicago, Chicago, IL, USA

Sekar S. Bhavani, MD
Institute of Anesthesiology, Cleveland Clinic, Cleveland, OH, USA

Steven Butz, MD
Associate Professor of Anesthesiology, Medical College of Wisconsin, Medical Director, Children's Hospital of Wisconsin Surgicenter, Milwaukee, WI, USA

Audrice Francois, MD
Associate Professor of Anesthesiology, Loyola University Medical Center, Maywood, IL, USA

Shuchita Garg, MD
Resident Physician, Department of Anesthesia, University of Iowa Hospitals and Clinics, Iowa City, IA, USA

Sherine Hanna, MD
Associate Professor of Anesthesiology, Loyola University Medical Center, Maywood, IL, USA
VA Hines Medical Center, Hines, IL, USA

Walter G. Maurer, MD
Section Chief, Ambulatory Anesthesia, Cleveland Clinic, Cleveland, OH, USA

Neal A. Mehta, MD
Resident Housestaff, Loyola University Medical Center, Maywood, IL, USA
VA Hines Medical Center, Hines, IL, USA

Johann Patlak, MD
University of Vermont College of Medicine, Burlington, VT, USA

Johan Raeder, MD, PhD
Director of Ambulatory Anesthesia, Oslo University Hospital and Professor of Anesthesiology, University of Oslo, Norway

Niraja Rajan, MBBS
Medical Director of Hershey Outpatient Surgery Center, Assistant Professor of Anesthesiology, Penn State Milton S. Hershey Medical Center, Hershey, PA, USA

Srikantha Rao, MD, MS
Associate Professor of Anesthesiology, Penn State Milton S. Hershey Medical Center, Hershey, PA, USA

Dawn Schell, MD
Department of General Anesthesiology, Cleveland Clinic, Cleveland, OH, USA

Fred E. Shapiro, DO
Assistant Professor of Anesthesia, Beth Israel Deaconess Medical Center, Boston, MA, USA

Jaspreet Somal, MD
Department of Anesthesiology, Cleveland Clinic, Cleveland, OH, USA

Ramprasad Sripada, MD, MMM, CPE
Clinical Associate Professor, Medical Director of
Acute Pain Service, Director of Regional Anesthesia
Fellowship Program, Department of Anesthesia,
University of Iowa Hospitals and Clinics, Iowa City,
IA, USA

Bobbie-Jean Sweitzer, MD
Professor of Anesthesia and Critical Care, Professor
of Medicine, Director of Anesthesia Perioperative
Medicine Clinic, University of Chicago, Chicago, IL,
USA

John E. Tetzlaff, MD
Professor of Anesthesiology, Cleveland Clinic Lerner
College of Medicine, Case Western Reserve
University, Cleveland, OH, USA

Richard D. Urman, MD
Director of Anesthesia Services – Ambulatory
Care Center (Chestnut Hill) and Associate
Professor of Anesthesia, Harvard Medical
School, Brigham and Women's Hospital, Boston,
MA, USA

Preface

Our goal with this book is to provide an up-to-date, practical guide for the practitioners of ambulatory anesthesia. Ambulatory anesthesia incorporates most anesthetic topics and knowledge, but the focus is shifted somewhat from looking solely at what happens in the operating room to encompassing the complete perioperative period. Although safety and quality in the operating room remain major goals, the ambulatory anesthesia provider should also plan to optimize the postoperative period. Our book includes a discussion of regional anesthesia techniques, anesthesia for subspecialty surgery, and multimodal approaches to pain and postoperative nausea and vomiting. We also included a chapter on practical anesthesia "recipes" to suggest different anesthetic options for commonly performed cases. This is not an exhaustive textbook, but rather a selection of topics that we think are important in this context for the anesthesia provider. The book is partly built on ideas from Raeder, J., *Clinical Ambulatory Anaesthesia* (Cambridge University Press, 2010), but we have expanded and updated it to reflect current US practice. We have also incorporated brief discussions on important aspects of organization, unit setup, and quality assurance, as the anesthesia provider often will be the perioperative physician involved throughout the patient's treatment, from start to finish. With this book, we hope to bring forward some issues related to, and evidence for, the pragmatic and evidence-based practice of ambulatory anesthesia. However, it is important to realize that in many cases, there is no firm evidence regarding different aspects of the case. As anesthesia providers must make decisions under these circumstances, we have tried to guide you based on many years of clinical practice in most kinds of ambulatory and office-based practice. We have also tried to incorporate knowledge from our own clinical research as well as the research and teaching by many of our colleagues working in the international ambulatory anesthesia scene. We wish to express our gratitude to everyone who has worked with us over the years, for all their unceasing inspiration and good ideas. We also would like to thank our chapter contributors who are recognized experts in the field of ambulatory anesthesia. Finally, we gratefully acknowledge our colleagues, families and Cambridge University Press for their encouragement and support.

Johan Raeder
Oslo, Norway

Richard D. Urman
Boston, Massachusetts, USA

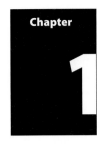

Chapter

1

Introduction to ambulatory surgery and anesthesia

Sherine Hanna, MD, Neal A. Mehta, MD, and Johan Raeder, MD, PhD

Ambulatory surgery rates have steadily increased around the world. In the United States, ambulatory surgical centers (ASCs) have seen a growth from only 2 in 1970 to 1556 in 1991.[1] Between 2004 and 2009, the number of Medicare-certified ASCs increased by 28%, growing from 4106 to 5260. Furthermore, the number of Medicare-certified ASCs grew by an average annual rate of 3.6% from 2006 through 2010.[2] This growth has been driven by improved patient safety outcomes, socioeconomic advantages, and increased patient and surgeon convenience. Studies have shown improved patient satisfaction, greater scheduling flexibility, lower morbidity and mortality, lower incidence of nosocomial infection, less dependency on hospital beds, less cognitive dysfunction, greater efficiency, and lower overall procedural costs with ambulatory surgery.[3]

As medical costs rise in the United States, third-party payers and the government are looking for cost-effective strategies to provide more economic healthcare. Physicians are also seeking facilities that provide modern equipment, easy access, and more personalized care for their patients. As the spectrum of surgeries performed in the ambulatory setting broadens, and patient complexity continues to increase, the adherence to guidelines set by the American Society of Anesthesiologists (ASA) as well as the Society of Ambulatory Anesthesia (SAMBA) is paramount. The advantages to ambulatory surgery must be coupled with a zero tolerance for mortality and severe morbidity. These are realistic goals; in two major surveys of a total of 85,000 patients from Denmark, the mortality and severe morbidity rates caused by ambulatory surgery per se were zero. As the envelope is continually being pushed, patient safety must remain a top priority.

Definitions

Ambulatory anesthesia can be defined as an anesthesiology subspecialty encompassing the preoperative, intraoperative, and postoperative anesthetic care of patients undergoing elective, same-day surgical procedures. This definition is focusing on length of hospital stay and the need for anesthetic care. Ambulatory care is different from inpatient care, as the latter is usually defined in any patient staying one or more nights in hospital.

In the US, in contrast to the rest of the world, the Centers for Medicare and Medicaid Services (CMS) State Operations Manual states that "patients admitted to an Ambulatory Surgical Center will be permitted to stay [no longer than] 23 hours and 59 minutes starting from the time of admission [to the time of discharge] after the surgical procedure".[4] Although a patient may have a 23-hour perioperative stay and still be considered "ambulatory," this black and white designation should not obscure the underlying goal of careful patient selection that ensures simple postoperative medical management at home without complications requiring intensive physician or nursing management. The goal of ambulatory surgery is to have the patient ready for discharge to a setting without healthcare staffing within the scope of a single workday. Hotel or hospital-hotel stay can be classified as "ambulatory" as long as dedicated healthcare staffing is not needed to routinely monitor the patient. Having a backup service, such as a receptionist or even a nurse when requested falls within the ambulatory concept.

Ambulatory anesthesia can also further be categorized into four types, according to the type of organization:[5]

Practical Ambulatory Anesthesia, ed. Johan Raeder and Richard D. Urman. Published by Cambridge University Press. © Cambridge University Press 2015.

1. Hospital-integrated (patients are managed in the same facility as inpatients);
2. Hospital-based (separate ambulatory surgical facility within a hospital);
3. Free-standing (surgical and/or diagnostic facility associated with a hospital without sharing space or patient-care functions);
4. Office-based (operating and/or diagnostic suites in conjunction with a physician's office).

Short history of ambulatory surgery and anesthesia

Modern ambulatory anesthesia in surgery has dated back over 150 years, with the development of general anesthesia. Actually, looking further back, the very few surgical procedures performed were usually ambulatory in the sense that they were done in private facilities – few hospitals were available, apart from in the military setting. Horace Wells first documented the use of nitrous oxide in the mid-1800s, with the first public demonstration of its use by William T.G. Morton in 1846. During the same period, while training in New York City, Crawford Long had utilized diethyl ether to anesthetize a patient for removal of neck tumors in 1842.[6] As the use of anesthetics in surgical procedures grew over the years, so did the integration of anesthesiology within office-based surgical practice.

Ralph Waters pioneered the utilization of a dedicated anesthesiologist in the office setting in 1919, which encompassed not only the delivery of anesthetics but also the organization of operating room and recovery room resources. His anesthetic practice, the Downtown Anesthesia Clinic (Sioux City, Iowa), responded to calls from healthcare providers such as dentists, and provided an operating room as well as a waiting room and small cot for recovery.[6] Decades later in 1968, an office-based anesthesia facility at the Dudley Street Facility (Providence, Rhode Island) attempted to incorporate a medical office building along with an operating suite with complete operating room facilities and recovery room. However, this setup was not supported by the state's regulatory agencies, which deemed the institution as simply another doctor's office. Shortly after, in 1969, Wallace Reed and John Ford established a free-standing ambulatory surgical center in Phoenix, Arizona, where they proved that minor surgical procedures could be completed successfully and more economically compared to hospital-based minor surgeries.[7]

Paving the way for office-based surgery and anesthesia

Within the last 200 years, the above-mentioned pioneers have laid the foundation for the mobilization of anesthesia delivery. As technology advances and the discovery of shorter-acting anesthetics with decreased side effects continues, the context in which an anesthetic can be safely and efficiently administered will continue to expand. A nice example of this is office-based anesthesia. Office-based anesthesia is a rapidly growing practice and subset of ambulatory surgery in which the operating suite is managed in conjunction with the physician's office. Although the concept of modern-day office-based anesthesia is relatively new in the United States, a model for office-based dental anesthesia has been in place for many decades in the United Kingdom, and has proven to be safe and successful. Currently, about 20% of outpatient surgical procedures in the US are performed in the office.[8]

Safety guidelines and checklists for the perioperative management of patients in the office setting have been extended from those made for free-standing ambulatory surgery centers. Office-based surgery practice guidelines have been established by the American Society of Anesthesiologists (ASA), the American Association of Nurse Anesthetists (AANA) and the The Joint Commission (TJC).[9,10]

Furthermore, checklists have been developed to ensure the safe practice of office-based anesthesia. These checklists incorporate verification of the facility (i.e., building codes, recovery area, backup power), equipment availability (i.e., backup oxygen source, Ambu-bag, emergency crash cart, patient monitors) and general preparedness (ACLS-trained staff, licensed medical doctors, quality assurance policies).[11]

The recent surge of ambulatory and office-based anesthesia centers is a testament to the feasibility of applying safe anesthetic practice to satellite locations outside of the hospital, and the increasingly "portable" nature of anesthetic delivery. However, this portability will require due diligence in assuring strict safety measures and quality control. There should also be zero tolerance for mortality and severe morbidity.

Zero tolerance for mortality/severe morbidity

When discussing the practicality of ambulatory anesthesia, as well as office-based anesthesia, it is important to touch upon the advantages and disadvantages from the perspective of: (1) safety; (2) quality; (3) economics; and (4) education and staff satisfaction.

Ambulatory surgery requires an established infrastructure within the ambulatory unit that demands a disciplined and efficient team effort. The healthcare staff needs to adopt new routines and tighter schedules, the patients need to be well informed and the surgical and anesthesia-related procedures may need to be modified to accommodate same-day discharge. The backup systems outside the hospital such as phone access, road communication, ambulance systems, and well-informed chaperones need to be functional and dependable. Adequate staffing of the recovery room is vital to a successful ambulatory surgical center, and this may be susceptible to failure given the current financial status of the institution or overall morale of the staff. In this sense, ambulatory care requires a healthy financial system that acts as an incentive for those involved rather than a disincentive, as is the case when hospital income is based on inpatient numbers.

A modern approach to ascertain whether a patient should have surgery in the ambulatory setting is to ask, "Is there any reason why this patient should stay overnight?" In doing so, criteria can be formulated that address key variables in ambulatory care such as safety, quality, and economy. Again, questions should be asked about the potential worst-case scenario and issues of perceived quality; namely, "Is the patient best served in the hospital or at home with a responsible chaperone?" An important part of this thinking is to realize that complications may arise both with an inpatient and ambulatory plan for the patient. The key question will be if the ambulatory setting increases the risk of an unfavorable outcome per se, and whether the cost–benefit of choosing an inpatient status is reasonable.

Safety in ambulatory care

Prior to scheduling an ambulatory surgical procedure, a thorough preoperative evaluation of the patient is necessary to determine if they are an appropriate candidate for ambulatory surgery. The following contraindications may warrant postponement of surgery or inpatient surgical intervention: anticipation of significant blood loss or postoperative complication, concurrent unstable or serious illness, poorly compensated systemic disease, need for invasive monitoring, and inability or unwillingness to understand perioperative instructions.[11] When appropriate

preoperative evaluation and patient selection occurs, ambulatory surgery has shown to be safe with low associated morbidity. Studies show that unanticipated admission to the hospital and return visits occur in less than 3% of ambulatory surgical procedures.[12] In a study of more than 45,000 patients for 30 days after an ambulatory surgical procedure, Warner et al. concluded that the major morbidity (i.e., respiratory, circulatory, cardiac) was similar to that in the general population not having surgery.[13] In a more recent study of 18,500 Danish ambulatory surgical patients, there were no cases of death or permanent disability that could be ascribed to the procedure during a 90-day follow-up.[14] However, such safety data are a result of qualified care with already high standards. In a study of ambulatory liposuction in Florida, Vila et al. found a 10-fold increase in mortality when these procedures were performed in physicians' offices with improper standards, compared with licensed ambulatory centers.[15] This study, however, likely overestimated patient mortality rates.

Summary of key points regarding safety in ambulatory care:

(a) The safety is very close to 100% when proper ambulatory care is undertaken, thus emphasizing the need for zero tolerance for serious errors in patient handling.

(b) Ambulatory surgery is safe because of high standards of care. If the standards are suboptimal, ambulatory surgery (as well as inpatient surgery) may not be safe and acceptable.

(c) Some procedures and patients will continue to have higher risks of rare and/or serious complications that may not be completely avoidable by doing the procedure either in an inpatient or in an ambulatory setting. Thus, care for ambulatory patients should be carried out using the same standards and necessary resources as care rendered to inpatients.

Quality assurance

Quality assurance and improvement play a key role in maintaining the high standards of outpatient care that allow for ambulatory anesthesia to be both safe and effective. In the US, quality standards for ambulatory centers are enforced by The Joint Commission (TJC), which is the same organization that accredits inpatient facilities. Both the ASA and Accreditation Association for Ambulatory Health Care (AAAHC) and the American Association for the Accreditation of Ambulatory Surgery Facilities (AAAASF) have established guidelines for ambulatory and office-based anesthesia as well.[16]

There are a number of quality of care considerations favoring ambulatory care, which are listed below:

(a) The risk of having a hospital infection is reduced as the patients are subjected to less of the hospital environment, both in terms of exposure duration and also because ambulatory surgery centers are usually less contaminated by seriously ill inpatients. In a study done by Grogaard et al., the rate of infection after mixed ambulatory surgery during a 30-day observation period was 3.4%, being mostly benign, superficial wound infections.[17] The infection rate in comparable inpatients was in the range of 5–15%. Also in a study by Holtz and Wenzel the infection rate was about 3 times higher in inpatients when compared with ambulatory surgery.[18]

(b) Reversible cognitive dysfunction for some weeks or even months after surgery may be seen in up to 20–40% of the patients, more frequently with older age and extensive surgery.[19] The risk of cognitive dysfunction 1 week after hernia repair in elderly patients was significantly reduced from 9.8% with inpatient care to 3.8% (similar to nonoperated) after ambulatory care.[20] This seems logical: elderly patients especially, as well as psychiatric patients, patients with cerebral dysfunction, and children, may all be stressed and confused by being subjected to an unfamiliar environment and unfamiliar people, and the longer the exposure and more strangers involved the worse the effect. Thus, it is beneficial for these types of patients to be discharged back to their familiar environment as soon as possible.[21]

(c) Less internal transport and fewer caregivers allow for a shorter chain of treatment in ambulatory care, usually involving the same caregivers throughout the duration of recovery. This increases continuity in terms of information provided and results in fewer miscommunications.

(d) Less bed rest and immobility allow for less post-operative morbidity. This contrasts with the inpatient setting, where being immobilized for extended periods of time may cause complications with gut function, lung function, deep vein thrombosis, and overall feelings of wellness.

(e) Fewer delays and cancellations occur in the ambulatory setting. The ambulatory surgical path is usually organized with its own nursing staff and dedicated facilities. The risk of a case being postponed because of an incidental burden from emergency care surgery or because there is no space in the post-anesthesia care unit (PACU) is decreased when compared to the mix of facilities with major inpatient surgeries.

(f) "Home is best." If you ask patients where they want to be after surgery, provided that they feel safe, have no nausea and have well-managed pain, they usually prefer to be in the comfort of their own home.

Economic considerations

It is beyond the scope of this book to discuss the economics of the ambulatory healthcare system in detail. In brief, however, it can help decrease expenses associated with nursing care and patient accommodation, especially in the late evening and overnight. The costs of doing the procedure, including all costs related to surgery and anesthesia, are basically the same as if the patient were an inpatient.

Still, the situation may not be so simple. For a single hospital or unit to achieve such savings, the ambulatory program needs to be large enough to produce reduced staffing levels. Alternatively, the program needs to be predictable enough to release beds to other patients, thus increasing hospital production rather than saving money. In order for patients to have a rapid and uneventful recovery, more expensive anesthetic drugs may have to be used, but this expenditure may be recouped in reduced length of time in the operating room and reduced stay and need for nursing care in the PACU. Furthermore, perioperative ambulatory stays usually tend to avoid the dogmatic use of routine laboratory testing that may be present in the inpatient setting, thus further reducing costs and resource expenditure. The involvement of fewer caregivers reduces the need for patient handover and reduces the extent of double documentation, which is often seen when many people are involved with one patient. Establishment of an ambulatory service may by itself improve the efficiency of the hospital, as a large amount of work occurs in a predictable manner with few cancellations and no interruptions or disputes over emergent cases.

A potential cost problem with ambulatory care occurs when very expensive equipment (e.g., laparoscopy racks, robots, etc.) is used only during the daytime. However, this may be solved by having dedicated afternoon surgical cases or by using the equipment in other places in the hospital when the ambulatory operating room is down. Ambulatory care may also become expensive when a large number of patients are unexpectedly admitted following surgery, if they need a lot of expert care after being sent home, or if there is a high rate of unplanned readmission.

Education and staff satisfaction

Healthcare staff, as most other people, are usually less inclined to work during evenings, nights, and weekends. Thus, staff recruitment and retention in ambulatory care units is usually very good. However, there is some concern that ambulatory surgery care units are too predictable and rarely present with emergencies and difficult situations, thus providing a less enriching and stimulating environment from an academic standpoint. This may be overcome by having personnel rotate in and out of the unit for those that are interested, and by having regular training in simulated emergency scenarios, such as advanced cardiopulmonary resuscitation. For the anesthesiologist, it may be useful to undergo these emergency-type simulations or to attend training sessions encompassing basic troubleshooting when managing patients with difficult airway, anaphylaxis, and invasive procedures.

As ambulatory surgery becomes more extensive, it is necessary to make the ambulatory unit an area of education and training for medical students, residents, surgeons, anesthesiologists, and nurses. This may be accomplished by requiring dedicated resources, such as instructors and time allotted for perioperative teaching. This can be accomplished without significantly delaying case performance, turnover times, or quality of care.[22]

References

1. Durant GD. Expanding the scope of ambulatory surgery in the USA. *Ambulatory Surgery* 1993;**1**:173–78.

2. Medicare Payment Advisory Commission. Report to the Congress: Medicare Payment Policy. Washington, DC, 2013.

3. Snyder DS, Pasternak LR. Facility design and procedural safety. In White PF, ed. *Ambulatory Anesthesia and Surgery*. London: WB Saunders; 1997.

4. Centers for Medicare and Medicaid Services. State Operations Manual: Appendix L – Guidance for Surveyors: Ambulatory Surgical Centers. Rev. **89**, 08-30-13.

5. White PF, ed. *Textbook of Ambulatory Anesthesia and Surgery*. London: WB Saunders; 1997.

6. Waters RM. The Downtown Anesthesia Clinic. *Am J Surg Anesthesia* 1919;Suppl **71**.

7. Reed WA, Ford JL. Development of an independent outpatient surgical center. *Int Anesthesiol Clin* 1976 Summer;**14**(2):113–30.

8. James DW. General anaesthesia, sedation and resuscitation in dentistry. *Br Dent J* 1991 Dec 7–21;**171** (**11–12**):345–47.

9. Boysen PG. Ancillary site and office based anesthetic care: 48th annual refresher course lectures and clinical update program. *ASA* 1997;**154**.1–7.

10. American Society of Anesthesiologists. Guidelines for Office-Based Anesthesia, 2009. Available at: https://www.asahq.org/For-Members/Standards-Guidelines-and-Statements.aspx (last accessed July 30, 2014).

11. Twersky RS, Philip BK, ed. *Handbook of Ambulatory Anesthesia*, 2nd ed. New York, NY: Springer; 2008.

12. Gold BS, Kitz DS, Lecky JH. Unanticipated admission to the hospital following ambulatory surgery. *JAMA* 1989;**262**:3008.

13. Warner MA, Shields SE, Chute CG. Major morbidity and mortality within 1 month of ambulatory surgery and anesthesia. *JAMA* 1993;**270**:1437–41.

14. Engbaek J, Bartholdy J, Hjortso NC. Return hospital visits and morbidity within 60 days after day surgery: a retrospective study of 18,736 day surgical procedures. *Acta Anaesthesiol Scand* 2006;**50**:911–19.

15. Vila H, Jr., Soto R, Cantor AB, Mackey D. Comparative outcomes analysis of procedures performed in physician offices and ambulatory surgery centers. *Arch Surg* 2003;**138**:991–95.

16. Frezza EE, Girnys RP, Silich RJ, Coppa GF. Commentary: Quality of care and cost containment are the hospital-based ambulatory surgery challenges for the future. *Am J Med Qual* 2000;**15**:114.

17. Grogaard B, Kimsas E, Raeder J. Wound infection in day-surgery. *Ambul Surg* 2001;**9**:109–12.

18. Holtz TH, Wenzel RP. Postdischarge surveillance for nosocomial wound infection: a brief review and commentary. *Am J Infect Control* 1992;**20**:206–13.

19. Rasmussen LS. Postoperative cognitive dysfunction: incidence and prevention. *Best Pract Res Clin Anaesthesiol* 2006;**20**:315–30.

20. Canet J, Raeder J, Rasmussen LS, *et al.* Cognitive dysfunction after minor surgery in the elderly. *Acta Anaesthesiol Scand* 2003;**47**:1204–10.

21. Ward B, Imarengiaye C, Peirovy J, Chung F. Cognitive function is minimally impaired after ambulatory surgery. *Can J Anaesth* 2005;**52**:1017–21.

22. Skattum J, Edwin B, Trondsen E, *et al.* Outpatient laparoscopic surgery: feasibility and consequences for education and health care costs. *Surg Endosc* 2004;**18**:796–801.

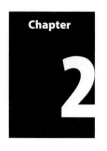

Organization of ambulatory surgery and anesthesia

Audrice Francois, MD, and Johan Raeder, MD, PhD

A. Physical organization

Ambulatory surgery centers (ASCs) are modern healthcare facilities focused on providing same-day surgical care, including diagnostic and preventive procedures. As there is a steadily increasing demand for ambulatory surgical procedures, there are different levels of organizing ambulatory surgery facilities; from a single ambulatory case performed between scheduled inpatient procedures in an inpatient organization, to hospital outpatient departments (HOPDs), to centers dedicated completely to ambulatory surgical care, Ambulatory Surgery Center (ASC), as well as Office-Based Surgery (OBS) centers.[1] There are as many ASCs as there are hospitals in the United States. The first ASCs were established in the early 1970s. ASCs numbered 1000 in 1988. In 2013, there were over 5000.

ASCs have transformed the outpatient experience for millions of people, providing them with a more convenient alternative to hospital-based procedures. The growth in ASCs parallels a historic shift away from hospital inpatient surgeries. Many factors have contributed to this growth in ASCs, including changes in population demographics, new surgical and diagnostic techniques, changes in population health guidelines for disease screening, shorter-acting anesthetic agents, consumer and physician preferences, and payer incentives and reimbursement decisions to pay for care in the most cost-effective settings. ASCs offer alternative sites for surgical care including diagnostic and preventive procedures that do not require an overnight stay.[2]

The single ambulatory patient integrated in an inpatient organization

In this instance, the patients are integrated within an inpatient organization. It is planned in advance that they are to be discharged home after surgery. This model may be the only option in hospitals where mainly inpatient care is provided, or in very small hospitals. This may also be the model used when trying to expand ambulatory care services to new patient categories, using it as a pilot project for expanding ambulatory care. If the patient's perioperative course is uneventful and the patient fulfils discharge criteria, the patient is sent home. If, however, care aspects such as analgesia, safety or anti-emesis are not met, the patient may be required to stay overnight. When it becomes evident that most of the patients in this new category actually go home, a new ambulatory patient treatment chain has been smoothly and effectively established.

The ambulatory program as part of an inpatient organization

When the ambulatory program is part of an inpatient organization, ambulatory care can be planned for the entire perioperative course. Preoperative instruction, intraoperative care such as choice of premedication, anesthetic, anti-emetic drugs, and minimizing opioids, as well as using cardiovascular, hormonal, and fluid therapies that focus on achieving an uneventful and fast recovery, can be tailored for an ambulatory patient. There should be an area as well as personnel dedicated fully to ambulatory care, with a phase 2 recovery room and a discharge area. The integration with inpatients usually occurs in the preoperative room and operating room which is part of the inpatient hospital facility. The hospital may attain better cost-efficiency through the fuller utilization of operating rooms and specialized equipment. These facilities can offer patients shorter waiting times. The downside is in coordinating those parts of the treatment pathways that are shared with inpatients. This includes having personnel who may not be wholly dedicated to providing ambulatory care.

The ambulatory unit integrated into an inpatient hospital

The ambulatory unit may be part of the hospital, but is run totally separate from the inpatient program. This occurs when there are enough ambulatory patients to run an ambulatory unit; however, major facilities are provided by the inpatient hospital. The unit runs five full days a week, with the hospital employing a dedicated ambulatory staff for all preoperative and postoperative care, and providing the patients with the comfort of not being exposed to the full hospital setting. Usually, this is a unit with a reception area, a preoperative holding area and a recovery area, and a discharge area. The integration with inpatients usually occurs in the operating rooms which is part of the inpatient hospital facility.

The benefit of this organization is that it enables the hospital to take full advantage of employing a dedicated ambulatory staff for all preoperative and postoperative care. The hospital may attain better cost-efficiency through the shared use of expensive operating rooms and specialized equipment for an increased total number of hours per week than can be achieved with two fully separate locations. The downside remains the demanding logistics implicit in coordinating those parts of the treatment pathways that are shared with inpatients. Problems may arise through having personnel who are not dedicated to ambulatory care and the potential for cancellation or delays of the ambulatory patient should the inpatient organization become overloaded with emergency cases.

The free-standing ambulatory unit inside the inpatient hospital

The ambulatory program has its own premises and dedicated perioperative staff, with the exception of maybe the anesthesiologists and the surgeons who are often employed by the mother hospital. The positive aspect of this model is that the hospital is readily available to provide backup for any extra testing, unplanned transition to inpatient care, for any prolonged recovery and unexpected emergencies. The doctors also have some flexibility in managing their

time across hospital tasks and ambulatory care. The negative aspects are that an ambulatory case may have to wait for a doctor who is not dedicated to the ambulatory program.

The free-standing ambulatory unit as a satellite of the inpatient hospital

In this model, the ambulatory unit is physically separate from the rest of the hospital, either at the end of a long corridor, or in a separate building some distance away, but still close enough for access to expertise or unplanned admissions. Being geographically distant protects the ambulatory personnel from being moved to provide inpatient care if the main hospital is experiencing staff shortages or other problems. The downside of being at a distance is the more demanding logistics for patient transportation when extra tests or evaluations are needed, or in cases of emergencies or unplanned admissions.

The free-standing ambulatory unit or hospital

The free-standing ambulatory unit has all the benefits of being a separate unit in terms of personnel, routines, productivity, and economy. Having a fully separate unit makes it easier for cost-efficiency measures and to have separate budgets and accounting. It is also easier to promote team-building and to allow everyone in the treatment chain to reap the benefits of working together efficiently to get the cases done without delay, so as to avoid having to remain after hours. Short turnaround times and specialized focus by nurses and other support staff increase the efficiency. These offer the patients shorter waiting times, more convenient locations, ease in scheduling surgeries, lower co-payments and overall higher patient satisfaction with their experience. Physicians may have better control over staffing decisions and the ability to better manage their work environment. A larger ambulatory unit may also have its own ancillary services such as radiology, cardiology, and laboratories. Although the ambulatory unit may screen the patients for appropriateness for day surgery procedures, there will always be the need for the patient with a rare or serious complication to be admitted to an inpatient hospital, and this should be included in the planning. There may be a need to establish connections with a neighboring inpatient hospital should such a need arise.

What is the optimal size of a unit?

Unit size is usually defined as the number of operating rooms and surgical teams working simultaneously within it. Two major aspects are important in this context: the bigger the unit's size, the greater the flexibility in the use of personnel and equipment, and the bigger unit's size requires more managerial work to organize, coordinate, and plan for maximum benefit. Bigger units may be better able to handle staff absences, unpredictable length of cases, and other unforeseen circumstances.

Having only one operating room may work well and efficiently if the turnover time between patients is not too great, and there are enough instruments so that delays are avoided while equipment is being sterilized. With two operating rooms, two teams may work in parallel or, if the cases are short, one surgeon may utilize both rooms to optimize time. In systems with nurse anesthetists, one anesthesiologist may supervise up to four operating rooms.[3]

Free-standing office-based practice

These units almost always concentrate on a narrow selection of procedures, for instance solely dental surgery, ear, nose and throat (ENT), plastic surgery, gastrointestinal endoscopies, and so on. Most of these will also place restraints on patient selection so as to avoid serious complications and problems. These units can be very efficient, having very stable teams as they are focused on one type of patient and surgery. However, they can be lulled into a false sense of security as a consequence of infrequent exposure to problems, and not have adequate safety measures, fully qualified staffing, and all the requirements for the safe running of the center. Should a rare and occasional serious complication occur, the whole clinic may be under threat and investigated to see whether formal safety aspects and backup routines were adequate.

There is a growing trend for surgeries to be done in a doctor's office.[4] This offers the convenience of having the procedure in what may be perceived as a more comfortable setting and with a quick return home. However, the procedure should be of a duration and degree of complexity such that the patient will recover and be discharged from the facility within a reasonably short period of time.

Surgical complexity in the office-based practice may range from Level 1 surgery, such as the excision of moles, warts, and cysts that require minimal preoperative sedation, to Level 3 surgery which includes procedures that would require general anesthesia or major conduction blocks. Healthcare practitioners themselves establish written policies regarding the specific surgical procedures that may be performed in their office. Procedures that involve significant blood loss, or major body cavities such as intra-abdominal or intra-thoracic, are not appropriate for the office setting.

Patient selection should be appropriate for the office setting. Although the lack of precise definitions for each ASA physical status can result in inconsistent ratings between practitioners, the ASA physical status of the patient should be considered, as it is the single most important predictor of morbidity and mortality for general surgery. Each office should establish guidelines that delineate criteria for patient selection for the office procedure, and should consider the patient's medical status and comorbidities, the degree of stability of the medical conditions, the psychological state of the patient as well as the support system in place for accompanying the patient from the office and caring for the patient postoperatively.

The anesthesiologist providing care in the office setting should follow the standards and guidelines adopted by the American Society of Anesthesiologists in order to ensure the same measures of safety to all patients regardless of the venue of their surgery. The same anesthesia techniques used in hospitals and ASCs are used in office-based surgery centers. Problems for such units are ensuring that they fulfill all the requirements for patient safety.

Non-operating room anesthetizing locations

In the United States, the ASA Standards Guidelines and Policies should be adhered to in all non-operating room settings, except where they are not applicable to the individual patient or care setting. The European Society of Anaesthesiologists (ESA) as well as the World Federation of Societies of Anaesthesiologists (WFSA) have similar standards for patient care. Prior to administering any anesthetic, the anesthesiologist should consider the capabilities, limitations, and accessibility of the oxygen sources, and adequate and reliable sources of suction. There should be adequate monitoring equipment to allow adherence to the ASA "Standards for Basic Anesthetic Monitoring" and sufficient electrical outlets to satisfy anesthesia machine and monitoring equipment requirements. Appropriate post-anesthesia care should be provided, and there should be adequate staff to provide support for the anesthesiologist. An emergency cart with a defibrillator should be available, as well as emergency drugs and other equipment adequate to provide immediate cardiopulmonary resuscitation if necessary.

B. What is needed to run an ambulatory anesthesia practice?

For further reference it may be recommended to check the rules of accreditation for your unit in your institution or state. The ASA has published practice guidelines for ambulatory settings that address all aspects of patient care and facility administration.[5]

Equipment

Basic monitoring equipment should be available in all facilities: noninvasive blood pressure monitoring, electrocardiography, pulse oximetry, capnography for all intubations and all types of anesthetics, suction, gas monitoring of oxygen and all inhalational gases and patient temperature monitoring.[5] Scavenger systems should be present for all inhalational anesthetics. Alarms to alert to problems of gas delivery and low oxygen content in the ventilation gas should be available. In units carrying out more extensive surgery and for fragile patients, the ability to measure blood pressure invasively should be an option. Appropriate anesthesia apparatus and equipment should allow monitoring consistent with Society of Anesthesia standards, and all equipment should be maintained, tested, and inspected according to the manufacturer's specifications, and documentation of regular preventive maintenance as recommended by the manufacturer should be followed.

Anesthesia professionals interact with many different types of monitors, machines, infusion pumps, and other equipment. Many of these devices have audible and/or visual alarms which are relied on to signal when set parameters and thresholds are violated, or when a potentially abnormal situation has occurred. Alarm systems must be such as to balance patient and provider safety risks against unintended consequences such as distraction, alarm fatigue, and intrusiveness. Alarm system settings in the equipment should be locally customized to reflect the patients and the practice, and should have an institutional

process for changing any default alarm settings. Individual anesthesia professionals should not be able to change default alarm settings of any anesthesia equipment. Anesthesia professionals should adjust alarm settings as appropriate for a particular patient prior to starting an anesthetic. Clinicians should not indefinitely silence or disable alarms on any given device, unless it is necessary either because the device or module is not in use, or has malfunctioned, or the patient's medical condition supports the AUDIO OFF or ALARM OFF modes.

Backup systems

Spare tanks of oxygen should always be ready for immediate use. In the case of emergencies, there must be fast access to a self-expanding ventilation bag with reservoir and extra oxygen supply, a defibrillator and emergency drugs, and intubation devices for difficult intubations: stylet, bougie, supraglottic airways, extra laryngoscopes, and fiber-optic or video laryngoscopic devices. Where neuraxial and regional blocks or extensive use of local anesthetics (e.g., liposuction) are being performed, there should be access to intravenous lipid emulsions for rescue in the event of local anesthetic-induced toxicity. Where inhalational anesthesia and/or succinylcholine are used, there should be medications, equipment, and written protocols to treat malignant hyperthermia (see chapter on Emergencies for details).

There should be backup electrical power sufficient to ensure patient safety in the event of an emergency and reliable means of two-way communication to request assistance. There should be written protocols for cardiopulmonary emergencies and other internal disasters such as a fire. All access to exit stairwells should be marked by illuminated signs that are on emergency power. The unit should have a written protocol in place for the safe and timely transfer of patients to a pre-specified alternate care facility when extended care or emergencies are needed in order to protect the health and well-being of the patient. For each location, all applicable building and safety codes and facility standards, where they exist, should be observed.[6]

Emergency procedures

Because disasters may occur, it is important that the ambulatory facility has written policies as to what should be done and who should do it. Disasters can be external, including tornado, hurricane, flood, earthquake, or war. Internal disasters include fire, bomb, explosion, loss of power, equipment malfunction, loss of oxygen, a hostage situation, or a disturbed employee, patient, or visitor. There should be a specific disaster manager or a designee to immediately assume responsibility for the implementation of the disaster plan to see that the police and fire departments are notified, coordinate information, and direct personnel. The designee will also determine whether evacuation of patients is necessary and by what route.

Security of medications

Safe storage and security of medications is a fundamental care process. A secure environment is needed for medication safety, including security of oral, sublingual, parenteral and inhaled drugs, and drugs used for elective and emergency patient care. Confirming that refrigerated items are stored under proper conditions is essential. Security of medications in the operating room suite is essential for patient safety. All schedule 3 and 4 medications must be kept in a locked, controlled area and only authorized persons should have access to controlled substances. A monitoring system for drug safety and security is an essential part of any ASC organization.

Education and training

Anesthesiology is the practice of medicine.[5] Clinical privileges in anesthesiology are granted to physicians who are qualified by training to render patients insensible to pain and to minimize stress during surgical and certain medical procedures using general anesthesia, regional anesthesia, or monitored anesthesia care. In the United States, and in accordance with the ASA Guidelines, criteria to be considered for privileges in anesthesia include the following.

1. Graduation from a medical school accredited by the Liaison Committee on Medical Education (LCME), from an osteopathic medical school or program accredited by the American Osteopathic association (AOA), or from a foreign medical school that provides medical training acceptable to and verified by the Educational Commission on foreign Medical Graduates (ECFMG).
2. Completion of an anesthesiology residency training program approved by the Accreditation Council for Graduate Medical Education (ACGME) or by the AOA.
3. Permanent certification by the American Board of Anesthesiology (ABA) or current recertification within the time interval required by the ABA.
4. Compliance with the ABA Maintenance of Certification in Anesthesiology program (MOCA).
5. Completion of Continuing Medical Education requirements (CME).
6. Compliance with relevant state or institutional requirements.
7. Demonstration of competence in Basic Life Support (BLS), Advanced Cardiac Life support (ACLS), and Pediatric Advanced Life Support (PALS) where applicable.
8. Current, active, unrestricted medical, or osteopathic license in a United States state, district, or territory of practice.
9. Current, unrestricted Drug Enforcement Administration (DEA) registration.

Subspecialty training is available for critical care medicine, pain medicine, pediatric anesthesiology, cardiothoracic anesthesiology, obstetric anesthesiology, and completion of the certification examination in perioperative trans-esophageal echocardiography.

Organizations may have a mixture of required and optional criteria and should determine which criteria to include and whether to include additional criteria based on the institution's individual requirements and preferences. Some facilities may decide that certification by the Board of Anesthesia (American Board of Anesthesiology or in Europe, the European Board of Anaesthesiology) is a requirement, while others may deem board certification to be desirable but not essential. Some organizations may require subspecialty fellowship training for certain clinical privileges. Some organizations may wish to recognize residency training or certification awarded outside of the United States.

Staff

Professional staff should include physicians and other practitioners and nurses. They should hold a valid license or certificate and be qualified to perform their assigned duties. The anesthesiologist must be personally responsible to each patient for the provision of anesthetic care. The physician anesthesiologist is responsible for performing and verifying an appropriate pre-anesthesia evaluation of the patient, medical management of the anesthetic procedure and of the patient during surgery, post-anesthetic evaluation and care, supervision of resident physicians, and medical direction of any non-physicians who assist in providing anesthesia care to the patient. This includes a review of any medically indicated studies and consultations, and abnormalities of major organ systems, and should develop a plan of anesthetic care.[7]

The anesthesiologist should be satisfied that the procedure to be undertaken is within the scope of practice of the healthcare practitioners and within the capabilities of the facility. The ASA believes that anesthesiologist participation in all office-based surgery is optimally desirable as an important anesthesia patient safety standard. Where anesthesiologist participation is not a practical matter, non-physician anesthesia providers must, at a minimum, be directed by a licensed physician or by the operating practitioner, who should be immediately available for diagnosis and management of any anesthesia-related complications.

In many countries, and also some US states, a nurse anesthetist or resident trainee will maintain the anesthetic assisted by the physician during induction and emergence, and in most countries nurses will take care of postoperative surveillance with the physician as a backup. In the cases of moderate or deep sedation administered by non-anesthesia providers, appropriate training and education should be mandatory for all cases where there is a risk of obstructed airway or apnea, and the provider should be dedicated to that task and the individual patient continuously. Non-anesthesia sedation with moderate doses of approved conventional opioids, benzodiazepines, and sometimes propofol is allowed to be given under the supervision of any doctor, who is ultimately responsible for that treatment. However, sedation is recognized by the ASA as a continuum ranging from anxiolysis to moderate sedation and analgesia, to deep sedation and analgesia, to general anesthesia. Therefore, the use of a pulse oximeter is required, as is the dedicated and continuous surveillance of the patient. Local anesthesia is often used by surgeons and proceduralists, but care should be taken to obey the rules of maximum dosing and toxicity, especially important in plastic surgery where large doses are sometimes used in tumescent solutions for liposuction.

The administration of regional anesthesia should generally be reserved for trained anesthesia providers, although some surgeons are adequately trained in dedicated blocks for eye surgery and hernia surgery as well as in intravenous regional anesthesia.

Neuraxial anesthesia, paravertebral blocks and deep plexus nerve blocks should be done by anesthesia providers and monitored by anesthesia-trained personnel. Continual patient monitoring is mandatory throughout these cases.[8]

In the post-anesthesia care unit (PACU), the patients should be monitored by nurses specially trained in the handling of emergencies of ventilation, circulation, and surgical complications such as bleeding. They are required to have appropriate knowledge of pain and nausea evaluation and treatment. A dedicated professional should monitor the patient continuously until the patient is discharged from the PACU. Immediate access to the anesthesiologist should be possible. The physician anesthesiologist is the key perioperative physician in facilitating the recovery phase and should play a pivotal role in establishment of guidelines for patient discharge criteria. Patients who receive anesthetics should be discharged with a responsible adult. Personnel with training in advanced resuscitative techniques, that is, advanced cardiac life support (ACLS) and, where children are treated, pediatric advanced life support (PALS) should be immediately available until all patients are discharged from the facility. The patient should have written postoperative and follow-up care instructions relative to the type of surgery and anesthesia that has been undergone. The patient should also be given information about important potential complications and how to get immediate and adequate contact with healthcare services on a 24-hour basis.

In the United States, the anesthesiologist is encouraged by the ASA to play a leadership role as the perioperative physician in all ambulatory surgical facilities and anesthetizing locations.[1] Specific anesthesia training for medically supervising is especially important in office-based centers where normal institutional backup or emergency facilities and capabilities are often not available. The anesthesiologist should participate in facility accreditation in order to have standardization of practice and to maintain a high quality of patient care that is consistent with industry standards. The physician in a leadership role who provides medical care in the facility should also be responsible for reviewing credentials, delineation of privileges of the professionals, and participation in quality assurance reviews. An ambulatory facility should have qualified staff available to handle emergencies and unforeseen contingencies, such as patient transfer to an emergency room or hospital.

C. Patient flow

In the ambulatory care unit, there is a need for separate areas for preoperative care, the operation, and for postoperative care. In the office-based setting, these may all be in the same office if the surgery is minor and the risk of contamination is minimal, which includes dental procedures, gastrointestinal endoscopies, or vaginal gynecologic procedures. Otherwise, the demands of minimal contamination will require a separate operating room with increased standards for hand washing, draping, wearing of masks and hygiene of the personnel.

In the operating room, there should be a dedicated telephone or calling system or emergency button for immediately summoning assistance in critical situations. In office-based settings it is especially important to pay attention to facilities for resuscitation, access to the emergency cart, and a method of enabling the transportation of the patient on a stretcher out of the unit and into an ambulance should the need arise. Also elevator breakdown should be considered, so there should be access to a stairway that is large enough for a stretcher to pass through, or for a semi-upright stretcher that may be taken down a narrow stairway.

The preoperative area may be divided into a reception area in which the patient arrives, a preoperative or holding area where the patient is dressed in a hospital gown and ready for surgery, and in some cases an induction room for anesthesia or establishment of blocks. The postoperative area may be divided into a PACU with monitoring of the patient's vital functions, and a phase II recovery with or without technical monitoring in which the patient sits in a chair waiting for discharge. There should be a room for private conversations and consultations with patients' families individually. In units with a mixture of children and adults, it is wise to have a separate area for children, and even further separation for children who are crying and distressed. Separate areas for children are also useful because of the need to involve parents more extensively in all phases of the stay, except the operation itself.[1]

The pre- and postoperative areas may follow different flow charts. In a pull-through organization, the patient comes into the facility via one route and leaves via a different one. In a race-track organization, the patient leaves one area for surgery and returns to it afterwards, thus coming into and leaving the facility via the same route. The benefits of the race-track organization are that the patients may be treated by the same nursing staff before and after surgery, the postoperative premises are familiar and the staff may be better employed throughout the day, with predominantly preoperative care early on and postoperative care at the end of the day. The benefits of a pull-through organization are that preoperative patients do not intermingle with postoperative patients and relatives, the premises and personnel can be more fully dedicated to either pre- or postoperative care, and it is easier to keep good track of where patients are in the perioperative process. Generally, a race-track organization is best for small units, whereas a pull-through organization may better serve the needs of big units.

Hospital hotels

Some large centers that attract patients from afar may utilize hospital hotels where general hotel amenities are offered and patient comfort and privacy are maintained. These serve as an extension of the hospital environment to welcome individuals who are visiting the facility, and to help accommodate patients and families who are coming from afar. They can also serve patients who may not need medical care continuously but who may need more support than can be given at home postoperatively after same-day surgery. The model is based on a system used in Scandinavia, with hotel chains running the service on hospital sites. In this way, patients' needs, clinical and otherwise, can be met, enhancing the patients' experience which is made a priority. They can afford quick access to specialist consultants should the patient need urgent treatment. Communication from the room to reception area may be by telephone or by emergency buttons, operated by the patient or a friend/relative staying with him/her. Basically the hotel is staffed with non-medical personnel, but there are also organizational models with nurses making rounds or special floors with enhanced nurse presence, representing a near-transition to ordinary hospital wards.

D. Accreditation and safe practice

ASCs are regulated in many ways and compliance to these regulations is a major focus of practice. They are subject to rigorous oversight and independent inspections to assess each center's level of compliance with both state and national standards. In the United States, most ambulatory surgery centers are licensed, certified, and accredited by one of the major healthcare accrediting organizations. Most ASCs provide care to Medicare beneficiaries, and thus must meet the standards of the Center for Medicare and Medicaid Services (CMS). In order to verify that standards are met, an ASC must have an inspection by representatives of an organization that is authorized to conduct such inspections. The accrediting organization focuses on multiple core standards related to facilities and environment, quality of care, documentation and clinical records, professional improvement and safety. The inspection process verifies compliance with established industry standards. The inspector also assesses the scope of procedures performed in the center to ensure that the surgeons and practitioners have comparable core hospital privileges for procedures that they perform at the center.

The Joint Commission

Founded in 1951 under the sponsorship of the American Hospital Association, the American Medical Association, the American College of Physicians, and the American College of Surgeons, The Joint Commission (TJC) is an independent, non-profit organization that accredits and certifies more than 20,000 healthcare organizations in the United States.[9] The American Dental Association was later added to the sponsoring group. Formerly called The Joint Commission on Accreditation of Healthcare Organizations, the organization underwent a major rebranding and simplified its name to The Joint Commission, with the tagline "Helping Healthcare Organizations Help Patients." The Canadian Medical association was also one of the original founding members, but departed to lead development of a national healthcare accrediting body in Canada. The stated mission of TJC is to "continuously improve healthcare for the public, in collaboration with other stakeholders, by evaluating the healthcare organization and inspiring them to excel in providing safe and effective care of the highest quality and value." Its major functions include developing organizational standards and performance measurement, awarding accreditation and certificates, and providing education and consult. TJC advocates the use of patient safety measures, the spread of information, the measurement of performance and the introduction of public policy recommendations.[9]

The Joint Commission International (JCI) was established in 1997 as a division of Joint Commission Resources. This is a private, not-for-profit affiliate of TJC, whose worldwide mission is to improve the quality of patient care by assisting international healthcare organizations, governments, public health agencies, and health ministries to evaluate, improve, and demonstrate the quality of patient care and enhance patient safety. It works to provide accreditation, education, and advisory services. JCI is involved in more than 60 countries in Asia, Europe, the Middle East, and South America. The World Health Organization partnered with JCI to establish the first WHO Collaborating Center for Patient Safety Solutions. The WHO has also established the check routines of "Safe surgery," which includes perioperative considerations for surgery, anesthesia, and nursing. In addition, the Agency for Healthcare Research and Quality (AHRQ) has launched a Safety Program in Ambulatory Surgery, including the development of an ambulatory surgery checklist.[10]

TJC has put forward National Patient Safety Goals (NSPGs) to promote specific improvement in patient safety. The Goals highlight problematic areas in healthcare and describe evidence and expert-based solutions to these problems. The NPSGs have become a critical method by which TJC promotes and enforces major changes in patient safety in healthcare organizations in the United States and around the world. As a result of the changes in healthcare environment that now include ambulatory surgery centers, TJC broadened its scope to include ambulatory care.

In 2001, TJC introduced standards and a survey process for smaller, office-based practice with an Office-Based Surgery (OBS) accreditation program. TJC accreditation and certification is recognized nationally, and reflects an organization's commitment to meeting certain performance standards. TJC has introduced national patient safety goals for ambulatory care for 2014, that include: correct identification of patients, using medications safely by labeling medication syringes to prevent errors in administration, using hand-cleaning guidelines from the Centers for Disease Control (CDC) or the World Health Organization (WHO), using proven guidelines to prevent infections after surgery, preventing mistakes associated with wrong site surgery, and using a safe surgery checklist.

Facilities undergo a three-year, periodic on-site accreditation cycle. Patient-focused functions and organization functions are assessed. They are assessed on several accountability measures of evidence-based care processes that are linked to positive patient outcomes. Considerable effort and resources are expended to prepare for and undergo Joint Commission surveys. TJC requires ongoing self-assessment and corrective actions between the three-year on-site surveys. The fees for accreditation visits are based on patient visits and types of services provided by the facility. Although it cites evidence-based medicine in its requirements, the criticism is that there is little evidence of any improvement in quality of care as a result of its efforts. However, many obvious and logical measures have not been subjected to prospective, randomized double-blind trials. Thus, even though there is no solid evidence for every practice guideline, educated decisions regarding best practices have to be made and implemented.

Some third-party payers and Medicare require that facilities be accredited in order to provide reimbursement of both the facility and the clinician. Accreditation by a recognized accrediting organization may also serve as a marketing tool for both patients and surgeons to assure that the facility has met and is in compliance with high standards. The drawback to accreditation is the cost involved.

Accreditation Association for Ambulatory Health Care (AAAHC) and American Association for Accreditation of Ambulatory Facilities (AAAASF)

These are other accrediting bodies that address aspects of ambulatory surgery: the facility's physical layout and environmental safety, patient records, personnel files, quality assurance reviews, and equipment safety similar to TJC.

Surgical Care Improvement Project (SCIP)

The Surgical Care Improvement Project is a national quality partnership of organizations focused on reducing the incidence of surgical complications. The SCIP program is sponsored by the Center for Medicare and Medicaid Services (CMS) in collaboration with several other national partners. They include the Centers for Disease Control and Prevention, the American Hospital Association

(AHA), the Institute for Health Improvement (IHI), and TJC. SCIP target areas are advised by a panel of experts and the measures are supported by evidence-based medicine. Current SCIP measures include prophylactic antibiotic administration within 1 hour prior to incision, 2 hours for vancomycin, hair removal with clippers and not razors, temperature management with immediate postoperative normothermia, B-blocker therapy within 24 hours of surgery for patients on B-blockers, and venous thromboembolism prophylaxis. These measures are also part of TJC core measures, as well as that of the American College of Surgeons National Surgical Quality Improvement Project (ACS/NSQIP).

Credentialing, privileges, and performance improvement

This is the process whereby the clinicians have their current medical or technical performance, patient care results, and competence evaluated and confirmed. The granting, reappraisal, and revision of clinical privileges should be awarded on a time-limited basis in accordance with the facility and governmental rules and regulations as applicable. Quality assurance and continuous quality improvement (CQI) programs are necessary to promote high quality patient care. This is in accord with TJC standards for Ongoing Professional Performance Evaluation (OPPE).[10] This is a peer-review process and is essential to ensure high-quality care in an environment where the impetus is on speed and efficiency. The process investigates and verifies the clinician's license status, continuing medical education hours, medical liability claims experience, risk adjusted for frequency and severity with respect to specialty and years of practice that is judged acceptable by the institution medical staff or peer review group. It also investigates technical capabilities and overall character and performance measures in comparison to benchmarks. It also determines the clinician's scope of practice, that they adhere to best-practice guidelines, and that they have acceptable clinical outcomes. The process of peer review is more difficult in smaller units due to the small number of clinicians available to perform a review which must be fair, equally applied, confidential, and well documented. The difficulty is compounded in situations where the providers do not practice in a hospital setting but only in an ASC or office-based facility.

Tracking patient outcome

An outcomes surveillance reporting system for ambulatory and office-based surgery is important. Patients should have a follow-up evaluation within 24 hours of surgery, and a tracking system in place for 30-day follow-up. Outcome indications include cancellation rates, re-intubations, infections, unplanned hospital admissions, falls, burns, pulmonary aspiration, pulmonary embolism, cardiopulmonary arrests, and death. Continuous quality indications should also be documented. They include cardiorespiratory complications, uncontrolled nausea/vomiting, uncontrolled pain, medication error, prolonged PACU stay, and injury to eye and teeth. Patient satisfaction is a hallmark of the ASC industry. Patient satisfaction is being recognized as a major continuous quality indicator and is a major component of pay-for-performance metrics. The CMS, hospitals, and insurance providers are striving to better define and measure quality of care. Patient outcomes and patient satisfaction are inextricably linked.

Risks and medico-legal issues

ASCs have a strong track record of quality care and positive patient outcomes. The great majority of data indicate that ambulatory procedures are safe, but there are inherent risks involved. Ambulatory surgery is not a totally non-risk entity, particularly in a surgery center that is physically separate from a hospital. When unexpected outcomes occur, access to care may be delayed by limitation in staffing models, facilities' technology status or location. ACS/NSQIP has recently introduced an online calculator for use by clinicians and patients in the perioperative assessment process (http://www.riskcalculator.facs.org).[11] This may improve shared decision-making and allow for patient-centered informed consent. The calculator is based on outcomes data collected prospectively by ACS/NSQIP from nearly 400 hospitals and 1.4 million patients, and generates an individualized percentage prediction of mortality and of eight important different postoperative complications. It takes into account the patient's risk factors and comorbidities. It also compares the patient's outcome to the average outcomes for that type of surgery.

Informed consent

Informed consent is the process whereby a fully informed patient can participate in choices about the patient's healthcare. It originates from the ethical and legal right the patient has to direct what happens to his body, and from the ethical duty of the physician to inform the patient about his healthcare. The patient therefore has an opportunity to be an informed participant in making decisions about their healthcare.

The informed consent has several important elements: it should include a discussion about the nature of the procedure in layman's terms, and reasonable alternatives to the proposed intervention. An overview of the risks and benefits of the procedure and alternatives should be a basic preoperative requirement, taking a collaborative approach with the patient towards the perioperative process.[12] Not all risks may be addressed, but priority should be made for any risk or complication which is fairly frequent (i.e., more than 1–10% of cases) as well as any risk of serious permanent disability, outcome, or death, beyond basic everyday living risks. Assessment of the patient's understanding of the process should be done before acceptance of the intervention by the patient. Patients will be asked to sign the consent form stating that they have received and understood the risks and benefits of anesthetic care.

Legal guardians are appointed by the courts to act as decision-makers on behalf of another, as for a minor child or incapacitated adult. Although physicians may deal primarily with parents and guardians in making decisions about their procedures, physicians should make an effort to make the discussions intelligible to children as a matter of prudence so as to gain the children's acceptance and willingness in the procedure.

Documentation

All facilities should have a regularly updated collection of documents relevant to their practice and should ensure that products and services are safe, reliable, and of good quality.

There should be a user manual for all equipment and backup systems in case of failure. The facility should also have routines for personnel to ensure proper standards, education, continuing education, emergency drills, descriptions of responsibilities, and procedures for reporting and documentation of problems. There should also be routines for running the unit and individual cases; what equipment, medications, personnel, and procedural requirements are necessary. There should be criteria for patient pre-operative preparation and documentation, PACU discharge and postoperative follow-up, as well as routines for potential medical emergencies.

Documentation of anesthetic care

Documentation is an important factor in the provision of quality care and is the responsibility of the anesthesiologist. There should be documentation to reflect pre-anesthesia evaluation, intraoperative anesthesia, and postoperative components.[5,7] These may be recorded on paper, electronically, or both according to the facility's practice. The CMS has specific requirements for the contents of perioperative documentation.

The preoperative evaluation with patient interview must include the patient and procedure, medical history, anesthetic history, medications, allergies, and time of last food or drink. A physical examination is necessary that includes vital signs and assessment of the airway. Any objective, pertinent laboratory data and medical records should be evaluated as well as any applicable medical consultations. Assignment of an ASA physical status should also be included. A discussion of the anesthetic plan, with discussion of risks and benefits, should be undertaken with the patient or guardian. An informed consent of the procedure should be documented. Some facilities have separate consents for surgery and anesthesia. The side and site of the procedure should be marked, where applicable, in order to prevent wrong side/site surgery.

Equipment, drugs, and gas supply check should be documented. Intraoperative and procedural documentation require a re-evaluation with a Time-Out process prior to the start of the procedure that includes verification of the procedure, the side and site of the procedure, attestation of administration of prophylactic antibiotics if necessary, re-iteration of patient allergies, and any other concerns. Monitoring of the patient requires documentation of the anesthesia technique, ventilator settings if a ventilator is used, documentation of vital signs and special monitors, patient position, doses, routes and times of administration of medications, intravenous fluids, any unusual events during the procedure, and the status of the patient at the end of the procedure.[5,7]

Post-anesthesia evaluation includes the documentation of vital signs on arrival in the PACU and the writing of postoperative orders. Documentation of the report given to the PACU nurse is vital. The PACU nurse records time-based vital signs and level of consciousness. A modified Aldrete score is widely used in many PACUs. It assigns a score of 0, 1, or 2 to activity, respiration, circulation, consciousness, and oxygen saturation over 92% on room air, giving a maximum score of 10 in the original setup, and a score of 14 when pain and nausea are added.[13] A time-based record of any drugs administered, their dosage, and routes of administration is done. Pain assessment and a satisfactory score on the pain scale in use at the facility should be documented, as well as assessment of any nausea or vomiting. Types and amounts of intravenous fluids are recorded, as well as any unusual events including post-anesthesia and post-surgical complications. The patient should be ambulatory without signs of orthostatic hypotension and this should be documented. If neuraxial anesthesia is used, the motor blockade should have regressed and the patient's motor strength should have returned to pre-anesthesia status. An anesthesia discharge note is essential. It should be dated, timed, and signed by the anesthesiologist. It should include the patient's level of consciousness, vital signs including temperature, the procedure performed, hydration status, pain control, any nausea/vomiting, and whether the patient is able to participate in the discharge.

The patient's caregiver should have written instructions regarding administration of any medications including analgesics and antibiotics, about important potential complications, and how to get immediate and adequate contact with healthcare services on a 24-hour basis. A follow-up post-procedure phone call is made within 24 hours to address issues of the patient's experience including pain, nausea, vomiting, and general satisfaction with the care received. All of these evaluations should be dated and timed. The names of all personnel involved and the name of the responsible anesthesiologist and surgeon should be documented. A copy of the written report from the surgeon should be in the patient's record at discharge.

In the event of any lawsuit, documentation will be essential. Medical malpractice cases are often tried years after the inciting incidents when memory has faded. The medical record is the care rendered. If it was not documented, it was not done.

Conclusions

Over the past three decades, the proportion of surgeries performed in an outpatient setting has increased dramatically. Contributing to this trend are factors such as improvements in anesthetic care, shorter-acting anesthetic agents as well as innovations in minimally invasive surgical techniques and healthcare economics. The steadily increasing demand for ambulatory surgical procedures has led to different levels of organization for ambulatory surgical care.

The Society for Ambulatory Anesthesia, the American Society of Regional Anesthesia, and the European Society for Regional Anaesthesia are growing anesthesia organizations responding to education and research needs, and they provide professional guidance to perioperative physicians practicing ambulatory anesthesia, improving healthcare by advancing innovations in anesthesia practice. They help ASCs to make valuable contributions to the evolution and improvement of healthcare. However, concern over patient safety remains as the outpatient surgery population has increased in volume, age, and complexity. Treatment options are becoming available to patients with far greater comorbidities. That the practice of outpatient/ambulatory surgery has increased tremendously is evident, for example, in pediatric otolaryngology. In children, adenotonsillectomy and myringotomy tubes are two of the most widely performed ambulatory operations in the United States. There are inherent risks. The American Academy of Otolaryngology – Head and Neck Surgery has published guidelines on the selection of appropriate patients for ambulatory adenotonsillectomy.[14] ASCs have led the advancement of technology to replace intraocular lens. Once an inpatient procedure, it is now done safely at an ASC at a much lower price. The explosion of ambulatory surgery centers (ASCs) has created a need to identify patients who are suitable for surgical procedures on an outpatient basis as they strive to deliver a quality of care that is equal to or better than that provided at a hospital.

References

1. Jarrett P, Roberts L. Planning and Designing a Day Surgery Unit In: Lemos P, Jarrett P, Philip B, eds. *Day Surgery – Development and Practice*, London: IAAS, 2006: 61–88.

2. ASCA Ambulatory Surgical Care Association. A Positive Trend in Health Care. http://www.ascaassociation.org.

3. Gisvold SE, Raeder J, Jyssum T, *et al.* Guidelines for the Practice of Anesthesia in Norway. *Acta Anaesthesiologica Scandinavica*, 2002 Sep;**46**(8):942–46.

4. Desai MS. Office-based Anesthesia; New Frontiers, Better Outcomes and Emphasis on Safety. *Current Opinion in Anaesthesiology*, 2008;**21**(6):699–703.

5. American Society of Anesthesiologists. Standards, Guidelines, Statements and Other Documents. Available at: https://www.asahq.org/For-Members/Standards-Guidelines-and-Statements.aspx. Last accessed July 30, 2014.

6. National Fire Protection Association. Healthcare facilities Code 99; Quincy, MA: NFPA 2012.

7. American Society of Anesthesia Guidelines for Ambulatory Anesthesia and Surgery. http://www.asahq.org/publicationsandservices/standards/04.pdf.

8. O'Donnell CD, Iohom G. Regional Anesthetic techniques for Ambulatory Orthopedic Surgery. *Current Opinion in Anaesthesiology*, 2008:**21**(6):723–28.

9. The Joint Commission. www.thejointcommission.org.

10. AHRQ Safety Program for Ambulatory Surgery. Available at: http://ascsafetyprogram.org. Last accessed November 2, 2014.

11. Moonesinghe SR. Individualised Surgical Outcomes. *Postgraduate Medical Journal*, 2013;**89**:677–78.

12. Social Psychology Network: Tips on Informed Consent, 1996–2004. www.socialpsychology.org/consent.htm.

13. White PF, Song D. New criteria for fast-tracking after outpatient anesthesia: a comparison with the modified Aldrete's scoring system. *Anesthesia and Analgesia*, 1999 May;**88**(5):1069–72.

14. Brigger MT, Brietzke SE. Outpatient Tonsillectomy in Children: A Systematic Review. *Otolaryngology Head and Neck Surgery*, July 2006;**135**(1):1–7.

Chapter 3

Patient and procedure selection

Jennifer M. Banayan, MD, Johan Raeder, MD, PhD, and Bobbie-Jean Sweitzer, MD

This chapter discusses patient selection and procedures that can be performed safely in an ambulatory setting. Even patients with multiple comorbidities can be cared for safely in ambulatory settings if they are undergoing anesthesia for a minor procedure such as cataract surgery. On the other hand, those patients undergoing more invasive surgery in an ambulatory setting should be stable and as optimized as possible. If information about comorbidities is obtained preoperatively, the anesthesiologist can plan ahead to safely care for the patient on the day of surgery.

When planning for ambulatory care it is important and useful to have a specified list of discharge criteria in mind. Both the Aldrete Scoring System[1] (Table 3.1) and the Post Anesthesia Discharge Scoring System (PADSS)[2] (Table 3.2) are widely accepted tools for evaluating patients for discharge. Among the various discharge assessment tools, most include the evaluation of vital signs, mental status/consciousness, pain, nausea, vomiting, mobilization, and ability to function in a home environment.

If a patient will not likely fulfill discharge requirements by the late afternoon or evening of the day of the operation, the procedure should not be performed in an ambulatory facility, although the 23-hour option and overnight stay is a rescue in some institutions. Complications that may arise during travel home also should be considered. These depend on the nature of the patient's surgery and anesthetic. Ambulatory settings range from free-standing centers remotely located to centers that are attached to larger hospitals with readily available resources. Each center will have different guidelines for managing discharge requirements.

According to the guidelines of the American Society of Anesthesiologists (ASA), "Patients who receive other than unsupplemented local anesthesia must be discharged with a responsible adult."[3] In other words, anyone who receives oral or intravenous anesthesia cannot be discharged without a companion.

Procedure selection

Suitability of a procedure depends on the resources within the ambulatory center, the patient's anticipated condition within the first few hours after the procedure and the risk for serious complications or need of professional health care within the next days. The objective should be to discharge the patient before the end of the day.

Procedures that open the abdomen, thorax, or skull may necessitate specialized postoperative care. Surgeries that lead to major blood loss or fluid shifts, cause severe postoperative pain, or require care of postoperative wounds or drains may be more safely managed in a non-ambulatory setting. For example, a urologist may perform a cystoscopy in an ambulatory setting but not a cystectomy. A general surgeon may perform a hemorrhoidectomy but not a colectomy. Procedures that leave a patient unable to ambulate, not fully awake, or unable to consume oral fluids by discharge are not suitable for ambulatory care. Some patients (i.e., orthopedic) may not be able to walk freely, but if they can manage at home with the help of a non-professional adult escort, day surgery is acceptable.

Similarly, some procedures may not be appropriate in an ambulatory setting because of a patient's comorbidities. A patient with severe obstructive sleep apnea may need close postoperative monitoring after a tonsillectomy, beyond the scope of an ambulatory center. Table 3.3 lists examples of some procedures that have been performed successfully in ambulatory settings.[4–7]

Practical Ambulatory Anesthesia, ed. Johan Raeder and Richard D. Urman. Published by Cambridge University Press.
© Cambridge University Press 2015.

Table 3.1 The Aldrete Scoring System.

Activity	
Moves all extremities	2
Moves two extremities	1
No movement	0
Circulation	
BP within 20% of normal	2
BP within 20%–50% of normal	1
BP > 50% of normal	0
Oxygen saturation	
> 92% on room air	2
> 90% with oxygen supplementation	1
< 90% with oxygen supplementation	0
Consciousness	
Awake, alert and oriented	2
Arousable	1
No response	0
Respiration	
Spontaneous breathing	2
Dyspnea or shallow breathing	1
Apnea	0

Add up score in left column and if total score is greater than 9, then okay to discharge

Adapted from Aldrete JA, Kroulik D. A postanesthetic recovery score. *Anesth Analg* 1970;49:924–34; Aldrete JA. The post-anesthetic recovery score revisited. *J Clin Anesth* 1995;7:89–91.

Table 3.2 The Postanesthetic Discharge Scoring System (PADSS).

Activity and mental status	
Oriented × 3 AND steady gait	2
Oriented × 3 OR steady gait	1
Neither	0
Intake and output	
Tolerated PO fluids AND voided	2
Tolerated PO fluids OR voided	1
Neither	0
Pain, nausea, and/or vomiting	
Minimal	2
Moderate	1
Severe	0
Surgical bleeding	
Minimal	2
Moderate	1
Severe	0
Vital signs	
Within 20% of preoperative value	2
20%–40% of preoperative value	1
> 40% of preoperative value	0

Add up score in left column and if total score is greater than 9, then okay to discharge

Adapted from Chung F, Chan VWS, Ong D. A post-anesthetic discharge scoring system for home readiness after ambulatory surgery. *J Clin Anesth* 1995;76:500–06.

Table 3.3 Examples of advanced procedures successfully carried out in ambulatory settings.

- Laparoscopic major gastric surgery: cholecystectomy,[4] fundoplication,[5] gastric banding
- Laparoscopic major gynecology: hysterectomy[6]
- Minimally invasive low-back surgery
- Breast surgery
- Bladder/prostate cancer surgery
- Cruciate ligament repair
- Open shoulder surgery
- Major plastic surgery: breast reduction, abdominal fat reduction
- Thyroidectomy
- Tonsillectomy[7]

Adapted from Raeder J. *Clinical Ambulatory Anesthesia*. New York: Cambridge University Press, 2010.

Patient selection

The ASA physical status classification is one component of risk assessment in choosing appropriate patients for ambulatory surgery (Table 3.4). ASA 1 and 2 patients are typically considered healthy enough to receive ambulatory care. ASA 3 and 4 patients are evaluated for possible suitability for ambulatory care. Stable ASA 3 and sometimes even ASA 4 patients may be treated in an ambulatory setting.[8] The concern is whether the patient's condition is stable and the effect of the added stress of surgery and anesthesia is compatible with same-day discharge.

Patient selection is also influenced by access to expert help and equipment and the logistics of an unplanned admission. If the ambulatory unit is within a large hospital, ambulatory surgery may proceed for patients who have a significant risk of needing inpatient care afterwards. Conversely, a free-standing unit located a great distance from a hospital generally only accepts patients with a very low risk of needing inpatient care after a procedure.

Table 3.4 The American Society of Anesthesiologists classification of general preoperative health.

ASA 1: A normal healthy patient
ASA 2: A patient with mild systemic disease
ASA 3: A patient with severe systemic disease
ASA 4: A patient with severe systemic disease that is a constant threat to life
ASA 5: A moribund patient who is not expected to survive without the operation
ASA 6: A declared brain-dead patient whose organs are being removed for donor purposes

Patient comorbidities

Difficult airway

Whether patients with a history of difficult ventilation and/or intubation should be managed in an ambulatory setting depends upon available resources, including airway equipment such as supraglottic airways, videolaryngoscopes, and fiberoptic bronchoscopes. Fiberoptic bronchoscopes and laryngeal mask airways have traditionally been the foundation for managing a difficult airway, but now videoloaryngoscopes are another popular alternative. Most importantly, access to personnel with experience dealing with a difficult airway is necessary. The ability to call upon another experienced provider to assist in an emergency situation is not always possible in an ambulatory setting. The important issue, however, is to ensure that the patient is adequately NPO, and to ascertain if the patient may potentially have a difficult airway, based on airway examination and/or prior anesthetic history.

Cardiovascular disease

The most recent consensus guidelines from the American College of Cardiology and the American Heart Association do not recommend routine cardiac testing, including ECG, especially in patients undergoing low-risk procedures. Because ambulatory surgery is low-risk surgery, it is rarely necessary for patients to undergo any preoperative cardiac testing. The exception is those individuals with active cardiac conditions such as decompensated or new onset heart failure, unstable or severe angina, a recent myocardial infarction (MI) (within 60 days), symptomatic arrhythmias, and severe aortic or mitral stenosis. These active cardiac conditions deserve further evaluation prior to proceeding with surgery.

Ischemic heart disease

It is no longer recommended to wait 6 months after an MI before having non-cardiac surgery. The function of the ventricles and the portion of myocardium at risk predict a further cardiac event, not the age of the infarction. It is recommended that patients delay surgery for at least 60 days after an acute MI.[9]

Patients with a history of coronary artery disease should be taking daily aspirin and a statin. If a patient is taking a beta-blocker, the beta-blocker should be continued. Whether a patient should begin taking a beta-blocker in the immediate preoperative period is controversial because the risk of a stroke may outweigh the benefits.[9]

Coronary intervention

It is recommended to delay surgery if a patient has undergone angioplasty within the last 2 weeks, a bare metal stent has been placed within the last 4–6 weeks, a drug-eluting stent has been placed within the last 12 months, or if the patient has undergone a coronary artery bypass graft within the last month.[9] If a procedure cannot be delayed, dual antiplatelet therapy is continued (aspirin and thienopyridine). If the surgeon believes that the patient will be at risk for bleeding and recommends discontinuing dual antiplatelet therapy, then the patient's cardiologist should be consulted. Every effort should be made to continue aspirin throughout the perioperative period, and the thienopyridine therapy should be discontinued for the shortest time possible.[10] The concern is acute stent thrombosis, which has been effectively treated with percutaneous coronary intervention (PCI). Therefore, in such situations, it would be best not to proceed with surgery in an ambulatory setting unless the operating room is in the same location as a 24-hour interventional cardiology laboratory.[11] The recommended time frame from "door-to-balloon" is 90 minutes to open an occluded vessel.[12]

Arrhythmias

For a patient with an arrhythmia preoperatively, efforts are made to rule out an MI, ischemia, drug toxicity, or metabolic cause. Patients with an atrioventricular block, atrial fibrillation with rapid ventricular response or a new onset, symptomatic bradycardia, or newly recognized ventricular tachycardia should be evaluated further before proceeding with surgery.[9] The risk of stopping or maintaining anticoagulant therapy should be considered individually. A 1–4 day interruption of warfarin with preoperative control of the INR should be considered, whereas a 1–2 day preoperative interruption of dabigatran will usually be appropriate, after considering the risk of bleeding versus thrombosis. Typically, anticoagulants are not interrupted before cataract procedures.

Implantable cardiac defibrillator (ICD)/pacemakers

Patients with a pacemaker or ICD whose condition is stable may safely undergo ambulatory surgery. Anesthesia providers should discuss with the patient's device cardiologist a perioperative plan including pacemaker dependency and response to magnets. A full device interrogation is not necessary as most cardiologists have detailed information on each device, and in many cases the pertinent information can be obtained by a phone call.

For a patient with an ICD/pacemaker, a magnet should be immediately available. Placing a magnet over the pacemaker will typically convert it to asynchronous mode; placing a magnet over an ICD will typically suspend tachyarrhythmia detection without affecting pacing function. The effects of a magnet, however, cannot be guaranteed. In some ICDs a magnet can turn off the antitachyarrhythmia detection permanently.

If a magnet has suspended tachyarrhythmia detection of an ICD, a plan of action is necessary if the patient suffers an unstable arrhythmia. The magnet is removed (if the ICD is not permanently disabled by a magnet) and a defibrillator is used for back up. It may be necessary to place defibrillator pads on a patient for easy defibrillation without contaminating the field or making position changes. A prone patient may be best managed with defibrillator pads because turning the patient supine in the middle of surgery is nearly impossible.[13] It is important to minimize the need for surgical electrocoagulation. Use of bipolar electrocautery minimizes interference with the implantable device. If unipolar electrocoagulation is needed, placing the grounding pad to avoid electrical current across the device is necessary.

Hypertension

A patient with stable hypertension (resting values up to 180 mmHg systolic or 110 mmHg diastolic) is usually acceptable for ambulatory care. Isolated systolic values of 180–200 mmHg may be acceptable in the elderly if the diastolic pressure is below 110 mmHg. Otherwise, patients with newly discovered hypertension, high values, or unstable high values should be evaluated and optimized before ambulatory care. Ideally, hypertensive patients should be well controlled and take their daily medication the morning of surgery. Angiotensin-converting enzyme inhibitors (ACEi) and angiotensin II receptor blockers (ARBs) may be interrupted in cases associated with significant hypotension, especially if neauraxial anesthesia is planned.

Heart failure

Patients with decompensated or Class IV (symptoms at rest) heart failure are not candidates for ambulatory care. In fact, studies suggest that patients with an ejection fraction less than 30% have increased mortality as compared to those with ejection fraction's greater than 29%. For minor surgery, the patient's medical condition can be optimized preoperatively with ACEi, diuretics, and beta-blockers.[9]

Valvular abnormalities

For patients with a history of valvular abnormalities, a thorough history is taken and the physical examination assesses for heart failure or ischemic symptoms. A preoperative echocardiogram within the last year to evaluate the valve is necessary in symptomatic patients or patients who are not physically active in whom symptoms cannot be assessed. Patients with known severe, symptomatic aortic or mitral stenosis are not candidates for ambulatory surgery. Patients with valvular abnormalities such as mild stenotic disease, mitral regurgitation, or aortic insufficiency can tolerate noncardiac surgery if left ventricular function is reserved and there are no heart failure symptoms.[14] Patients with murmurs of unclear etiology should have an evaluation by a cardiologist or an echocardiogram preoperatively to define any pathology.

Pulmonary disease

For patients with severe airway or pulmonary disease, the history and physical examination should focus on the patient's need for home oxygen, use of inhalers and other medications, including how often one uses their rescue inhaler, the ability to walk up two flights of stairs, the frequency of coughing and secretions, and the episodic changes versus stability of their condition. Other useful tests are preoperative chest radiographs, arterial blood gas, and spirometry including vital capacity and forced expiratory volume in one second (FEV_1), with and without a bronchodilator. Generally, a vital capacity of less than 1.5–2 liters in an adult or an FEV_1 of less than 1–1.5 liters indicates an increased likelihood of the need for ventilatory support and inpatient status postoperatively. Nevertheless, some patients with severe pulmonary disease may be stable in their daily functions and are candidates for outpatient surgery. Still, transferring such patients postoperatively to an inpatient facility should be anticipated as an option.

Smoking

Smoking increases the risk of perioperative complications: pneumonia, unplanned intubation, mechanical ventilation, cardiac arrest, myocardial infarction, stroke, sepsis, infection, septic shock, and death.[15] Smokers should be strongly advised not to smoke on the day of surgery as a small amount of carbon monoxide reduces the oxygen-binding capacity of hemoglobin for hours. However, an anticipated surgery provides an opportunity to convince patients to stop smoking. Abstinence from smoking can decrease wound infection and promote healing. Oxygen carrying capacity increases within 12 hours of smoking cessation and abstinence for at least 4 weeks before surgery reduces respiratory complications.[16]

Obstructive sleep apnea

Obstructive sleep apnea (OSA) is underdiagnosed but may be found in 4% of middle-aged men and in 2% of middle-aged women. It is most often associated with increased age, obesity, and the presence of redundant pharyngeal tissue including large tonsils and adenoids,[17] although it can also be seen in the pediatric population who have large tonsils and recurrent upper respiratory infections, which may be a particularly high-risk group (see also Chapter 8). The symptoms of OSA almost always include snoring, episodes of apnea, and tiredness in spite of a normal night's sleep. A formal diagnosis can be made with polysomnography, a sleep study in which a patient is monitored continuously for a full night with pulse oximetry, an electroencephalogram (EEG), electro-oculogram (EOG), capnography, airflow sensors, noninvasive blood pressure, and electrocardiogram (ECG). Throughout the night, the number and length of apnea episodes (cessation of airflow for longer than 10 seconds) and hypopnea episodes (marked reduction in tidal volumes) are recorded. More than 30 episodes of hypopnea or apnea per hour signal a serious condition; fewer than 15 episodes indicate a mild condition.[18]

A diagnosis of OSA can lead to a variety of complications for patients undergoing ambulatory surgery. Among them are difficult/failed mask ventilation, difficult/failed tracheal intubation, need for reintubation, obstruction during spontaneous ventilation, delayed discharge, postoperative admission, cardiac complications, and even death.[19] Because OSA impacts anesthetic management, it is reasonable to screen for OSA. One screening tool, the STOP-BANG questionnaire, contains eight questions (Table 3.5). If a patient answers yes to more than five questions, there is a high risk of moderate to severe OSA.[20]

Patients with OSA may be more sensitive than others to sedatives and hypnotic agents. Therefore, administration of anesthetics without proper monitoring postoperatively may be dangerous. Anesthetics can decrease pharyngeal muscle tone and exacerbate

Table 3.5 Sleep apnea screening survey (STOP-BANG Questionnaire).

Please answer the questions with a yes or no answer:		
Do you snore loudly?	Yes	No
Do you often feel sleepy during the daytime?	Yes	No
Has anyone ever told you that you stopped breathing during your sleep?	Yes	No
Do you have high blood pressure?	Yes	No
Is your BMI > 35 kg/m^2	Yes	No
Are you 50 or older?	Yes	No
Is your neck circumference greater than 40 cm?	Yes	No
Are you a male?	Yes	No

Adapted from Chung F, Subramanyam R, Liao P, et al. High STOP-BANG score indicates a high probability of obstructive sleep apnoea. Br J Anaesth 2012;108:768–75.

Table 3.6 Approach to managing patients with OSA in an ambulatory setting.

Access to CPAP[a] after discharge and optimized comorbidities[b] →	Proceed with ambulatory surgery with CPAP in the postoperative period
Unable or unwilling to use CPAP after discharge →	Proceed with ambulatory surgery if postoperative pain relief provided without opioids[c]
If patient's comorbidities[b] not optimized →	Not suitable for ambulatory surgery
Upper airway surgery →	Per surgeon's and anesthesiologist's discretion

[a] CPAP, Continuous Positive Airway Pressure.
[b] Comorbidities include hypertension, heart failure, cerebrovascular disease, and metabolic disease.[19]
[c] Options for postoperative pain relief limiting opioid use include regional and/or local analgesia, non-steroidal anti-inflammatory drugs, cyclooxygenase-2 specific inhibitors, acetaminophen, and/or dexamethasone.[22]

airway obstruction, which may lead to hypoxia, hypercarbia, and even death.[18] Although fatalities are rare, eight cases were reported in one large survey[21] which may have been prevented with admitting the patient for continuous monitoring overnight.

A rational approach to patients with OSA scheduled to undergo ambulatory surgery is shown in Table 3.6.

Patients who use continuous positive airway pressure (CPAP) at home should be instructed to bring their device with them on the day of surgery. They are encouraged to use their CPAP diligently for several days after surgery including during daytime naps.[19] If patients with a history of, or risk for, OSA are to be managed in an ambulatory setting, CPAP devices should be available.

Obese patients

Body mass index (BMI) is the most common way of classifying obesity, although it underestimates obesity for short people and overestimates for tall, muscular, or heavily built individuals. BMI is calculated from the weight and square of the height: weight (in kg) ÷ height (in meters) squared. Some BMI classifications appear in Table 3.7.

Patients who have a BMI > 30 and < 50 without other comorbidities do not appear to be at increased risk for adverse postoperative outcomes while undergoing noncardiac surgery,[23] other than venous thromboembolism. Consequently, obesity itself is not a reason to deny ambulatory care. On the other hand, obese patients with metabolic syndrome, characterized by central obesity, hypertension, hyperglycemia, and dyslipidemia are at increased risk for cardiac events and acute kidney injury. Therefore, it is prudent to evaluate obese patients for comorbidities

Table 3.7 BMI classifications.

Underweight	BMI < 18.5 kg/m^2
Normal weight	BMI ≥ 18.5–24.9 kg/m^2
Overweight	BMI ≥ 25.0–29.9 kg/m^2
Obesity	BMI of 30.0–39.9 kg/m^2
Extreme obesity	BMI 40.0–49.9 kg/m^2
Super obesity	BMI ≥ 50 kg/m^2

that contribute to risk, such as metabolic syndrome, diabetes mellitus, OSA, and coronary artery disease. Many of these conditions may be undiagnosed before surgery.

Comorbidities and ASA status dictate patient selection for ambulatory surgery not BMI. Consequently, there is not an accepted BMI or weight cut-off for patients undergoing ambulatory surgery. Instead, one must determine the feasibility of managing obese patients by considering availability of difficult airway equipment and the weight limits of the operating table and carts. Because obese patients may have redundant airway tissue, a difficult airway, or suffer from OSA, arrangements should be made for advanced emergency airway equipment and CPAP. More recent studies have shown super-obesity to have a higher risk of complications, and this subset of patients may not be candidates for any procedure other than minor ambulatory surgery.[24]

Diabetes mellitus

Diabetic patients can usually be cared for in ambulatory settings if their disease is well controlled. Potential comorbidities are cardiovascular disease, kidney failure, neuropathy, and morbid obesity, which may require a higher level of care.

Table 3.8 Insulin recommendations for day of surgery.

Insulin medication	Instructions
Insulin pump	Set to basal rate
Long-acting, peakless insulins (glargine or detemir)	75–100% of morning dose
Intermediate acting insulins (NPH)	50–75% of morning dose Reduce nighttime dose if concern for morning hypoglycemia
Fixed combination insulins	50–75% of morning dose
Short and rapid-acting insulin	Hold the dose

Adapted from SAMBA Consensus Statement on Perioperative Blood Glucose Management in Diabetic Patients Undergoing Ambulatory Surgery.[26]

An important preoperative test is the fasting blood sugar which should be checked in the preoperative holding area. There is no specific blood glucose level that is found to be optimal for ambulatory surgery, but the consensus statement from the American Association of Clinical Endocrinologists recommends a blood sugar of <180 mg/dl or 10 mmol/l.[25] Surgery should be postponed in patients with complications of hyperglycemia such as ketoacidosis or hyperosmolar nonketotic states.

In the days before surgery, diabetic patients are advised to continue taking diabetic medication, including insulin. On the morning of surgery the patient can consume water until 2 hours before surgery but skip oral diabetic medications. Contrary to previous recommendations, there is no need to stop metformin earlier than the day before surgery because there is no evidence that metformin leads to lactic acidosis. Nevertheless, metformin can affect patients with renal dysfunction or those receiving intravenous contrast.[26] Table 3.8 contains recommendations for managing insulin dosing on the morning of surgery.

Pregnancy

Anesthesia has not been shown to cause significant risk for either mother or child during pregnancy, yet elective surgery in pregnant women, especially during the first and third trimesters, is not encouraged to limit the risk of miscarriage or preterm labor. If malignancy is suspected or if a condition will deteriorate left untreated, an anesthetic may be given at any time during pregnancy. If surgery is performed for a patient with a viable fetus, fetal monitoring is necessary. An ambulatory setting is appropriate if fetal monitoring is available. At the very least, pre- and post-procedure fetal heart rate and contractions are monitored to assess fetal well-being and to verify the absence of contractions before sending the patient home.[27]

Breastfeeding patients

Breastfeeding is fully compatible with any surgery and anesthesia. For mothers who would like to continue breastfeeding perioperatively, a plan should be discussed. There are studies that suggest breast milk contains low levels of anesthetic agents within 24 hours of general anesthesia and breast feeding can continue unchanged.[28,29] Other studies find repeated and high doses of benzodiazepines and opioids may accumulate to dangerous levels in milk,[30] suggesting mothers may need to pump and discard milk prior to breastfeeding.

End-stage renal disease

Patients with end-stage renal disease (ESRD) on dialysis can be cared for in an ambulatory setting if they have received their dialysis in a timely manner, preferably the day before surgery, and have no acidosis, volume overload, or electrolyte abnormalities. Whether laboratory test results should be obtained before proceeding with surgery is controversial. Some advocate checking the potassium level. The ambulatory facility should be equipped to determine laboratory results quickly if needed.

Liver disease

Patients with acute liver disease such as acute hepatitis or fulminant hepatic failure are not candidates for elective surgery. For patients with chronic liver disease, more information is needed before proceeding to the operating room. Two different scoring systems, Child–Turcotte–Pugh and the Model for End-Stage Liver Disease (MELD), can help risk stratify for such patients (see Tables 3.9–3.12). Patients with MELD scores ≤ 15 can most likely be safely cared for in an ambulatory setting. Patients with MELD scores > 30 are generally not good candidates.[31]

Table 3.9 Child–Turcotte–Pugh Score.[29]

	1 point	2 points	3 points
Total bilirubin concentration (mg/dl)	< 2	2–3	> 3
Serum albumin concentration (g/dl)	> 3.5	2.8–3.5	< 2.8
International normalized ratio	< 1.7	1.7–2.2	> 2.2
Ascites	None	Medically controlled	Poorly controlled
Encephalopathy	None	Medically controlled	Poorly controlled
Add up the points for each category to calculate one's score.			

Table 3.10 Calculating Model for End-stage Liver Disease (MELD).[29]

Lab values needed to calculate MELD:

- INR
- Serum total bilirubin
- Creatinine

$(9.6 \times \log[\text{creatinine mg/dl}]) + (3.8 \times \log[\text{bilirubin mg/dl}]) + (11.2 \times \log[\text{INR}]) + 6.4$
Visit online calculator at: http://reference.medscape.com/calculator/meld-score-end-stage-liver-disease

Comments

- Lab values should be obtained within 24 hours of surgery.
- The final score should be rounded to the nearest whole number.
- The maximum score is 40.
- Scores larger than 40 are assigned a value of 40.
- For any laboratory values less than 1.0 a value of 1.0 is used.
- The maximum creatinine concentration used is 4.0 mg/dl.
- If a patient has had dialysis twice within the previous week, the creatinine value used should be 4.0 mg/dl.

Table 3.11 Recommendations for surgery based on Child–Turcotte–Pugh Score.[29]

Score	Recommendations
5–6	May undergo elective surgery
7–9	May undergo elective surgery with caution
10–15	Should not undergo elective surgery

Table 3.12 Recommendations for surgery based on MELD score.[29]

Score	Recommendations
< 10	May undergo elective surgery
10–15	May undergo elective surgery with caution
> 15	Should not undergo elective surgery

Thyroid disorders

The presence of a goiter may cause a difficult airway. A radiograph (anterior and lateral projections) or a computed tomography (CT) scan of the neck should be examined if a displaced or compressed upper airway is suspected. Hyperthyroidism should be corrected before elective surgery, otherwise arrhythmias and unpredictable anesthetic drug dosing may result. Thyroid hormone replacement therapy should be instituted to achieve stable levels in patients with hypothyroidism.

Rheumatoid arthritis

Patients with rheumatoid arthritis may present potential airway or intubation challenges and require special anesthetic consideration. Neck mobility is assessed and documented in the chart. There is a disagreement about which patients need radiographs to document upper neck anatomy and detect atlantoaxial subluxation. Some providers advocate a history and physical examination for clicking or neurologic deficits during flexion or extension of the neck. Others recommend that rheumatoid patients, even if asymptomatic, have 5-view radiographs, including flexion and extension views, especially those with potential difficult airways who may undergo procedures requiring neck manipulation. Other manifestations that can complicate mask ventilation and intubation include temporomandibular joint involvement, crico-arythenitis, or chest stiffness.[32] It is important to carefully evaluate the patient's mouth opening and range of motion of neck.

Neurologic diseases

Any patient who has experienced an acute stroke within the last 30 days is not a good candidate for any surgery, especially one performed in an ambulatory setting as he/she should be in close proximity to a neuro-interventionalist in case of an emergency. It is important to evaluate if there is symptomatic carotid stenosis which requires neurologic consultation preoperatively.

For others with neurologic diseases ambulatory care is usually well tolerated, but paresis must be documented. Regional anesthesia and the implications of neuroaxial blockade should be discussed thoroughly with the patient preoperatively. Uneventful regional anesthesia has not been shown to cause deterioration in neurologic symptoms.

Myasthenia gravis

Generally, patients with severe myasthenia gravis are better cared for in an inpatient hospital setting where they can easily be transported to an intensive care unit postoperatively for positive pressure ventilation if necessary. Patients in the early stages of myasthenia gravis can be managed in an ambulatory setting, and they are directed to continue their daily medication. Ideally, all muscle relaxants should be avoided. A peripheral nerve block may offer a safer alternative if it is appropriate for the scheduled procedure. Minor procedures which do not require general anesthesia or the use of neuromuscular blocking agents may be done safely in an outpatient setting.

Seizure disorders

Patients with epilepsy having procedures in an ambulatory center should continue epileptic medications preoperatively. Patients who have frequent seizures in spite of medications may still be scheduled for ambulatory care, provided they are returning to a care environment on the day of surgery (parents, spouse, specialized institution) where seizures can be handled adequately.

Malignant hyperthermia

Patients at risk for malignant hyperthermia (MH) are identified with a thorough preoperative history. Patients with personal or family histories of MH may be treated in an ambulatory setting as long as the center is able to provide a trigger-free anesthetic.

A surgery center that provides inhalational agents or succinylcholine for anesthesia must be prepared to manage an MH crisis. Dantrolene must be available and administered quickly with enough healthcare providers available to dilute the numerous vials needed, obtain arterial blood gas results, and transfer patients to an inpatient setting for monitoring and ongoing treatment.

Children
The newborn infant

There does not seem to be a consensus regarding the youngest age for a procedure in an ambulatory setting. Full-term infants do not seem to be at greater risk from surgery in an ambulatory setting. Nevertheless, most centers will not treat patients younger than 4–6 weeks old because of concerns of apnea or respiratory complications. On the other hand, prematurely born infants are at higher risk than full-term infants of developing apnea during the first day after anesthesia, intravenous sedation, or any opioid administration. Consequently, the vast majority of centers will not accept infants younger than 54–60 weeks post-conception due to the need to admit them for postoperative apnea monitoring.

Upper respiratory infection

Many children, especially during the winter season, display upper respiratory symptoms. The concern with such patients is a reactive airway and copious secretions, yet delaying surgery until the child is symptom-free may not always be possible. A thorough history and physical examination should be taken to document the child's level of activity, appetite, and presence of fever. If the child is functioning normally, playing and eating as usual, does not show signs of lower airway infection or wheezing, does not have purulent discharge, and is afebrile most centers would agree that the case can safely proceed.[33] Not using an endotracheal tube and limiting anesthesia to a mask or supraglottic airway with sevoflurane may also reduce complications.

Asthma

Patients with mild asthma who experience symptoms infrequently and do not require daily medications are excellent candidates for ambulatory surgery. If a patient with moderate asthma is to undergo ambulatory surgery, it must be adequately controlled on the day of surgery. In other words, the patient should not have wheezing, coughing, or upper respiratory symptoms. Patients with severe asthma are best managed in non-ambulatory settings. For patients undergoing ambulatory surgery who have asthma, it is best to refrain from using endotracheal tubes or stimulating the airway.[34] Patients are encouraged to use their regular prophylactic asthmatic medications on the morning of surgery, even if used "as needed."

The elderly

Age, specifically over the age of 70, seems to affect outcomes in outpatient surgery and increases the risk of perioperative complications.[35] In one study of unplanned hospital admission within 7 days of outpatient surgery, age (the highest risk being over age 85 years) led to a greater likelihood of unanticipated inpatient admission. Other risk factors included admission to a hospital in the last 6 months and type of procedure. The highest-risk procedures were radical mastectomy, arteriovenous graft placement, and transurethral resection of prostate and laparoscopic cholecystectomy. Elderly patients may benefit from ambulatory surgery by having a reduced chance of cognitive dysfunction or delirium when compared with the inpatient setting. When managing elderly patients in outpatient settings, a plan should be in place to transfer them to an inpatient setting in the event perioperative complications occur.[36]

Preoperative information

Preoperative information provided by the patient

A standard self-administered questionnaire before ambulatory surgery can be useful (Table 3.13). Not only may it save time in documenting the patient's health status, but it also may reveal areas of general health and give the patient an opportunity to provide important information. It is best if the questionnaire is completed before the day of surgery so that it can be reviewed and necessary tests and information can be gathered preoperatively.

Preoperative information given to the patient

It is important that the patient receives written and oral instructions about food and liquid intake limits and medication usage before surgery (Table 3.14).

Medication recommendations

The general rule for most medications is to continue them as usual, including any morning dose, which should be taken with enough water to comfortably swallow pills (Table 3.15). The following exceptions apply.

Anticoagulants

Dabigatran (Pradaxa), an FDA-approved drug for atrial fibrillation, is an alternative to warfarin for stroke prevention. The duration for which the drug should be discontinued before a procedure depends on renal function, creatinine clearance, and risk of bleeding during the procedure (Table 3.16). A 24-hour discontinuation is sufficient in most cases, unless contraindicated because of a high risk of bleeding or thrombosis.

Warfarin (Coumadin) needs to be discontinued 5 days prior to surgery (if INR between 2 and 3) except for patients having cataract surgery, dental procedures, gastrointestinal endoscopies, colonoscopies, and minor foot procedures. For patients who discontinue warfarin but require anticoagulation, typical bridging is with low-molecular-weight heparin (LMWH). The dose is best determined in consultation with the physician who prescribes the anticoagulant. The timing of the first dose of LMWH depends on

Table 3.13

SAMPLE QUESTIONNAIRE[a]

Patient's Name _____ Age_____ Sex _____

Date of Surgery_____

Proposed operation_____

Primary Care physician name/phone #_____

Cardiologist/phone #_____

1. Please list all previous operations (and approximate dates)

a. _____c. _____

b. _____ d. _____

2. Please list any Allergies to medications, latex, food or other (and your reactions to them)

a. _____ c. _____

b. _____ d. _____

3. Circle TESTS that you have already completed, list where and when you had them. Please bring all existing reports for your visit. We are NOT suggesting that you require (or need to have) these tests.

a. ECG   d. BLOOD WORK

b. STRESS TEST   e. SLEEP STUDY

c. ECHO/ultrasound of heart   f. Other

4. Please list all Medications you have taken in the last month (include over-the-counter drugs, inhalers, herbals, dietary supplements and aspirin)

Drug Name / Dose and how often

a. _____ e. _____

b. _____ f. _____

c. _____ g. _____

d. _____ h. _____

(Please check YES or NO and circle specific problems)

5. Have you taken steroids (prednisone or cortisone) in the last year? ....YES NO

6. Have you ever smoked? (Quantify in ____ packs/day for ____ years ....YES NO

        Do you still smoke? (Quantify in ____ packs/day).........................YES NO

        Do you drink alcohol? ....YES NO

        (If so, how much?) _____

        Do you use or have you ever used any illegal drugs? ....YES NO

7. Can you walk up one flight of stairs without stopping? ....YES NO

Table 3.13 (cont.)

8. Have you had any problems with your heart? (circle all that apply) ....YES NO

(Chest pain or pressure, heart attack, abnormal ECG, skipped beats, murmur, palpitations, heart failure)

9. Do you have high blood pressure?...YES NO

10. Do you have diabetes?...YES NO

11. Have you had any problems with your lungs or your chest? ....YES NO

(circle all that apply) (shortness of breath, emphysema, bronchitis, asthma, TB)

12. Are you ill now or were you recently ill with a cold, fever, chills, flu or productive cough?

....YES NO

Describe recent changes _____

13. Have you or anyone in your family had serious bleeding problems? ....YES NO

(circle all that apply) (Prolonged bleeding from nose, gums, tooth extractions, or surgery)

14. Have you had any problems with your blood ? ....YES NO

(circle all that apply) (anemia, leukemia, lymphoma, sickle cell disease, blood clots, transfusions)

15. Have you ever had problems with your: (circle all that apply)

Liver (Cirrhosis; Hepatitis A, B, C; jaundice)?...............................YES NO

Kidney (Stones, failure, dialysis)?...YES NO

Digestive system (frequent heartburn, hiatus hernia, stomach ulcer)?.............YES NO

Back, Neck or Jaws (TMJ, rheumatoid arthritis, Herniation)?.........................YES NO

Thyroid gland (under active or overactive)?......................................YES NO

16. Have you ever had: (circle all that apply)

Seizures?...YES NO

Stroke, facial, leg or arm weakness, difficulty speaking?...................................YES NO

Cramping pain in your legs with walking?...YES NO

Problems with hearing, vision or memory?...YES NO

17. Have you ever been treated with chemotherapy or radiation therapy?..........YES NO

List indication and dates of treatment: _____

18. Women: Could you be pregnant?...YES NO

Last menstrual period began: _____

19. Have you ever had problems with anesthesia or surgery?...............................YES NO

(circle all that apply) (Severe nausea or vomiting, malignant hyperthermia (in blood relatives or self), breathing difficulties, or problems with placement of a breathing tube)

Table 3.13 (cont.)

20. Do you have any chipped or loose teeth, dentures, caps, bridgework, braces, problems opening your mouth or swallowing, or choking while eating? (circle all that apply)

21. Do your physical abilities limit your daily activities?...................................YES NO

22. Do you snore?..YES NO

23. Do you have sleep apnea?... YES NO

24. Please list any medical illnesses not noted above:

_____

_____

25. Additional comments or questions for the anesthesiologist?

_____

_____

I confirm that I have read through the form and that the information I have provided is correct.

Signature _____

Date _____

[a] Questionnaire created by Bobbie Jean Sweitzer at University of Chicago, used with permission.

Table 3.14 Patient instructions.

On the day *before* your surgery, you should take all of your regular medications unless instructed otherwise. For medications taken on the morning of surgery, take enough water to swallow your medications.

Please refrain from eating any food within 6 hours of your surgery unless directed otherwise. You can drink water up to two hours before you are scheduled for surgery.

You must have an adult escort to take you home. This individual must be here with you or readily available if you are receiving anesthesia the day of your surgery. A taxi driver is not an escort. You will not be able to drive yourself home, walk home, or take a bus after receiving anesthesia.

Please leave all jewelry, cash and other valuables at home. This includes rings in your belly button, ears, nose, tongue, and/or face. Please do not wear make-up to the hospital.

how quickly the INR declines. In general, the first dose can be administered 36 hours after the last dose of warfarin, but an INR should be checked to ensure that it is subtherapeutic. The last dose of LMWH needs to be 24 hours before surgery (Table 3.17).

Antiplatelet agents

Aspirin. Most surgeries can be performed for patients taking low-dose aspirin prophylaxis without major bleeding concerns. Patients taking aspirin for primary prophylaxis (no diagnosis of vascular disease) should discontinue aspirin 7 days before surgery. For patients taking aspirin for secondary prevention (known vascular disease such as for a history of coronary artery disease, transient ischemic attack, peripheral arterial disease, or percutaneous coronary intervention), daily aspirin is continued even on the day of surgery.[37] Some surgeons believe there is a benefit if the dose of aspirin is decreased

Table 3.15 Medications to continue on the day of surgery.

Anti-depressants, anti-anxiety, psychiatric medications[a]

Anti-hypertensives[b]

Anti-seizure medications

Aspirin and clopidogrel (Plavix)[c]

Asthma medications (oral and inhaled)

Oral contraceptives

Cardiac medications (i.e., digoxin)

COX-2 inhibitors

Ophthalmic drops

Heartburn or reflux medications

Pain medications

Statins

Steroid medications (oral and inhaled)

Thyroid medications

[a] Monoamine oxidase inhibitors (MAOIs) are continued but important adjustments in anesthesia may be necessary.
[b] Angiotensin-converting enzyme inhibitors (ACEi) and angiotensin II receptor blockers (ARBs) may be the exception.
[c] Exceptions apply.

Table 3.16 Dabigatran (Pradaxa) instructions.

Creatinine clearance	Discontinue
> 50 ml/min	24 hours before procedure
30–50 ml/min	48 hours before procedure
< 30 ml/min	2–5 days before procedure

*Those patients at high risk of bleeding should be off dabigatran for longer than the above recommendations, sometimes up to 7 days.

from 325 mg to 81 mg for the week before surgery for patients who have passed the high-risk time after stents.

Clopidigrel or Ticlopidine. For patients taking clopidogrel or ticlopidine who have had a myocardial infarction in the previous 6 weeks, angioplasty within the last 2 weeks, a bare metal stent in the previous 4 weeks, or a drug-eluting stent within 12 months, surgery should be performed only if they continue antiplatelet therapy. All other patients who are taking clopidogrel or ticlopidine should discontinue these medications 7 days before surgery.[38]

Oral hypoglycemics and insulin (see diabetes mellitus).

Angiotensin-converting enzyme inhibitors (ACEi), angiotensin II receptor blockers (ARBs)

Advice on whether to discontinue these agents varies. A pragmatic view is that if a patient needs an ACEi for heart failure, the need will persist in the perioperative phase and the drug should be continued. If the drug is used to control hypertension, the medication may be discontinued on the evening before surgery and/or the morning of surgery and hypertension can be controlled with a beta-blocker or other antihypertensive if needed. Other antihypertensives, especially beta-blockers, should be continued.

Estrogen compounds

Estrogen-containing medications may increase the risk of thrombosis slightly, and the general rule is to advise the patient to discontinue this medication 3–4 weeks before surgery. These drugs may be continued if used for birth control or as part of cancer therapy.

Herbals and other supplements should be discontinued 7 days before surgery.

Vitamins, minerals, iron should not be taken the day of surgery.

Some drugs should certainly NOT be discontinued or reduced, but rather should be reinforced perioperatively. Among them are the following:

Anti-asthmatics

These drugs, sprays, and aerosols are often used intermittently. If patients are taking such drugs, they may be advised to take them prophylactically, starting the day before surgery and then again on the morning of surgery.

Beta-blockers

The benefit of starting beta-blockers in at-risk patients before major surgery remains controversial. However, there is no debate about the potential harmful effects of discontinuing beta-blockers just before surgery. Patients should be asked specifically if they have taken their beta-blockers.

Statins, cholesterol-lowering agents

There is good documentation for the potential benefits of continuing these drugs perioperatively. Because these drugs have an anti-inflammatory

Table 3.17 Peri-procedural bridging protocol.

Day before surgery	Warfarin use	INR recommendations	Enoxaparin use
		Start the protocol by checking an INR	
7	Last day of warfarin if INR is 3.0–3.5	Repeat INR on Day 5	Begin enoxaparin when INR is subtherapeutic
6	Last dose of warfarin if INR is 2.5–3.0	Repeat INR on Day 4	Begin enoxaparin when INR is subtherapeutic
5	Last dose of warfarin if INR is 2.0–2.5	Repeat INR on Day 4	Begin enoxaparin when INR is subtherapeutic
4	No warfarin		Continue enoxoparin
3	No warfarin		Continue enoxoparin
2	No warfarin		If surgery scheduled before noon on Day 0, last dose of enoxaparin must be taken before 2100
1	No warfarin	Order INR[b]	If surgery scheduled after noon on Day 0, last dose of enoxaparin at 0900
0[a]	Resume warfarin after surgery if okay with surgeon	STAT INR one hour prior to surgery	Resume enoxaparin 12–72 hours post-procedure/surgery depending on surgical recommendations

[a] Day 0 = Day of surgery.

If INR on Day 1 is above 1.5, administer oral vitamin K 2.5 mg × 1 and recheck INR.

For those patients who have a contraindication to enoxaparin, such as allergies to heparin, history of heparin-induced thrombocytopenia, or renal insufficiency, they can be reversed with vitamin K. Their management includes taking their last dose of warfarin three days before surgery. Two days before surgery, they will hold their warfarin and take 5 mg of oral vitamin K. The day before surgery they should have their INR checked and repeat a dose of vitamin K if their INR remains above 1.5.

Table 3.18 Risks associated with anesthesia.

- Sore throat, hoarse voice, vocal cord trauma
- Postdural puncture headache
- Minor, transient pain localized in the back after spinal or epidural needle puncture
- Urinary retention after spinal or epidural anesthesia
- Stiffness or slight aching in the muscles for 1–2 days
- Anaphylaxis or allergic reactions to anesthetic drugs or adjuvants (dressings, fluids, antibiotics)
- Injuries to teeth and mouth
- Temporary soreness and discoloration at the site of intravenous access
- Deep venous thrombosis or pulmonary embolism
- Cardiopulmonary complications including cardiopulmonary arrest
- Coma
- Death

effect that is beneficial for lessening cardiovascular risk, discontinuing them on the day before surgery may result in severe rebound inflammatory effects.

Risks and benefits

It is important to discuss with the patient the risks, benefits, and complications that may occur before, during, and after surgery. Some risks of anesthesia can be seen in Table 3.18.

References

1. Aldrete JA, Kroulik D. A postanesthetic recovery score. *Anesth Analg* 1970;**49**:924–34.

2. Chung F, Chan VWS, Ong D. A post-anesthetic discharge scoring system for home readiness after ambulatory surgery. *J Clin Anesth* 1995;**7**:500–06.

3. American Society of Anesthesiologists Committee on Ambulatory Surgical Care. Guidelines for ambulatory

anesthesia and surgery. Available at www.asahq.org/standards-Guidelines. Accessed January 22, 2014.

4. Mjaland O, Raeder J, Aasboe V, *et al.* Outpatient laparoscopic cholecystectomy. *Br J Surg* 1997;**84**:958–61.

5. Trondsen E, Mjaland O, Raeder J, Buanes T. Day-case laparoscopic fundoplication for gastro-oesophageal reflux disease. *Br J Surg* 2000;**87**:1708–11.

6. Levy BS, Luciano DE, Emery LL. Outpatient vaginal hysterectomy is safe for patients and reduces institutional cost. *J Minim Invasive Gynecol* 2005;**12**:494–501.

7. Gravningsbraten R, Nicklasson B, Raeder J. Safety of laryngeal mask airway and short-stay practice in office-based adenotonsillectomy. *Acta Anaesthesiol Scand* 2009;**53**:218–22.

8. Ansell GL, Montgomery JE. Outcome of ASA III patients undergoing day case surgery. *Br J Anaesth* 2004;**92**:71–74.

9. Fleisher LA, Fleischmann KE, Auerbach AD, *et al.* 2014 ACC/AHA Guideline on Perioperative Cardiovascular Evaluation and Management of Patients Undergoing Noncardiac Surgery: Executive Summary: A Report of the American College of Cardiology/American Heart Association Task Force on Practice Guidelines. *Circulation.* 2014;**64**:e77–e137.

10. Grimes CL, Bonow RO, Casey DE, *et al.* Prevention of premature discontinuation of duel antiplatelet therapy in patients with coronary artery stents. *J Am Coll Cardiol* 2007;**49**(6)734–39.

11. Newsome LT. Anesthetic considerations for the patients with coronary stents part II. *Curr Rev Clin Anesth* 2009;**30**:49–50.

12. Nallamothu BK, Bradley EH, Krumholz HM. Time to treat in primary percutaneous coronary intervention. *N Engl J Med* 2007;**357**:1631–38.

13. Crossley GH, Poole JE, Rozner MA, *et al.* The Heart Rhythm Society (HRS)/American Society of Anesthesiologists (ASA) expert consensus statement on the perioperative management of patients with implantable difibrillators, pacemakers and arrhythmia monitors: Facilities and patient management: Executive summary. *Heart Rhythm* 2011;**8**:e1–e18.

14. Bach DS, Eagle KA. Perioperative assessment and management of patients with valvular heart disease undergoing noncardiac surgery. *Minerva Cardioangiol* 2004;**52**:255–61.

15. Turan A, Mascha EJ, Roberman D, *et al.* Smoking and perioperative outcomes. *Anesthesiology* 2011;**114**:837–46.

16. Wong J, Lam DP. Short-term preoperative smoking cessation and postoperative complications: a systematic review and meta-analysis. *Can J Anesth* 2012;**59**:268–79.

17. Flemons WW. Obstructive sleep apnea. *N Engl J Med* 2002;**347**:498–504.

18. Benumof JL. Obstructive sleep apnea in the adult obese patient: implications for airway management. *J Clin Anesth* 2001;**13**:144–56.

19. Joshi GP, Ankichetty S, Gan TJ, Chung F. Society for Ambulatory Anesthesia consensus statement on preoperative selection of adult patients with obstructive sleep apnea scheduled for ambulatory surgery. *Anesth Analg* 2012;**115**:1060–68.

20. Chung F, Subramanyam R, Liao P, *et al.* High STOP-Bang score indicates a high probability of obstructive sleep apnea. *Br J Anaesth* 2012;**108**:768–75.

21. Lofsky A. Cases of sleep apnea syndrome. *Anesth Pt Safety Found News* 2002;**17**:24–25.

22. Joshi GP. Multimodal analgesia techniques and postoperative rehabilitation. *Anesthesiol Clin N Am* 2005;**23**:185–202.

23. Klasen J, Junger A, Hartmann B, *et al.* Increased body mass index and peri-operative risk in patients undergoing non-cardiac surgery. *Obes Surg* 2004;**14**:275–81.

24. Joshi G, Ahmad S, Riad W, *et al.* Selection of obese patients undergoing ambulatory surgery: a systematic review of the literature. *Anesth Analg* 2013;**117**:1082–91.

25. Moghissi ES, Korytkowski MT, DiNardo M, *et al.* American Association of Clinical Endocrinologist and American Diabetes Association consensus statement on inpatient glycemic control. *Endocr Pract* 2009;**15**:353–69.

26. Joshi GP, Chung F, Van MA, *et al.* Society for Ambulatory Anesthesia consensus statement on perioperative blood glucose management in diabetic patients undergoing ambulatory surgery. *Anesth Analg* 2010;**111**:1378–87.

27. ASA Committee on Obstetrical Anesthesia. Statement on nonobstetric surgery during pregnancy, 2009. Available at www.asahq.org/Standards/guidelines. Accessed January 22, 2014.

28. Dalal PG, Bosak J, Berlin C. Safety of the breast-feeding infant after maternal anesthesia. *Ped Anesth* 2014;**24**:359–71.

29. Nitsun M, Szokol JW, Saleh HJ, *et al.* Pharmacokinetics of midazolam, propofol, and fentanyl transfer to human breast milk. *Clin Pharmacol Ther* 2006;**79**:549–57.

30. Berlin CM, Jr., Paul IM, Vesell ES. Safety issues of maternal drug therapy during breastfeeding. *Clin Pharmacol Ther* 2009;**85**:20–22.

31. Hanje AJ, Patel T. Preoperative evaluation of patients with liver disease. *Nat Clin Pract Gastroenterol Hepatol* 2007;**4**:266–76.

32. Samanta R, Shoukrey K, Griffiths R. Rheumatoid arthritis and anaesthesia. *Anaesth* 2011;**66**:1146–59.

33. Tait AR, Malviya S. Anesthesia for the child with upper respiratory infection: still a dilemma? *Anesth Analg* 2005;**100**:59–65.

34. Lindeman KS. Anesthesia, airways, and asthma. *Semin Anesth* 1995;**14**:221–25.

35. Polanczyk CA, Marcantonio E, Goldman L, *et al.* Impact of age on perioperative complications and length of stay in patients undergoing noncardiac surgery. *Ann Intern Med* 2001;**134**:637–43.

36. Fleisher LA, Pasternak LR, Herbert R, Anderson GF. Inpatient hospital admission and death after outpatient surgery in elderly patients: importance of patient and system characteristics and location of care. *Arch Surg* 2004;**139**:67–72.

37. O'Riordan JM, Margey RJ, Blake G, O'Connell R. Antiplatelet agents in the perioperative period. *Arch Surg* 2009;**144**:69–76.

38. Chassot PG, Delabays A, Spahn DR. Perioperative antiplatelet therapy: the case for continuing therapy in patients at risk of myocardial infarction. *Br J Anaesth* 2007;**99**:316–28.

Chapter 4

Pharmacology

Claude Abdallah, MD, MSc, Richard D. Urman, MD, and Johan Raeder, MD, PhD

Anesthetic techniques are tailored to provide smooth-onset, adequate depth of anesthesia and minimal secondary effects on organ function while ensuring a quick emergence and a prompt recovery with no or minimal unpleasant side effects.[1] The selection of inhalational or intravenous anesthetic agents or the combination of different agents is based principally on the different properties, pharmacokinetic and pharmacodynamic characteristics of these agents.

General aspects

Liposolubility of anesthetic drugs allows penetration through the blood–brain barrier which results in effect at the central nervous system (CNS). However, this characteristic results also in extensive diffusion, distribution, and binding to other tissues and inside cells.

Distribution volume may be calculated by dividing the dose by the plasma concentration after diffusion has taken place. The speed and amount of drug diffusion into different organs depend upon the blood flow to those organs, the plasma concentration (or partial pressure for inhalational agents), the concentration gradient between the blood and tissue, and drug solubility in the tissues. Some medications, such as neuromuscular blocking agents and reversal agents, do not need to be lipid-soluble, because their receptors are on the surface of the muscle membranes and thus accessible to water-soluble drugs. Although some of these drugs are partly degraded in the liver, they do not diffuse readily through membranes and into cells, thus their distribution volumes are lower than for lipid-soluble drugs.

Clearance is defined as the amount of blood that is fully cleared from drug per unit time. Elimination of anesthetic drugs may occur by exhalation

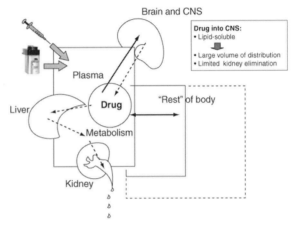

Figure 4.1. Anatomical model of anesthesia pharmacology.

(inhalational agents), by enzymatic elimination, or by liver metabolism and renal excretion. The maximum potential clearance of a liver-metabolized drug equates to the liver blood flow. For some drugs, such as propofol, there is extrahepatic metabolism (enzymes in lung, intestines, etc.), thus the clearance may be somewhat higher than liver blood flow. Another mode of drug clearance, independent of liver degradation, may provide rapid drug elimination such as in the case of remifentanil, which is degraded by tissue esterases very rapidly and extensively.

Metabolism may occur as a zero-order metabolism, in which a constant amount of drug is metabolized per unit time, or a first-order metabolism in which a constant fraction of drug is being metabolized per unit of time. All modern intravenous anesthetics have first-order metabolism, which protects somewhat against unlimited accumulation with overdose. This is because metabolism (i.e., amount of drug cleared) increases as drug levels in the plasma accumulate.

Practical Ambulatory Anesthesia, ed. Johan Raeder and Richard D. Urman. Published by Cambridge University Press. © Cambridge University Press 2015.

Table 4.1

Partition coefficients of inhaled agents	Desflurane	Nitrous oxide	Isoflurane	Sevoflurane
Blood/gas	0.42	0.47	1.43	0.69
Fat/blood	27.2	2.3	44.9	47.5
Brain/blood	1.29	1.1	1.57	1.70
Muscle/blood	2.02	1.15	2.92	3.13
Heart/blood	1.29	1.13	1.61	1.78
Liver/blood	1.31	0.92	1.75	1.85
Kidney/blood	0.94	–	1.05	1.15

Desflurane and Isoflurane prescribing information. Baxter Pharmaceuticals Products Inc., New Providence, NJ.

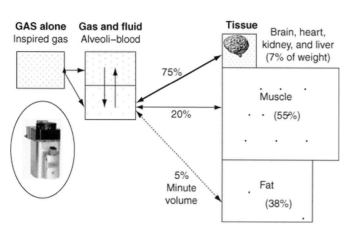

Figure 4.2. The gas molecules are delivered to the alveoli via the endotracheal tube, LMA, or mask and equilibrate (to equal partial pressure) with the lung blood. In a sleeping patient about 75% of the cardiac output will go to the brain, heart, kidney, and liver, which are only about 7% of the total body mass; 20% of the minute volume will go to the 55% of body mass which is muscle and 5% will go to fat. Thus the brain cells will fairly rapidly receive a large dose of drug, whereas the muscle and fat will continue to take up molecules for a very long time before equilibrium.

Inhalational drugs: pharmacokinetics

The partial pressure of an inhalational agent is responsible for the anesthetic effect. Although partial pressure is correlated to concentration for individual agents, the agents differ in terms of solubility: high solubility means that a large number of molecules are needed in the blood or tissue in order to build up a given partial pressure and effect. The partial pressure of an inhalational agent is dictated by the amount the patient inhales, equilibration between alveoli and blood, the binding of drug molecules to fluid and cells, and duration of exposure (Figure 4.2). A low solubility in blood means a more rapid establishment of a high partial pressure by induction, and a more efficient exhalation at the end of anesthesia, thus a more rapid induction and emergence (Table 4.1). For procedures of 1–2 hours in duration the *blood solubility* is the most important determinant of emergence speed, but with prolonged cases the *tissue solubility* and amount of gas dissolved in the tissue will be increasingly important. Nitrous oxide is the

least blood- and tissue-soluble and will be rapidly exhaled. Desflurane is less soluble in tissues than sevoflurane and will result in a more rapid emergence after procedures lasting more than 2–3 hours (Figure 4.3). In patients with a high fatty tissue component, there is a greater amount of inhalation agent distributed in these tissues, thus emergence from sevoflurane, for example, may be slower even after relatively short anesthetic duration.

Hyperventilation may create a more efficient wash-in and wash-out of inhalational drugs in blood, but this effect will be counteracted by a decrease in arterial partial pressure of carbon dioxide (pCO_2) and subsequent cerebral vasoconstriction, which would slow down the shift of inhalational drug into or out of the brain.

With a high flow of fresh gas into the ventilation system, the difference in partial pressure between inspiratory and expiratory alveolar gas will not be extensive; thus turning the vaporizer setting to 1 MAC (minimum alveolar concentration) may be

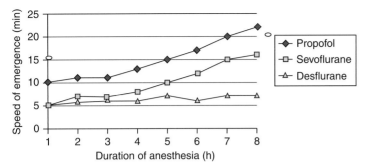

Figure 4.3. Speed of emergence (min) after different hypnotic, anesthetic agents have been given for standardized maintenance (x-axis) of general anesthesia over 1–8 hours without tapering of dose before stopping it: a patient given propofol will wake up at 10 min after 1 hour of anesthesia, and at 20 min after 7 hours of anesthesia, whereas a patient given desflurane will wake up at 7 min after 7 hours and at 5 min after 1 hour.

expected to deliver close to 1 MAC in end-alveolar gas with a fresh gas flow of 6–8 l/min during induction. However, low-flow circular systems are encouraged for maintenance from economical, humidity, and temperature regulation. Inhalational agents can be monitored in individual patients by end-tidal measurement, although this end-tidal concentration is not always exactly the same as the partial pressure in arterial blood. In all patients there will be a slight delay in the change of partial pressure in blood and a further delay in brain changes compared with alveolar changes. End-tidal values will be slightly higher than blood and brain values during induction and slightly lower during emergence. These discrepancies are exaggerated when a patient lies flat on an operating table and when the patient is elderly, obese, or ventilated by overpressure. This is related to alveolar shunting of blood through the non-ventilated alveoli. The discrepancy between brain and blood measurements may be in the range of 10–50%, the higher values with prolonged procedures, obese patients, and elderly. The shunting and discrepancy may be reduced when positive end-expiratory pressure (PEEP) is used.

The metabolism of modern inhalational drugs is negligible and does not contribute quantitatively to the amount of drug in the body.

Inhalational drugs: pharmacodynamics

The relationship between stable levels of an inhalational drug in blood as described by stable end-tidal values and the effect is very well established by the MAC concept, where 1 MAC is the partial pressure needed for 50% of patients to not move upon surgical stimulation. In order to have 95% of patients non-moving, a concentration of 1.3 MAC is needed.

Another MAC value may also be defined as the end-point at which 50% of the patients are asleep, i.e., MAC_{sleep}. MAC_{sleep} in 50% of patients is about 0.33 MAC for all the potent inhalational agents, and about 0.67 MAC for nitrous oxide. In order to have 95% of the patients asleep a further 30% should be added, thus $MAC_{sleep95}$ will be about 0.45 MAC for the potent inhalation agents. Thus, in order to ensure that patients stay safely asleep in 95% of cases, stable brain values of 1.0 kPa (or 1%) sevoflurane, 3 kPa desflurane, or 0.6 kPa isoflurane are needed. For nitrous oxide this value (50% of MAC + 30%) will be 90 kPa, which is impossible to administer. Nevertheless, at 67% nitrous oxide may have a "hypnotic" contribution equal to that of 1 $MAC_{sleep50}$, which may be added to other inhalational drugs or hypnotics. The high MAC and MAC_{sleep} of nitrous oxide means that it is used as an adjunct to the potent drugs, but the additive value of 67% nitrous oxide is slightly less than 1 $MAC_{sleep50}$ when used in children and with desflurane. For a 95% chance of being asleep with 67% nitrous oxide the concentration of sevoflurane should be 0.5%; of desflurane, 1.5%; and of isoflurane, 0.3%. Table 4.2 shows that the MAC reducing effect of nitrous oxide is attenuated in the presence of less soluble inhalational anesthetics.

Similarities exist between potent inhalational agents, in their effect-versus-side-effect profile, but some differences exist at equipotent doses. Desflurane has been shown to be less of a respiratory depressant than sevoflurane (and isoflurane) at equipotent concentrations.[2] When a high concentration of desflurane (1 MAC or more) is given without titration, it may result in airway irritation and sympathetic stimulation leading to a rise in heart rate and blood pressure. As to cardiovascular effects, isoflurane seems to be the strongest vasodilator whereas halothane seems to be the most cardiodepressive (at equipotent

Table 4.2

Minimum alveolar concentration (MAC) for desflurane by age (year)	100% O_2	With 60% N_2O
< 1	9.2–10%	7.5%
1–12	8.1–9.1%	6.4%
18–30	7.3%	4%
31–60	6%	2.8%
> 60	5.2%	1.7%

doses), with sevoflurane and desflurane being intermediate on both measures. Sevoflurane and desflurane are regarded as safe for not being vasodilatory [potentially increasing the intracranial pressure (ICP)] in the brain when given at less than 1 MAC. All potent inhalational agents have been shown to induce preconditioning, with a relative protection of cardiac cells against damage during episodes of hypoxemia. Potent inhalation agents may provide some degree of muscle relaxation. A high dose level (2–3 MAC) is needed to keep the laryngeal muscles relaxed during intubation with inhalational agents alone.

Sevoflurane is the least irritating potent volatile inhalational induction agent available and its use in high dose (i.e., 6–8% inspired) results in a rapid and smooth induction in pediatric patients. Sevoflurane has a low blood/gas partition coefficient, and therefore induction and loss of consciousness are very rapid (Table 4.1). In children, the time from application of the face mask to loss of the eyelash reflex and intubation increase with increasing age. The MAC of sevoflurane is similar for neonates and infants of less than 6 months of age, 3.2%, and then decreases to 2.5% in older children. The occurrence of hypotension is more probable at induction in the neonate and infant group, whereas older children are less prone to it. The quality and speed of induction is better when 8% sevoflurane is applied than when sevoflurane is introduced progressively with increased increments. In older children, the use of the "double-breath" technique with 8% sevoflurane can result in a very fast onset with fewer side effects.[1]

All the inhalational agents seem to have the potential to induce emesis postoperatively, when compared to propofol for maintenance.

Dynamic interactions with intravenous agents

The intravenous (IV) opioids and hypnotics will interact with inhalational agents: the combination of an inhalational agent with an IV hypnotic will provide additive hypnotic effect, but not much more analgesic effect. The combination of an inhalational agent with an IV analgesic will provide additive analgesic effect, but only slightly increased hypnotic effect.[3–5]

a. The MAC_{sleep} may be reduced for a given drug in a linear manner by adding increasing amounts of the hypnotics propofol or midazolam. With midazolam 0.1 mg/kg IV, MAC_{sleep} for a potent inhalational agent will be reduced by about 50%; similar results are achieved with a propofol plasma level of 1.5 µg/ml.

b. The MAC_{sleep} is reduced by only 10–20% after a 0.2 mg dose of fentanyl in the adult, corresponding to a target of 7–8 ng/ml remifentanil or an infusion of 0.3 µg/kg per min. Some patients may be fully asleep on a high opioid dose alone; however, there is a large inter-individual variation, thus an average reduction in MAC_{sleep} of 50% demands a very high dose of opioid (fentanyl 0.6 mg or other opioid in an equipotent dose) and the effect is unpredictable.

c. The MAC to achieve an analgesic effect will be reduced by 60% after a fentanyl dose of 0.2 mg in an average adult, and by 75% by doubling this dose.

d. The MAC to achieve an analgesic effect will be reduced by hypnotics by 30–40% by adding midazolam (0.1 mg/kg bolus) or by a propofol plasma level of 1.5 µg/ml. The effect of adding further hypnotics iv is infra-additive. Nevertheless, very high (intoxicating) doses of hypnotics actually have an anti-nociceptive clinical action.

Intravenous drugs: pharmacokinetics

The plasma concentration of intravenous drugs is determined by the administered dose, tissue distribution, and elimination. A physiological model may be used (Figure 4.1), but for dosing and calculation, a mathematical model, derived from measurements in volunteers or patients, may be more practical. The distribution and elimination of IV drugs after dosing follow logarithmic laws, and usually can be described in a

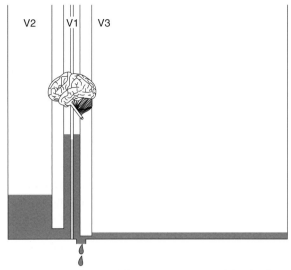

Figure 4.4. Mathematical three-compartment model with effect compartment embedded in volume 1 (V1). In the middle is V1, which receives drug and may be analogous to plasma and surrounding fluids. The level of black corresponds to drug concentration. From V1 there is good diffusion (a large opening) of drug into V2, which equilibrates with V1 within 10–30 min. A much slower diffusion takes place into V3 (a narrow opening), which is the larger part of the body and relatively poorly circulated. We may also note a constant "leakage" of drug from V1, which represents the clearance, inactivation, and/or excretion of the drug. The small gray compartment inside V1 is the CNS or effect compartment. The level of drug (black; gray in the brain) is an example of simulation 10 min after a bolus dose of propofol (from Tivatrainer®).

three-compartment model (Figure 4.4). The mathematical construct of V1 may be regarded as analogous to plasma plus extracellular fluids in very well vascularized tissues and organs, whereas V2 represents cells of the body receiving an intermediate proportion of the cardiac output, while V3 has a poor vascular supply, such as fat and bone tissue.

A bolus dose will result in a very high initial plasma concentration (in V1), which subsequently diffuses into V2 and V3. Because both V2 and V3 receive drug down a high concentration gradient initially, the decline in concentration in both plasma and V1 is rapid, but then slows as V2 equilibrates with V1. The third compartment (V3) fills very slowly due to its lower perfusion with blood. Constant metabolism (in terms of fraction of plasma drug metabolized, first order per unit time) will start immediately and continue, but is responsible for only a small fraction of the total decline in plasma concentration initially. An infusion is, in principle, multiple, very rapidly repeated small bolus administrations of a constant amount of a drug at a constant interval. After 3–5 times the elimination half-life of a drug, all

compartments (V1–V3) in the body are in diffusion equilibrium and the amount of drug metabolized is equal to the amount given per time unit if the concentration is steady. At this point a constant relationship is given for the time taken to reduce the plasma level of drug by 50% after cessation of dosing (the $T_{1/2}$ steady state or $T\frac{1}{2}_{\text{beta/gamma}}$), according to the formula:

$$T_{1/2} = V_D/\text{clearance} \times k$$

With a model such as that in Figure 4.4, and data for V1, V2, V3, clearance, and speed of equilibration between the compartments, computerized modeling may be used to predict the relevant plasma concentration in any patient at any time after a given setup for dosing [bolus(es) and/or infusion(s)]. Examples of such modeling are presented in the Stanpump® (http://anesthesia. stanford.edu/pkpd), RUGLOOP® (http://users.skynet. be/fa491447/index.html) and Tivatrainer® (www.euro siva.eu) simulation programs, which are very helpful for understanding intravenous dosing and predicting plasma levels.

The modeling of a fixed IV drug dose depends on the patient's weight, thus weight is always included in such models although often in quite simple ways: doubling the weight means doubling the dose in order to achieve the same plasma concentration. Taking other patient features into account may increase the precision of prediction, but these are not often included so far. Examples are: age, fat or lean (relationship between weight and height), gender, changes in liver or kidney function, etc.

With most IV anesthetic drugs (except remifentanil, stable after 20–30 min) it takes several hours to reach this level of steady state by continued, stable dosing or infusion (Figure 4.5). One very important concept for the anesthetist is derived from the pharmacokinetics described above, namely *context-sensitive elimination time*. Context-sensitive half-time predicts the time necessary to achieve a 50% decrease in drug concentration in the plasma after continuous infusion to a steady-state drug level in plasma. The "context" is the duration of a continuous infusion (Figure 4.6). Context-sensitive half-time provides information about drug offset time that is not reflected in the terminal elimination half-life or other pharmacokinetic parameters. Context-sensitive elimination time is the time taken to achieve a predefined reduction of drug in plasma.

Figure 4.7 shows the context-sensitive elimination half-life for propofol and other relevant opioids (see later for individual drug descriptions).

$$T_{1/2} = (V_D/\text{clearance} \times k_1)$$

$$\div \, (\text{diffusion from V1 to V2} + \text{V3}) \times k_2$$

Intravenous drugs: pharmacodynamics

a. Timing of onset/offset of effect.
b. Strength of effect.
c. Type of effect.

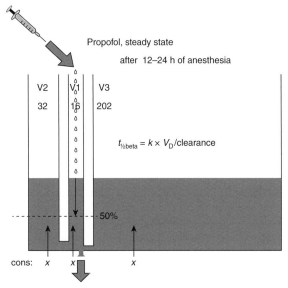

Figure 4.5. Steady-state picture of propofol in a three-compartment model, 70 kg adult patient. Note that the volume of V2 and V3 are upgraded in order to contain propofol at the same concentration (x) as in plasma. In a pure anatomical model (total volume= 70 liters) the V2 would be 16 liters and propofol concentration 2x, whereas the V3 would be 38 liters and propofol concentration about 6x.

Timing of onset/offset of effect

The following steps must take place for a drug to take effect.

- Diffusion out of blood vessels (through the blood–brain barrier).
- Diffusion into extracellular fluid.
- Diffusion to the surface of the effector cell.
- Bind to a receptor or cell surface or intracellular structure.
- Exert biologic effect.

The biologic effect may be fast, such as opening an ion channel; slower, such as activating protein synthesis [e.g., non-steroidal anti-inflammatory drugs (NSAIDS)]; or slower still, such as activating deoxyribonucleic acid (DNA) and protein synthesis (e.g., corticosteroids). As drugs differ both in their mechanism of biologic effect and in the time taken to get from the plasma to their effect site, they vary in time to onset. This difference may be expressed by a constant, k_{eO}, where a high constant means a rapid onset, or by $T_{1/2}\,k_{eO}$, which is the time taken for 50% equilibration from plasma to effect site. Both these terms are theoretical, based on the assumption of a stable plasma concentration, whereas the time to peak effect after a bolus dose is the result of both effect delay and the concentration gradient between the plasma and the brain, which reduces as the drug is distributed (Figure 4.8). With intravenous infusion without bolus start, the time to peak effect will be prolonged, but this is due to the slow increase in plasma concentration rather than the fixed delay to reach the effect site (Figure 4.9).

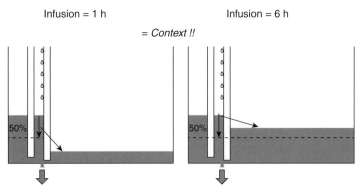

Same clearance – different distribution potential
→ *Different $T_{1/2}$ related to "context" !*

Figure 4.6. The same model as in Figure 4.5, but the propofol has been given for 1 h (left panel) or for 6 h (right panel). Note that in both cases the V2 is in equilibrium with the V1, but the V3 is "filled" less after 1 h than after 6 h. When the infusion stops the time to a 50% drop in plasma concentration (= V1) will be shorter after the 1-h infusion because the diffusion gradient to V3 is large.

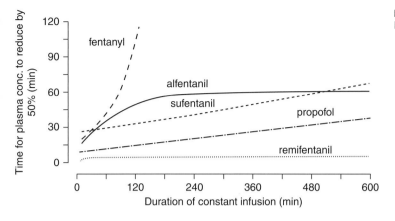

Figure 4.7. Context-sensitive elimination half-life.

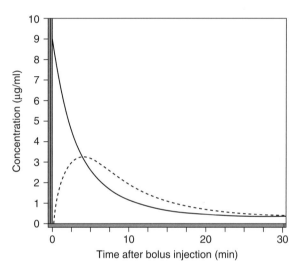

Figure 4.8. Propofol plasma concentration (solid line) after a 2 mg/kg bolus dose in a 70-kg adult. The dotted line is a qualitative estimation of strength of hypnotic effect. The peak effect is about 3–4 min after the start of bolus injection, and depends on: (1) the time taken to diffuse from the plasma to the CNS, and (2) the reducing concentration gradient as the drug is distributed.

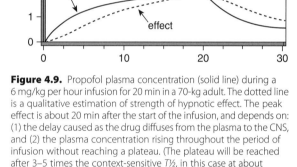

Figure 4.9. Propofol plasma concentration (solid line) during a 6 mg/kg per hour infusion for 20 min in a 70-kg adult. The dotted line is a qualitative estimation of strength of hypnotic effect. The peak effect is about 20 min after the start of the infusion, and depends on: (1) the delay caused as the drug diffuses from the plasma to the CNS, and (2) the plasma concentration rising throughout the period of infusion without reaching a plateau. (The plateau will be reached after 3–5 times the context-sensitive *T½*, in this case at about 30–40 min.)

$T½$ k_{eO} values and time to peak effect for some drugs are given in Table 4.3.

Knowing the time to peak effect after bolus administration is useful in three important contexts:

1. Aim to achieve the maximum effect when the stress is maximal, such as during intubation or the start of surgery.
2. Titrate a drug to the appropriate concentration. Titration involves giving a dose and waiting to observe its full effect. If the full effect is insufficient, a new dose is given and its effect assessed, and so on. The shorter the time to peak effect, the quicker the process of titration.

3. Anticipate the risk of side effects. For instance, with a slow-acting drug such as morphine, the event of respiratory depression will evolve slowly. Patients become gradually drowsy, then reduce breathing frequency before eventual apnea at the peak effect after 15–20 min. With alfentanil or remifentanil, the maximal effect occurs much more rapidly, with sudden apnea occurring earlier after a bolus. Thus, for safety issues, with a slow-acting drug, titration is relatively slow and a longer observation is required.

Table 4.3. Delay (min) from drug administration to plasma to onset of effect.

	$T\frac{1}{2}$ for equilibration between plasma and effect site ($T\frac{1}{2}$ keO) (min)	Time to maximal effect after a bolus dose (min) alone
Barbiturates	1.2	1.0–2.0
Propofol	2.6	1.5–3.5
Midazolam	5.6	5–7
Diazepam	2	1–3
Opioids:		
Remifentanil	1.2	1–2
Alfentanil	1.1	1.5–3
Fentanyl	5.8	4–5
Morphine	?	10–20
NSAID	?	15–30
Corticosteroid	?	60–120

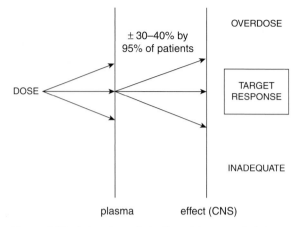

Figure 4.10. A dose (in mg/kg) will result in a spread of plasma concentrations of about ±30–50% around an average, for reasons of pharmacokinetics. Even when a specific plasma target is achieved, there will be a further spread of effect, due to pharmacodynamics.

Strength of effect

Computer programs will usually simulate the time course and changes in relative strength of effect, but not the actual level of clinical effect. For instance, with remifentanil the young and the elderly will have a fairly similar effect site curve, but in the elderly the actual clinical effect may be twice as strong.[6] This is probably due to increased CNS sensitivity to opioids in the elderly and should be taken into account when choosing a dosing level or target plasma or effect-site level. Females may need a little more hypnotic agent than males in order to be asleep; again the plasma or effect-site levels of drug may be similar, but the brain sensitivity may differ.[7]

The strength of effect for intravenous anesthetics may be expressed in ways analogous to the MAC: the ED50 or EC50. Effective dose, ED50, is the dose needed in order to bring about desired effect (e.g., sleep, no movement on incision) in 50% of patients; the effective concentration, EC50, is the plasma concentration needed. Generally there is a larger spread of inter-individual effects with IV drugs compared with inhalational drugs; in order to move from the EC50 to EC95 (effective concentration in 95% of patients), the dose needs to be increased by 40–50%; to move from ED50 to ED95, an increase of dose by 60–80% may be needed. The spread of ED will always be larger than the spread of EC, because a dose may result in a variety of plasma concentrations (Figure 4.10). The inter-individual variability in EC is generally greater for opioids than for hypnotic agents. The range may be fivefold, i.e., the patient with minimal opioid need will require one-fifth of the dose required by a patient with maximal need for the same standardized stimulus.

Type of effect – side effects

The intravenous anesthetic drugs also have side effects, the most important and frequently occurring of which are circulatory and respiratory in nature. These different effects arise from a variety of organs and effector cells, and each has a specific time–effect profile and delay (k_{eO}), which differ from those for the basic effects of general anesthesia, hypnosis, and anti-nociception.

Respiratory effects

Opioids cause a dose-dependent reduction in breathing frequency, culminating in apnea. Patients becoming drowsy with a respiratory rate below 8–10 breaths per minute should raise the suspicion of emerging apnea. An inability to maintain a free airway may occur before apnea is present.

Respiratory depression, being CNS-driven, usually follows the analgesic and sedative effects fairly closely. Respiratory depression may be counteracted by stimulation – verbal or (more efficient) tactile/painful or by naloxone, which will also reverse the analgesia abruptly. The respiratory depression caused by hypnotics is clinically evident as an inability to maintain a free airway and shallow tidal volumes, whereas the spontaneous ventilation frequency may be normal or low. Propofol will always result in apnea with high doses. Full reversal of the effects of benzodiazepines is possible with flumazenil.

Circulatory effects

The net circulatory effects are due to a combination of drug effects in the CNS and the periphery (directly in the heart and vessel walls, e.g., vasodilatation), as well as the physiologic effect of a reduction in sympathetic nerve tone. A drop in blood pressure (BP) and heart rate during general anesthetic induction is often seen (except with ketamine/etomidate), unless the surgery or other stimulation starts concomitantly. Kazama and coworkers have shown that the maximal drop in BP is delayed for 2–3 min when compared with the maximal hypnotic effect of propofol. The BP decrease is even more delayed (5–6 min) and more intense in the elderly.[8]

Intravenous drug interactions: opioids and hypnotics

General anesthesia may be achieved with a very high dose of hypnotic drug alone. Propofol at a dose five-fold higher than that required to induce sleep may achieve the same effect, but this is not practical in terms of drug economy, cardiovascular depression, and speed of recovery. Opioids, in contrast, provide excellent pain relief at high enough doses, but they are not reliable as hypnotics. Thus, general anesthesia with IV drugs only, total intravenous anesthesia (TIVA), is usually achieved with a combination of opioid and hypnotic drugs, most often propofol.

Opioids reduce the dose of propofol needed for sleep by 20–50% at fairly low doses, such as alfentanil 1–2 mg in an adult, or a remifentanil plasma level of 2.5–5.0 ng/ml.

Propofol reduces the need for opioids for antinociception in a dose-dependent manner: from a 10–20% reduction with a sleeping dose (6 mg/kg per hour or a target concentration of 3 µg/ml) to almost 90–100% if the dose is 5–6 times higher (target dose of 15–20 µg/ml).

The practical approach depends on the type of opioid in use as demonstrated by Vuyk and colleagues: EC50 and EC95 values for propofol + opioid combination in open gastric surgery (Table 4.4).

The main aim with the opioid/propofol combination is to use a high dose of the drug with the shorter context-sensitive elimination half-life. With remifentanil, that means having a low and stable concentration of propofol to ensure sleep and then adjust the opioid dose according to the strength of nociceptive stimulation. Of note is that concerning respiratory depression, the opioid/propofol combination is synergistic (see "Sedation" in Chapter 5).

Target control infusion[9]

Target control infusion (TCI) is a device to deliver a *plasma target concentration* of intravenous drugs with increased precision by adjusting to the patient's weight (Marsh) (Figure 4.11), and in other models also, to weight versus height ratio and other covariates such as age (Minto, Schnider, Schuttler, Paedfusor, etc.). A major limitation with all plasma models in how to achieve a target plasma level is that there is no account to the delay in drug equilibration between plasma and CNS. For propofol, for example, as the anesthetic drug effect is not in plasma, but in the CNS, it would be preferable to have an *effect-site TCI system* that delivers a preset concentration to effector sites in the CNS, taking into account the delay of diffusion and effect from plasma to CNS. A problem with effect-site modeling is that the delay until an effect is seen is quite variable between individuals, and also somewhat dependent on the rate of bolus/dosing, the dose level (high or low), the patient's cardiovascular status, etc. Also, the delay is hard to measure exactly and the relationship depends on both arterial and venous drug concentrations, which vary with changes in dosing. Plasma-concentration TCI and effect-site TCI are also being used with remifentanil, and for other opioids, such as alfentanil, fentanyl, and sufentanil. For remifentanil, for example, the Minto model hits the target well on average, but a ±30–50% deviation may be observed between individual patients.[10,11] When used in the effect-site mode, it will only deliver a drug "concentration" in the CNS and will not be adjusted for the patient's sensitivity to drug concentration (dynamics). Using plasma-concentration TCI, if overshooting with the target at

Table 4.4

		Drug			
		Alfentanil	**Fentanyl**	**Sufentanil**	**Remifentanil**
Optimal target with propofol (ng/ml) (EC95)		**130**	**1.6**	**0.2**	**8.0**
Manual dosing for target	1. Bolus (μg/kg) in 30 s	35	3	0.25	2
	2. Infusion (μg/kg per hour)	75 in 30 min	2.5 in 30 min	0.15	22 for 20 min
	3. Infusion thereafter	42	2 for 150 min	Same	19
	4. Adjustment	none	to 1.4 after 150 min	None	none
Optimal propofol target (μg/ml) with the opioid (EC95)		**4.4**	**5.4**	**4.5**	**2.8**
Manual dosing for target	1. Bolus (mg/kg) in 30 s	2.8	3.0	2.8	1.5
	2. Infusion (mg/kg per hour) for 40 min	12	15	12	8
	3. Infusion continued for 150 min	10	12	10	6.5
	4. Infusion thereafter	8	11	8	6

(Adapted from Vyuk J et al., Anesthesiology 1997:**87**:1549–62.)
Combinations of propofol + opioid in adults:
The bold font indicates the appropriate target concentrations required, whereas the bolus + infusion figure shows the relevant manual dosing for reaching and maintaining that target.

The figures are based on measurements of plasma concentrations of different combinations of alfentanil and propofol during open abdominal surgery, and the optimal combination for the most rapid emergence after 3 h of anesthesia. EC95 figures are the dose combinations needed to keep 95% of the patients completely immobile all the time.

The figures for the other opioids are extrapolated from the alfentanil clinical tests.

Comment: As these figures are based on open laparotomy in curarized patients, in the ambulatory setting we generally give even lower propofol doses (to 1.8–2.2 μg/ml) together with remifentanil unless the patient is paralyzed, but the target level of 2.5–2.8 μg/ml may be appropriate during phases of deep relaxation (i.e., being unable to move).

the start and when a rapid increase in effect may be required to achieve more rapid effect, it should be remembered that a higher bolus dose may exert a stronger effect on breathing and hemodynamics (Figure 4.12, Figure 4.13).

Computer-assisted Personalized Sedation (CAPS)

SEDASYS is an example of a CAPS system that is FDA-approved in the US to administer propofol sedation during gastrointestinal procedures by non-anesthesiologists. The system is intended to deliver moderate sedation to ASA class 1 and 2 patients undergoing a colonoscopy or an upper endoscopy, allows for only a small initial bolus of fentanyl, and requires that an anesthesia professional be "immediately available." CAPS is not a true closed-loop system because it cannot automatically increase the propofol infusion rate but only decrease or stop it based on a patient's physiologic response.[12]

Summary

Pharmacology is especially important in ambulatory anesthesia. The knowledge of the relationship between a given dose of medication and plasma level (pharmacokinetics) and between plasma level and effect(s) (pharmacodynamics) as well as the side effects of medications is crucial to insure safety and an efficient turnover for different types of ambulatory surgeries. The goal is to achieve an effective depth of anesthesia with limited perioperative adverse effects.

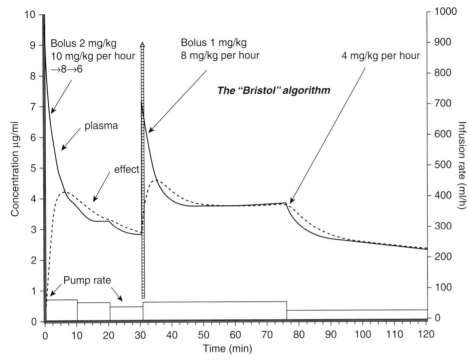

Figure 4.11. Plasma concentration (solid line) and relative strength of hypnotic effect (dotted line) for a manual propofol regime of starting bolus, followed by infusion adjusted at 10 and 20 min. Also shown are an increase in dosing at 30 min and a decrease at 75 min (Marsh kinetic/dynamic model, Tivatrainer®).

Anesthesiology drugs; some practical comments

This section does not provide thorough, systematic information about the indications, contraindications, and dosing for drugs as provided in a drug manual or a textbook of pharmacology. The idea is to provide some personal, practical clinical comments.

Inhalational agents

These should only be used where an appropriate scavenger system is present. In situations where there is a need for a rapid inhalational effect, high fresh gas flow of oxygen or oxygen–air at 6–8 l/min should be used.

In general, it may be wise to use a high fresh gas flow (6–8 l/min in adults) for 5–15 min during induction and at the end of the case, otherwise reducing to a fresh gas flow of 1.5–2 l/min for reasons of economy and improved humidity and temperature regulation. With low flow, the use of an end-tidal gas monitor is mandatory.

Sevoflurane is the routinely used potent gas, because of its low irritation and pungency.

Desflurane is not suited for induction secondary to its pungency, but it is well suited for maintenance. Desflurane is well suited for optimal emergence (faster than propofol) after prolonged procedures. One study also suggests that desflurane may result in less "sleepiness" in the days following cholecystectomy, compared with propofol maintenance.[13] With prolonged use (< 2–3 hours, less in the obese), desflurane has a more rapid emergence than sevoflurane. Desflurane is also reported to have less emergence delirium in children when compared with sevoflurane.[14]

Isoflurane is a well-documented and cheaper alternative to sevoflurane and desflurane. The recovery is slower, but with careful down titration towards the end of the procedure, emergence may be rapid.[15]

Nitrous oxide is less potent and also associated with nausea and vomiting, as with other inhalational agents. The potential of nitrous oxide to cause postoperative nausea and vomiting (PONV) is especially

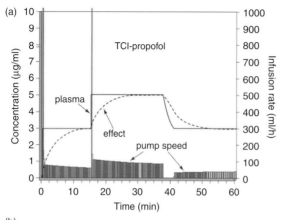

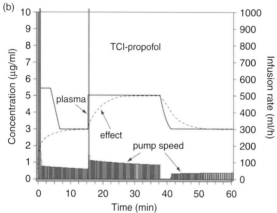

Figure 4.12 (a) Plasma target control infusion, TCI (pump rate indicated by black columns) for a target of 3, then 5, then back to 3. Note that the pump gives a short-lasting bolus injection both at the start and when increasing the dose, and decreases the dose through temporary stoppage. Also note that the pump rate is adjusted far more frequently (= more accurately) than is the case with a manual regimen (as in Figure 4.11). Also note the delay in effect, the patient is probably not asleep until 5–7 min. (b) Same as in (a), except for "cheating" with a plasma target of 5.5 µg/min during induction, in order to obtain a more rapid effect (dotted curve); the patient will probably be asleep at 2–3 min.

high in patients with a high baseline PONV risk. Its advantages are its rapid on–off effect, its minor influence on ventilation and circulation, and the resulting 20–40% reduction in dose of other drugs which may be achieved by simultaneous administration of nitrous oxide. When given together with an IV technique, the propofol dose may be reduced by one-third.

Intravenous hypnotics

Barbiturates

Rarely used in modern ambulatory anesthesia.

Thiopental sodium

Although thiopental sodium is used for fast induction with a fast onset of effect, its elimination is very slow. In some places it is still preferred for electroconvulsive therapy (ECT), because the visible convulsions are more easily triggered and evident than with propofol. Currently, it is not available in the US for patient use.

Methohexital

This is fairly rapidly cleared and eliminated. It is somewhat challenging to titrate as the patients may experience involuntary movements and quite strong pain associated with intravenous injection, as well as hiccups.[16,17]

Benzodiazepines

Diazepam

Has a slow elimination rate and active metabolites, but seems to be a little less hypnotic and thus more anxiolytic than midazolam. It is a good choice for premedication, 5–10 mg orally, especially if the patient needs an anxiolytic for more than 1–2 h ahead of surgery.

Midazolam

Hypnotic, anxiolytic, and amnesic. Midazolam is short-acting with no active metabolites, and has a clear drop in effect after 2 h. It is well suited for premedication when there is less than 2 h until the start of anesthesia, either orally or intravenously.

Propofol

Propofol is the "gold standard" hypnotic for ambulatory anesthesia. In low doses it will have anxiolytic, amnesic, and anti-emetic properties, and is also the drug of choice for sedation. Propofol has rapid metabolism and rapid recovery, although emergence may take a few minutes more than with sevoflurane or desflurane, unless the propofol dose is tapered carefully down by the end of anesthesia. However, recovery is pleasant, almost euphoric; it has an anti-emetic effect and a low incidence of shivering.

Propofol may ache in thin veins at the start of dosing; the aching may be avoided by using a large vein, for instance in the elbow. Propofol in medium-chain triglyceride solute and in diluted doses is less

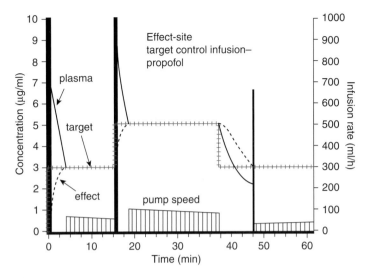

Figure 4.13. Effect-site TCI for propofol. The pump is programmed to deliver an effect-site level of 3, then 5, then 3 again. Note the differences from Figure 4.12 and plasma-concentration TCI. At the start and when increasing the dose there will be a plasma "overshoot" created by a faster bolus infusion, followed by cessation for proper equilibration with the effect site. To decrease the effect-site concentration, the pump is stopped and the plasma concentration allowed to fall below the new target level, after which a small bolus is given to "catch up" with the effect curve and maintain the new level stable.

painful on injection. Further tricks to reduce aching may be to inject lidocaine 10 mg/ml, 2–3 ml first (best with a tourniquet for 1–2 min, but it also works without a tourniquet), to give an IV opioid first, or to mix lidocaine 10 mg/ml, 1 ml into 10 ml propofol shortly before injection. Such lidocaine-mixed propofol should be used within a few hours, otherwise the lipid emulsion will become unstable. It has also been shown that using a local anesthesia pad (e.g., EMLA®) may further reduce the incidence of aching from propofol in the same area. Although propofol contains soybean oil, this is treated and free of antigens, thus hardly any cases of true propofol allergy or cross-reactions with soybeans or peanuts are reported in the literature.

In a situation that has been stable since the previous dose adjustment (more than 15–20 min), a propofol infusion of 6 mg/kg per hour will correspond to a target (plasma or effect site) of about 2.5 µg/ml.

Dexmedetomidine[18]

Dexmedetomidine is a highly selective α2 adrenoreceptor agonist with both sedative and analgesic effects with minimal respiratory depression. Dexmedetomidine induces a physiologic-like sleep.[19] It may induce hypotension, bradycardia, and a dry mouth, and has an anti-shivering effect. It may be a valuable drug in terms of sedation and opioid-sparing effects perioperatively; however, it has a slower onset and offset than propofol, which may not be ideal in the ambulatory setting.

Opioids

Fentanyl

Fentanyl is a favorite opioid for postoperative pain relief within the first 1–2 h, as it works fairly rapidly in 0.05-mg increments (0.5 µg/kg in children) with a weaning off effect and side effects after 20–30 min. There is no rationale for using fentanyl together with remifentanil at induction or for maintenance during a case; a better choice is to dose only remifentanil as needed.[20] Fentanyl may result in prolonged emergence and thus more PONV when used in high doses. Used together with remifentanil it is our routine to give 0.05–0.1 mg (adults, children 1 µg/kg) by the end of remifentanil-based anesthesia, in order to avoid having a patient wake up with no opioid effect and strong pain.

Alfentanil

It may be an alternative to remifentanil for short cases and for handling strong and short-lasting nociceptive stimulation. Alfentanil has a peak effect at 1–2 min and declines after 10–15 min. It may induce a stiff chest if dosed beyond 2–3 mg in an adult who has not received hypnotics first.[21]

Remifentanil

Remifentanil has gained a lot of interest for use as an opioid for ambulatory care; its rapid peak of effect occurs within 1–2 min and it never takes longer than

3–4 min for 50% recovery following cessation of administration even after very prolonged dosing.[22] Remifentanil has to be prepared from a powder, and given by an infusion pump. With an infusion of less than 0.1 µg/kg per minute there is a fair chance of maintaining spontaneous breathing, but for surgery usually a dose of 0.2–0.5 µg/kg/min is needed. It may also be given in bolus doses, 0.5–1 µg/kg, repeated every 5 min. One should be aware of the risk of a stiff chest with any dose of more than 1 µg/kg given rapidly (within 1 min) to a patient if no hypnotic drug has been given first, the elderly being more prone to a stiff chest. In a stable situation (more than 5–10 min after the last adjustment) a remifentanil infusion of 0.1 µg/kg per min will correspond to a target (plasma or effect-site concentration) of about 2.5 ng/ml.

Concern has been raised over the hyperalgesic effects of remifentanil, seen experimentally after only 30 min of infusion, and clinically after 2–3 h of infusions of more than 0.3 µg/kg per min. These patients have a lowered pain threshold postoperatively, with increased need for opioid and non-opioid analgesics. Experimental data suggest that in such cases hyperalgesia may be prevented effectively with a low-dose infusion of ketamine,[23] and probably partially by NSAIDs or cyclooxygenase inhibitors given preoperatively or a potent inhalational agent given perioperatively.

Sufentanil

Sufentanil behaves fairly similarly to fentanyl for limited use, as in ambulatory care, but has a slightly slower onset and no specific features for use in this setting.

Oxycodone

Oxycodone is the opioid with the highest and most predictable bioavailability (70–80%) after oral dosing. It is well suited for extra analgesia after discharge for 1–3 days in patients who have pain problems in spite of optimal non-opioid medication. It may be used in sustained-release tablet form twice a day. Oxycodone may also be used intravenously, and is probably slightly more (+25–50%) potent than morphine. Some studies suggest that oxycodone has a little less-sedative profile compared with morphine and may be better for visceral postoperative pain.[24] Oxycodone may also be supplied orally together with a small dose of naloxone in order to reduce constipation. This combination tablet is effective with prolonged therapy for cancer pain, but has not proved any benefits for a short 2–3-day use in ambulatory patients.

Codeine

Codeine has a lower bioavailability than oxycodone (50–60%) and works through degradation by cytochrome P-450 type 2D6 to morphine in the body. Some 5–10% of Caucasians have a failure of this enzyme and codeine will have almost no clinical effect for them. In contrast, 0.5–1% of Caucasians may be extensive metabolizers and for them codeine has a very strong effect, and may be dangerous. For these reasons the effect of codeine may be unpredictable, and it should not be used repeatedly in lactating females as lethal morphine concentrations may rarely occur in the milk of extensive metabolizers.

Codeine is still very popular as an oral opioid, often in conjunction with acetaminophen. When giving the combination of acetaminophen and codeine to supplement an optimal dose of acetaminophen alone, care should be taken to avoid an acetaminophen overdose.

Non-opioid analgesics

These are dealt with in more detail in Chapter 6. In order to avoid opioid-induced side-effects postoperatively, it is important to provide optimal non-opioid analgesia before transfer to the post-anesthesia care unit (PACU). The cornerstones are acetaminophen, NSAIDs or cyclooxygenase inhibitors, glucocorticoids, and local anesthesia applied directly to the wounds.

Neuromuscular blockers and reversal agents

In modern anesthesia and ambulatory care in particular, the use of neuromuscular blockers has declined. The use of muscle relaxants necessitates extra drugs, which has implications for cost and potential side effects. Very often reversal and anticholinergic agents are also needed and there is a rare risk of serious awareness, which is not seen in non-curarized patients who would move if they are in discomfort.[25]

Indications for neuromuscular blockers are as follows.

a. The surgeon needs strong muscle relaxation of the patient in order to access anatomic structures.

This may be the case with laparotomies, thoracotomies, and major joint surgery. In ambulatory cases this need is rare, but may be indicated in some cases of laparoscopy, e.g., in the obese or patients with many adhesions.

b. The surgeon sometimes needs the patient to lie completely still; even a small movement may ruin the result. This may be the case for some ambulatory procedures, such as microsurgery on vessels, the middle ear, or the eye. In these cases a TOF guard should always be used and one should maintain a dosing that ensures either one or no twitches during the critical periods and be prepared to use reversal agents to end the case.

c. The anesthesiologist needs to do a rapid sequence induction in the acutely ill or non-fasting patient in order to secure the airway rapidly. This indication is virtually nonexistent in ambulatory care; if there is a suspicion of non-fasting status, the patient's surgery should be postponed until an empty stomach is assured.

d. The anesthesiologist needs a neuromuscular blocker for routine elective intubation. Example: an obese patient for laparoscopy. In fairly healthy patients the intubation may be done with a combination of a narcotic such as remifentanil and propofol (see Chapter 7). There are very few reports of serious problems or prolonged disability due to this approach.[26–28]

e. The anesthesiologist needs a neuromuscular blocker for gentle induction (i.e., lower dose of opioid needed) with intubation in the elderly or otherwise fragile patient. This indication is also advantageous in that the use of an otherwise high-dose opioid (remifentanil) plus propofol in elderly patients may result in an unpredictable drop in blood pressure; thus, concomitant use of neuromuscular blocker allows more stable vital signs during intubation.

f. The anesthesiologist needs to use neuromuscular blockers to resolve a stiff chest (high-dose remifentanil or alfentanil in a non-sedated patient) or laryngospasm (in a child during induction or emergence, or patient with sudden, strong surgical perioperative stimulation).

Succinylcholine

Succinylcholine is a cheap, fast-onset, and short-acting drug with no need or effect of reversal.

Use in ambulatory patients may result in minor muscular pain for 1–2 days. There is an additional risk of anaphylactic reaction, hyperkalemia, and complications in the case of an undiagnosed neuromuscular disease. About 1 in 4000 patients may also have an unexpected metabolic degradation deficiency that calls for antiserum or ventilation and sedation for 3–4 h until the block resolves. Succinylcholine is also usually involved in the rare, but potentially lethal, cases of malignant hyperthermia (see Chapter 16).

Mivacurium

A fairly short-acting (20–40 min), nondepolarizing drug that does not require reversal routinely, and that has organ-independent metabolism. Cases of degradation enzyme deficiencies occur as with succinylcholine. It has a fairly slow onset, over 3–4 min. This drug is now rarely used in the US.

Vecuronium, cisatracurium

Well-established, safe alternatives for nondepolarizing block, fairly slow onset (3–4 min) and offset, should always be used in conjunction with TOF monitoring. These drugs usually have to be combined with neostigmine + glycopyrrolate reversal, which should only be attempted when two to three twitches are registered on the TOF guard.

Rocuronium

Acts faster than other nondepolarizing agents, especially at higher dosage; onset down to 1 min, comparable with succinylcholine. The downside of such dosing is its prolonged effect, which may be counteracted efficiently with a new reversal agent, sugammadex. However, sugammadex is not available in the US. Discussion about the more frequent anaphylaxis seen with rocuronium in some countries (France and Norway) is not fully conclusive,[29] but seems to be a local phenomenon due to cross-allergy with other common local drugs.

Neuromuscular reversal

Reports of serious clinical problems of residual neuromuscular block during recovery exist, with an increased incidence of pulmonary complications in the elderly with poor reversal of block.[30] Newer studies suggest that a TOF ratio of anything less than 0.9 (i.e., the fourth twitch strength is 90% that of the first twitch) may interfere with normal swallowing and thus lead to risk of aspiration,[31] although real clinical outcome data have not been produced.

Neostigmine

Even with a partial block, i.e., one or two twitches on the TOF guard, it takes 10–20 min for full reversal of block in some patients.[32] The dose of neostigmine should be 50–70 µg/kg in order to be adequate. With this dose the risk of nausea and vomiting is increased, almost doubled in one study,[33] and also other side effects may be seen (such as bronchial constriction or defecation).

Sugammadex

Sugammadex has been reported to provide rapid reversal for rocuronium and vecuronium, but is still not yet available in the US. Reversal within 1–2 min may be achieved at any level and duration of muscle relaxation. This may be relevant when the surgeon finishes suddenly (microsurgery) or even in the case of difficult intubation, when a high dose of rocuronium may be reversed by a high dose of sugammadex. Other indications are poor pulmonary function and the very obese patient, for whom complete and rapid reversal may reduce the risk of complications. The main problem is the cost, about 100 USD for a standard dose of 2 mg/kg and 2–4 times greater if a high dose is used for profound block. Nevertheless, unpublished work suggests that a small dose of 0.5 mg/kg may be sufficient for an average block and may even be combined with neostigmine for dose reduction.

Ketamine[23]

Ketamine is an N-methyl-D-aspartate (NMDA) receptor blocker with dose-dependent analgesic, hypnotic, and some muscle relaxant effects. Spontaneous breathing is maintained. In contrast with other general anesthetics, ketamine stimulates the sympathetic nervous system to maintain blood pressure and heart rate when the patient falls asleep. For this reason, ketamine is often the routine induction drug of choice in hypovolemic or severely bleeding patients. Because of its simplicity of use, ketamine is also much used in field situations or in places with limited resources. A problem with ketamine is the significant occurrence of bad dreams and hallucinations during emergence, which may be partly, but not completely, counteracted by a benzodiazepine given before the start of the ketamine.

As ambulatory anesthesia is particularly concerned with achieving rapid and uneventful recovery and is rarely undertaken in hypovolemic patients or field situations, ketamine traditionally has a limited role in ambulatory care. Nevertheless, two recent issues have challenged this view: one is the claim that ketamine is an ideal sedative when given in conjunction with propofol, and the other is research on the role of the NMDA receptor in hyperalgesia and chronic pain.

a. Although ketamine is traditionally associated with slow emergence and some incidence of unpleasant hallucinations, even when given in moderate doses for sedation,[34] Friedberg et al. have repeatedly reported a high success rate for ketamine-induced sedation during plastic surgery under local anesthesia. Propofol, increasingly supplemented with ketamine for light or profound sedation during spontaneous ventilation, gave no hallucinations and virtually no postoperative nausea and vomiting.[35,36] Recent publications in the ambulatory setting partly support this conclusion.[37] However, Aouad et al. reported increased agitation,[38] Goel et al. reported delayed recovery,[39] and a review by Slavik and Zed concluded that there are no specific benefits of this technique.[40] Regarding this controversy, it should be noted that this technique is mainly reported when carried out with sedation for plastic surgery and thorough local anesthesia infiltration to provide basic analgesia. The propofol doses have been fairly generous and the ketamine doses fairly low. To date, one randomized, double-blind study on the benefit of this technique has demonstrated improved cardiovascular stability when a single dose of ketamine (0.3 mg/kg) is compared with fentanyl (1.5 µg/kg) during propofol sedation.[37]

b. Recent interest has also been shown in low-dose ketamine infusion for the reduction of postoperative pain and hyperalgesia.[41,42] As NMDA activation appears to be involved in the development of opioid-induced hyperalgesia, low-dose ketamine infusion has proven efficacious at blunting hyperalgesia.[42] For this antihyperalgesic effect a continuous infusion (1–2 µg/kg per minute, throughout the whole perioperative period including up to 1–2 days postoperatively) seems to be best, although the clinical relevance of hyperalgesia in ambulatory anesthesia is not well documented. However, ketamine also has direct analgesic effects, given as a single bolus dose (0.15–0.5 mg/kg) or as a perioperative infusion. The meta-analyses of both Bell *et al.*[43] and Elia and Tramér[44] concluded on a postoperative opioid-sparing effect and no significant side effects from using a ketamine adjunct. One study of 0.15 mg/kg given preoperatively also suggests a pre-emptive effect after gynecologic surgery, as the group receiving the preoperative dose had better analgesia than the postoperative dosing group.[45] Nevertheless, while some studies are positive,[46] others do not find any effect apart from short-lasting analgesia together with increased post-operative sedation.[47]

In conclusion, ketamine may be a promising alternative to low-dose opioids as an adjunct to propofol sedation with safe, spontaneous breathing. However, more studies are needed on both this issue and the clinical benefits of ketamine for analgesia after ambulatory surgery. As ketamine is a racemic mixture, the more potent *S*-ketamine isomer has been isolated and marketed in Europe with good success. *S*-ketamine has a slightly faster onset of effect and seems to have reduced incidence of postoperative hallucinations.

Anti-emetics

These are dealt with in Chapter 7, in the section on postoperative nausea and vomiting (PONV).

References

1. Abdallah C, Hannallah R. Inhalation versus intravenous anesthetics. *Curr Rev Clin Anesth* 2009;**30**(3):25–36.

2. Einarsson SG, Cerne A, Bengtsson A, *et al.* Respiration during emergence from anaesthesia with desflurane/N$_2$O vs. desflurane/air for gynaecological laparoscopy. *Acta Anaesthesiol Scand* 1998;**42**:1192–98.

3. Katoh T, Ikeda K. The effects of fentanyl on sevoflurane requirements for loss of consciousness and skin incision. *Anesthesiology* 1998;**88**:18–24.

4. Albertin A, Dedola E, Bergonzi PC, *et al.* The effect of adding two target-controlled concentrations (1–3 ng ml^{-1}) of remifentanil on MAC BAR of desflurane. *Eur J Anaesthesiol* 2006;**23**:510–16.

5. Inagaki Y, Sumikawa K, Yoshiya I. Anesthetic interaction between midazolam and halothane in humans. *Anesth Analg* 1993;**76**:613–17.

6. Minto CF, Schnider TW, Egan TD, *et al.* Influence of age and gender on the pharmacokinetics and pharmacodynamics of remifentanil. I. Model development. *Anesthesiology* 1997;**86**:10–23.

7. Hoymork SC, Raeder J. Why do women wake up faster than men from propofol anaesthesia? *Br J Anaesth* 2005;**95**:627–33.

8. Kazama T, Ikeda K, Morita K, *et al.* Comparison of the effect-site k(eO)s of propofol for blood pressure and EEG bispectral index in elderly and younger patients. *Anesthesiology* 1999;**90**:1517–27.

9. Absalom AR, Struys MRF. *An overview of TCI and TIVA*. Ghent: Academia Press, 2005.

10. Hoymork SC, Raeder J, Grimsmo B, Steen PA. Bispectral index, predicted and measured drug levels of target-controlled infusions of remifentanil and propofol during laparoscopic cholecystectomy and emergence. *Acta Anaesthesiol Scand* 2000;**44**:1138–44.

11. Minto CF, Schnider TW, Shafer SL. Pharmacokinetics and pharmacodynamics of remifentanil. II. Model application. *Anesthesiology* 1997;**86**:24–33.

12. Urman RD, Maurer WG. Computer-assisted personalized sedation: friend or foe? *Anesth Analg* 2014;**119**:207–11.

13. Mjaland O, Raeder J, Aasboe V, *et al.* Outpatient laparoscopic cholecystectomy. *Br J Surg* 1997;**84**:958–61.

14. Beskow A, Westrin P. Sevoflurane causes more postoperative agitation in children than does halothane. *Acta Anaesthesiol Scand* 1999;**43**:536–41.

15. Seitsonen ER, Yli-Hankala AM, Korttila KT. Similar recovery from bispectral index-titrated isoflurane and sevoflurane anesthesia after outpatient gynecological surgery. *J Clin Anesth* 2006;**18**:272–79.

16. Raeder JC, Misvaer G. Comparison of propofol induction with thiopentone or methohexitone in short outpatient general anaesthesia. *Acta Anaesthesiol Scand* 1988;**32**:607–13.

17. Lee JS, Gonzalez ML, Chuang SK, Perrott DH. Comparison of methohexital and propofol use in ambulatory procedures in oral and maxillofacial surgery. *J Oral Maxillofac Surg* 2008;**66**:1996–2003.

18. Carollo DS, Nossaman BD, Ramadhyani U. Dexmedetomidine: a review of clinical applications. *Curr Opin Anaesthesiol* 2008;**21**:457–61.

19. Sanders RD, Maze M. Alpha2-adrenoceptor agonists. *Curr Opin Investig Drugs* 2007;**8**:25–33.

20. Lenz H, Raeder J, Hoymork SC. Administration of fentanyl before remifentanil-based anaesthesia has no influence on post-operative pain or analgesic consumption. *Acta Anaesthesiol Scand* 2008;**52**:149–54.

21. Raeder JC, Hole A. Alfentanil anaesthesia in gall-bladder surgery. *Acta Anaesthesiol Scand* 1986;**30**:35–40.

22. Raeder J. Remifentanil, a new age in anaesthesia? In: Vuyk J, Engbers F, Groen-Mulder S, eds. *On the Study*

and Practice of Intravenous Anaesthesia. Dordrecht: Kluwer Academic, 2000: 249–60.

23. Raeder JC, Stenseth LB. Ketamine: a new look at an old drug. *Curr Opin Anaesthesiol* 2000;**13**:463–68.

24. Lenz H, Sandvik L, Qvigstad E, *et al.* A comparison of intravenous oxycodone and intravenous morphine in patient-controlled postoperative analgesia after laparoscopic hysterectomy. *Anesth Analg* 2009;**109**:1279–83.

25. Sandin RH, Enlund G, Samuelsson P, Lennmarken C. Awareness during anaesthesia: a prospective case study. *Lancet* 2000;**355**:707–11.

26. McNeil IA, Culbert B, Russell I. Comparison of intubating conditions following propofol and succinylcholine with propofol and remifentanil 2 µg kg^{-1} or 4 µg kg^{-1}. *Br J Anaesth* 2000;**85**:623–25.

27. Mencke T, Echternach M, Kleinschmidt S, *et al.* Laryngeal morbidity and quality of tracheal intubation: a randomized controlled trial. *Anesthesiology* 2003;**98**:1049–56.

28. Stevens JB, Wheatley L. Tracheal intubation in ambulatory surgery patients: using remifentanil and propofol without muscle relaxants. *Anesth Analg* 1998;**86**:45–49.

29. Harboe T, Guttormsen AB, Irgens A, *et al.* Anaphylaxis during anesthesia in Norway: a 6-year single-center follow-up study. *Anesthesiology* 2005;**102**:897–903.

30. Berg H, Roed J, Viby-Mogensen J, *et al.* Residual neuromuscular block is a risk factor for postoperative pulmonary complications. A prospective, randomised, and blinded study of postoperative pulmonary complications after atracurium, vecuronium and pancuronium. *Acta Anaesthesiol Scand* 1997;**41**:1095–103.

31. Eriksson LI, Sundman E, Olsson R, *et al.* Functional assessment of the pharynx at rest and during swallowing in partially paralyzed humans: simultaneous videomanometry and mechanomyography of awake human volunteers. *Anesthesiology* 1997;**87**:1035–43.

32. Kirkegaard H, Heier T, Caldwell JE. Efficacy of tactile-guided reversal from cisatracurium-induced neuromuscular block. *Anesthesiology* 2002;**96**:45–50.

33. Lovstad RZ, Thagaard KS, Berner NS, Raeder JC. Neostigmine 50 µg kg^{-1} with glycopyrrolate increases postoperative nausea in women after laparoscopic gynaecological surgery. *Acta Anaesthesiol Scand* 2001;**45**:495–500.

34. Strayer RJ, Nelson LS. Adverse events associated with ketamine for procedural sedation in adults. *Am J Emerg Med* 2008;**26**:985–1028.

35. Friedberg BL. Propofol-ketamine technique. *Aesthetic Plast Surg* 1993;**17**:297–300.

36. Friedberg BL. Propofol ketamine anesthesia for cosmetic surgery in the office suite. *Int Anesthesiol Clin* 2003;**41**:39–50.

37. Messenger DW, Murray HE, Dungey PE, *et al.* Subdissociative-dose ketamine versus fentanyl for analgesia during propofol procedural sedation: a randomized clinical trial. *Acad Emerg Med* 2008;**15**:877–86.

38. Aouad MT, Moussa AR, Dagher CM, *et al.* Addition of ketamine to propofol for initiation of procedural anesthesia in children reduces propofol consumption and preserves hemodynamic stability. *Acta Anaesthesiol Scand* 2008;**52**:561–65.

39. Goel S, Bhardwaj N, Jain K. Efficacy of ketamine and midazolam as co-induction agents with propofol for laryngeal mask insertion in children. *Paediatr Anaesth* 2008;**18**:628–34.

40. Slavik VC, Zed PJ. Combination ketamine and propofol for procedural sedation and analgesia. *Pharmacotherapy* 2007;**27**:1588–98.

41. De Kock MF, Lavand'homme PM. The clinical role of NMDA receptor antagonists for the treatment of postoperative pain. *Best Pract Res Clin Anaesthesiol* 2007;**21**:85–98.

42. Stubhaug A, Breivik H, Eide PK, *et al.* Mapping of punctuate hyperalgesia around a surgical incision demonstrates that ketamine is a powerful suppressor of central sensitization to pain following surgery. *Acta Anaesthesiol Scand* 1997;**41**:1124–32.

43. Bell RF, Dahl JB, Moore RA, Kalso E. Peri-operative ketamine for acute post-operative pain: a quantitative and qualitative systematic review (Cochrane review). *Acta Anaesthesiol Scand* 2005;**49**:1405–28.

44. Elia N, Tramér MR. Ketamine and postoperative pain – a quantitative systematic review of randomised trials. *Pain* 2005;**113**:61–70.

45. Kwok RF, Lim J, Chan MT, *et al.* Preoperative ketamine improves postoperative analgesia after gynecologic laparoscopic surgery. *Anesth Analg* 2004;**98**:1044–49, table.

46. Roytblat L, Korotkoruchko A, Katz J, *et al.* Postoperative pain: the effect of low-dose ketamine in addition to general anesthesia. *Anesth Analg* 1993;**77**:1161–65.

47. Mathisen LC, Aasbo V, Raeder J. Lack of pre-emptive analgesic effect of (R)-ketamine in laparoscopic cholecystectomy. *Acta Anaesthesiol Scand* 1999;**43**:220–24.

Chapter 5

Anesthetic techniques

Niraja Rajan, MBBS, Richard D. Urman, MD,
and Johan Raeder, MD, PhD

In this chapter, we will discuss the following anesthetic techniques: general anesthesia, monitored anesthesia care (MAC), and local anesthesia, specifically tailored to ambulatory surgery.

The emphasis will be on the goals of the ideal ambulatory anesthetic, quick recovery with minimal adverse effects, and short times to discharge readiness. (Also see Chapter 7.)

Preoperative logistics

The techniques and agents discussed in this chapter will therefore focus on short-acting agents, agents with minimal or easily treatable side effects, and the use of a combination of agents (multimodal) to minimize adverse effects and maximize therapeutic effects.

General anesthesia

General anesthesia is a medically induced reversible coma accomplished by administering a combination of anesthetic drugs and agents for achieving amnesia, analgesia, hypnosis, and skeletal muscle relaxation. General anesthesia consists of the following phases.

Induction

This could be inhalational or intravenous.

Inhalational induction

Inhalational induction may be achieved with a mixture of oxygen/nitrous oxide (30/70) with added sevoflurane, all administered via a face mask to the patient until loss of consciousness. The airway and ventilation are supported as needed. Sevoflurane is non-irritating and has a low solubility which makes it the anesthetic of choice for inhalational induction. One option is to start with a nitrous oxide induction, wait for 1–2 min and then introduce sevoflurane 8%. Another option is to start both simultaneously, or eventually sevoflurane 8% may be used as the only agent. There are no major documented benefits or drawbacks to any of these options, and the choice of one may depend on local tradition and experience. Inhalational induction is typically used in infants and children, or in the needle-phobic adult who will not allow the placement of an intravenous line preoperatively. After loss of consciousness and placement of an IV, the airway device of choice is inserted. At this point, the patient may be given IV propofol (1 mg/kg) to achieve an adequate depth of anesthetic for insertion of a laryngeal mask airway (LMA).

The advantages of inhalational induction are ease of administration and widespread acceptance in the pediatric population. Disadvantages include unpleasant odor, claustrophobia, and prolonged induction in larger and older patients with the potential for complications such as breath-holding or laryngospasm and increased incidence of PONV. Therefore, inhalational induction is reserved for patients in whom obtaining preoperative IV access would be difficult or unduly traumatic. Some short procedures (such as myringotomies) may not require IV access or airway instrumentation, and can be completed with inhalational induction and maintenance with a facemask.

IV induction

In most patients, IV access is established preoperatively. For ambulatory procedures, propofol is the induction agent of choice due to its speed of onset, adequate depth for LMA insertion, and favorable recovery profile with decreased PONV and very low emergence delirium rates. It is administered in the dose of 1.5–2 mg/kg and usually combined with an analgesic (short-acting opioid) for induction. Some will also use

Practical Ambulatory Anesthesia, ed. Johan Raeder and Richard D. Urman. Published by Cambridge University Press.
© Cambridge University Press 2015.

a small dose of midazolam as a part of the induction, but this has no documented benefit in the stable, elective ambulatory patient. (Please also see Chapter 7 for details on premedication.)

In older patients with prolonged circulation times, pretreatment with 5–10 mg of ephedrine IV before the administration of propofol may result in less hypotension after induction.

Maintenance

After induction, the airway device of choice is inserted (LMA or ETT, see Chapter 7). Maintenance of anesthesia is achieved by inhalational agents or intravenous agents or a combination of the two. In either technique of maintenance, other IV adjuncts are used, primarily opioids, muscle relaxants, and analgesics to supplement the IV or inhalational agents.

Inhalational anesthetic

Maintenance of anesthesia is by inhalation of a mixture of air, oxygen, and sevoflurane or desflurane (at 1 MAC concentration). The use of nitrous oxide is controversial. The advantages of using nitrous oxide are that it is non-irritating, reduces the amount of halogenated agent required for maintenance, and due to reduced solubility, allows for quicker emergence. The disadvantages to using nitrous oxide are an increased incidence of PONV and relative contraindications in patients undergoing certain surgeries (tympanomastoidectomy) or coexisting medical illnesses such as pulmonary hypertension or anemia (secondary to vitamin B12 cyanocobalmin deficiency).

For a healthy individual undergoing intermediate extensive surgery, who is at a low risk for PONV, nitrous oxide could be a useful adjunct in the maintenance of general anesthesia.[1]

IV and inhalational anesthetic combination

IV induction with propofol is followed by maintenance of GA using either air–oxygen with inhaled agent (sevoflurane or desflurane) or with nitrous oxide–oxygen with an inhaled agent at half a MAC plus a propofol infusion at 50–100 µg/kg/min. The advantage of a combination of using half a MAC of each agent is one of smooth onset during induction, PONV prophylaxis, and a smooth emergence.

TIVA technique

IV induction is achieved with propofol 1.5–2 mg/kg followed by maintenance of GA with air–oxygen and an IV propofol infusion at 150–200 µg/kg/min for the first 10–15 min, and then titrated to surgical anesthesia, often in the range of 100–150 µg/kg/min. This technique of Total Intravenous Anesthesia (TIVA) completely avoids inhalational anesthetics and is useful in patients at high risk for postoperative nausea and vomiting (PONV) or patients who are susceptible to malignant hyperthermia (MH). TIVA is also very practical in areas or rooms not equipped with a full inhalational setup, anesthetic machine, vaporizer or scavenger.

TCI refers to target controlled infusion, where a microprocessor-controlled syringe pump controls and varies automatically the rate of infusion of a drug, to attain a target level (set by the operator) in the patient's blood (see also Chapter 4 on Pharmacology). These devices are so far not FDA-approved in the United States.

Airway management

The LMA is the mainstay of airway devices commonly used for GA and is discussed in detail in Chapter 7. There are several other supraglottic airway devices available that could be used as alternatives. Keep in mind that the LMA is a supraglottic airway device and therefore does not completely isolate the upper airway tract. An endotracheal tube is preferred in patients where there is a potential risk for aspiration, such as patients with severe untreated/symptomatic gastroesophageal reflux disease, massive trauma, pregnancy, and other conditions associated with delayed gastric emptying. However, some of these concerns regarding gastric fluid and reflux may be resolved with an LMA equipped with a gastric tube line (e.g. LMA-Proseal®). An endotracheal tube may otherwise be needed in case of consistent inspiratory leakage with the LMA, as well as in cases with high airway pressure and/or resistance, such as in some morbidly obese patients.

The patient may be allowed to breathe spontaneously or controlled ventilation may be used depending on the requirement of the procedure. Both spontaneous ventilation and controlled ventilation are possible with an LMA, depending on the requirements of the procedure. Newer modes of ventilation available on current anesthesia machines include Pressure Support mode where the patient initiates the breath but the tidal volume is increased by additional positive pressure provided by the ventilator. The PRVC™ mode of ventilation (Pressure Regulated Volume Control), called other names by the machine manufacturers, ensures an adequate (preset) tidal volume while staying within preset pressure parameters and adapts to varying chest and abdominal wall compliance of the patient.

For procedures requiring skeletal muscle relaxation to improve surgical exposure, or procedures requiring isolation of the upper respiratory tract, endotracheal intubation is the preferred technique of airway management. However, if appropriate ventilation and a good LMA seal are present, there is no contraindication for using LMA even during moderate muscle relaxation.

Endotracheal intubation may be facilitated by muscle relaxation, but it is not always required. The choice of muscle relaxant, if used, depends on the type and duration of the procedure. For a short procedure, where continuous muscle relaxation is not required, the lowest effective dose of a short-acting agent should be used. The degree of muscle relaxation and adequacy of reversal should be monitored with a neuromuscular monitor that records muscle response to a peripheral nerve using acceleromyography. Muscle relaxation should be completely reversed using neostigmine at the end of the procedure, before extubation. If the extent of spontaneous recovery of muscle function is greater than 90%, neostigmine need not be given. Given the mixed evidence of the effect of neostigmine on PONV, reversal of residual skeletal muscle paralysis using neostigmine should take precedence over the potential risk of PONV associated with its use.

Succinylcholine is a depolarizing muscle relaxant and does not need to be reversed.

Endotracheal intubation may also be achieved with a combination of propofol induction and high-dose remifentanil without paralysis. Usually, a remifentanil dose of 3–4 µg/kg given within 1–3 min (bolus or infusion) will render the vocal cords fairly relaxed and non-responsive for endotracheal intubation. This method works well, although there have been rare reports of mucus membrane damage in healthy patients, and it may also result in bradycardia and significant hypotension, the latter being move common in an elderly patient.

Emergence

As the surgical procedure approaches an end, the agents used for maintenance of the anesthetic are decreased in dose and then discontinued. Neuromuscular blockade is reversed with appropriate doses of neostigmine and glycopyrrolate as described above. Sugammadex is theoretically a better alternative of reversing rocuronium or vecuronium (see page 50, Chapter 4), but the high cost of this drug should be weighed against very marginal everyday clinical benefits. The patient is allowed to breathe spontaneously. The airway device (LMA or ETT) is removed once ventilatory parameters are satisfactory and protective airway reflexes have returned.

Monitored anesthesia care (MAC)

MAC refers to a type of anesthesia service rather than an anesthetic technique. MAC is a service where an anesthesiologist has been requested to participate in the care of a patient undergoing a procedure.[2] MAC does not refer to the depth of anesthesia required for safe and successful completion of the procedure. Patients receiving MAC, depending on the type of procedure and depth of stimulation, may be at different points along the continuum of depth of sedation. This continuum has been defined by the ASA Committee on Quality Management and Departmental Administration.[3]

Minimal sedation

Patients receiving minimal sedation have usually received an anxiolytic. They are able to respond appropriately to verbal commands. They may have mild impairment of cognition and coordination but airway reflexes, respiratory, and cardiovascular functions are unaffected. Examples include a patient undergoing surgery for cataract extraction who has received intravenous midazolam.

Moderate sedation/analgesia

Patients have received an anxiolytic combined with a sedative-hypnotic and an analgesic. They are able to respond to verbal commands alone or if accompanied by light tactile stimulation. They are able to maintain a patient airway and adequate ventilation without assistance; cardiovascular function remains unaffected.

Deep sedation/analgesia

The patient has a depressed level of consciousness from which they can be aroused by repeated or painful stimuli. Maintenance of a patent airway, airway reflexes, and adequate ventilation are impaired, cardiovascular function is maintained.

General anesthesia

Patients are unconscious and do not respond even to painful stimulation. Patients require assistance with maintaining a patent airway and ventilation. Cardiovascular function may be depressed.

Because MAC is a service, not a technique, patients receiving "MAC" could be at any point on the continuum of depth of sedation. Also the components of sedation may vary as a result of the choice of drugs and the need of the individual patient. It is always wise to define in each case what the patient needs: anxiolysis, amnesia, hypnosis, analgesia, or some combination thereof. For example, analgesia may be achieved by loco-regional techniques, ketamine or remifentanil infusions; amnesia by midazolam or propofol; anxiolysis by diazepam, midazolam, or propofol; hypnosis by propofol or ketamine.

The response of a patient to drugs varies depending on various factors including age, weight, medications, and comorbidities. Therefore, all anesthetic agents must be titrated to effect. The anesthesia practitioner must be vigilant, and able to recognize at what point on the depth of sedation continuum the patient is located, at any given time. He or she must be prepared and qualified to convert to general anesthesia if the procedure or patient warrants it. He or she must be equipped to provide airway and ventilator support as needed.

MAC therefore refers to anesthesia service and could include a range of techniques from local anesthesia with minimal sedation at one end to general anesthesia at the other end.

For any given procedure, the depth of the sedation required depends on the following.

- The nature of the procedure itself. For example, superficial procedures or procedures amenable to regional anesthesia (or field block) may be performed with minimal sedation.
- Patient preference. Some patients do not want to be awake even during minimally invasive procedures. Others have severe anxiety or are uncooperative. These patients may require deep sedation or general anesthesia even for minimally invasive procedures. On the other hand, some patients have severe comorbidities which necessitate avoidance of general anesthesia or deep sedation.
- Surgeon preference. An effective local anesthetic technique is of utmost importance to ensure that the procedure can be completed with minimal sedation. Not all surgeons are willing or able to perform an effective field block, and to continue to

supplement local anesthesia throughout the procedure. Therefore, in some situations deep sedation or general anesthesia may be required.

Safety considerations with MAC

OR fires

Analysis of the ASA closed claims database since 1985 for fire-related claims was published in 2013.[4] The results helped identify causes of OR fires. The take home points from this study are:

- electrocautery was the ignition source in 90% of these fire claims;
- most fires (81%) occurred during MAC;
- most fires occurred in head, neck, and chest procedures;
- oxygen (especially via open delivery systems) served as the oxidizer in 95% of electrocautery-induced fires;
- OR fire claims more frequently involved older outpatients.

For preventing OR fires, the authors recommend:

- identifying high-risk procedures (head, neck, and chest procedures);
- recognizing the fire triad; oxidizer – oxygen, especially via open delivery system; fuel – alcohol-based prep, patient hair, surgical drapes; and ignition source – electrocautery;
- Take steps to mitigate risk:
  - avoid open oxygen deliver systems. This means having the patient awake enough not to require continuous supplemental oxygen throughout the procedure on one hand, or a closed oxygen delivery system with general anesthesia via an LMA/ETT on the other.
  - Use draping techniques that avoid pooling of oxygen.
  - Communication with the surgeon if continuous supplemental oxygen is being used, to shut off oxygen one minute before the use of electrocautery.
  - Allow alcohol-based prep solutions to dry completely before draping.
  - Have a basin of sterile water or saline available on the back table.
  - Know the location of the shut-off valve for oxygen.

Respiratory depression

More than 70% of surgical procedures are ambulatory and many are being performed on older and sicker patients.[5] A lot of these procedures are minimally invasive and performed with "MAC." Analysis of surgical anesthesia claims associated with MAC since 1990 showed that more than 40% of these claims involved death or brain damage, with respiratory depression secondary to a relative or absolute overdose of sedatives or opioids being the most common mechanism. The patients were usually older and sicker, and were undergoing elective eye surgery or facial plastic surgery. About half the time, these complications were deemed avoidable by using better monitoring and vigilance.[6] It is important to emphasize constant vigilance during "MAC" and understand that "MAC" is a dynamic spectrum of sedation. With benzodiazepines alone respiratory depression will usually be modest, with maintained respiratory frequency but reduced tidal volume. With propofol, respiratory frequency will be reduced and with higher doses, apnea may ensue. Opioids typically result in reduced respiratory frequency, but fairly maintained tidal volume until apnea. Ketamine and dexmedetomidine can result in a very modest respiratory depression in sedative doses.

A combination of sedatives and opioids can be synergistic in affecting respiratory function. Pulse-oximetry should always be used with sedation. Changes in respiratory frequency should be noted. The goal should be oxygen saturation above 92% and respiratory frequency of more than 8–10/min. Trends of declining oxygen saturation and reduced respiratory frequency can be important signs of deepening sedation. It is sometimes debated whether oxygen supplementation should be used. Without supplemental oxygen, desaturation will occur faster thus allowing earlier detection, but the overall level of oxygenation during the procedure may be lower. Generally, it is best to maintain a low-flow oxygen supplementation for a target saturation of 92–96%, with an alarm for reduced respiratory frequency or hypoventilation.

Commonly used drugs for MAC

Anxiolytics

Usually short-acting benzodiazepines like midazolam administered intravenously in titrated doses to achieve anxiolysis.

Analgesics

Short-acting opioids such as fentanyl, alfentanil, or remifentanil are used to supplement local or regional anesthesia.

IV induction agents

Usually propofol is the mainstay of IV induction agents used for sedation. The method of administration, intermittent boluses or continuous infusion, depends on the procedure, patient, and the need for continued sedation throughout the procedure. Procedures which are amenable to regional anesthesia or an effective field block or local infiltration may not require continued sedation throughout the procedure. In these situations a small bolus of propofol 0.5–1 mg/kg is administered IV prior to the field block or local infiltration. Once a satisfactory block is achieved, the patient is allowed to awaken. Supplemental propofol, 0.15–0.25 mg/kg, can then be administered as needed throughout the procedure.

Summary

- MAC is a service, not a technique.
- MAC includes a spectrum of sedation techniques with local anesthesia alone at one end and general anesthesia at the other end.
- Depth of sedation required for a procedure depends on procedural factors as well as patient and surgeon preference.
- The anesthesia provider must be qualified to recognize depth of sedation and provide airway and ventilator support as needed.
- The anesthesia provider must be qualified to convert to general anesthesia if necessary.
- The risk of OR fire with certain procedures must be kept in mind and measures taken to prevent it.

Local anesthesia (see also Chapter 6)

This section discusses local anesthetic techniques such as field blocks, local infiltration, topical anesthesia, and intravenous regional anesthesia (IVRA). Regional anesthetic techniques and neuraxial anesthesia will be discussed in a separate chapter.

Field block

Local anesthetic is infiltrated around the surgical field with the intention of blocking nerves supplying the surgical field. Field blocks last longer than local infiltration of the incisional area and do not obscure anatomy in the surgical field. Field blocks are useful in head and neck surgeries, abdominal wall surgeries, and surgeries on the extremities.

There have been reports of the use of transversus abdominis plane block for hernia repairs, abdominoplasties, and laparoscopic procedures.[7]

Local infiltration anesthesia

This involves injection of local anesthetics at the surgical site, usually by the surgeon. Various techniques of infiltration anesthesia include subcutaneous, submucosal, in the wound, or intra-articular.

Topical anesthesia

This includes application of the local anesthetic to the cleaned site without the need for injection. Topical anesthetics are available in several forms: gels, sprays, creams, drops, patches, ointments. They are poorly absorbed through intact skin with the exception of EMLA® (Eutectic mixture of Lidocaine and Prilocaine). Because absorption varies greatly depending on the surface area and site of use, these agents must be used with caution to avoid local anesthetic toxicity. Prilocaine can cause methemoglobinemia with increased doses and should be used with caution.

Intravenous regional anesthesia (see also Chapter 6 on regional anesthesia)

Intravenous regional anesthesia (IVRA) was first described by the German surgeon August Bier in 1909 and is also called a Bier block.[8] There are multiple mechanisms of action producing surgical anesthesia after IVRA.

- Initial conduction block of small nerves and nerve endings along the veins filled with the local anesthetic.
- Intraneural distribution of local anesthetic (via vasa nervosum which provides blood supply to the endoneureum).
- Ischemia plays a major role in conduction blockade especially after 12–15 min of tourniquet inflation.
- Compression of nerves under the tourniquet (this is a more delayed block).

Technique

Successful IVRA requires a cooperative patient, a surgeon who is experienced in the use of the technique, and an amenable procedure. At our center, patients are consented for the procedure and an IV cannula is inserted into the operative hand. In the OR the limb is exsanguinated by combination of limb elevation and an Esmarch bandage. A double tourniquet is used for procedures over 45 min and a simple tourniquet is sufficient for procedures under 45 min. After exsanguination, the tourniquet is inflated. The optimal tourniquet inflation pressure for upper extremity procedures is 50–100 mmHg above the patient's systolic BP, and for lower extremity procedures it is 100 mmHg above the patient's systolic blood pressure. Once the tourniquet is inflated, absence of peripheral pulses is confirmed by palpation. The local anesthetic agent typically used for this block is 0.5% lidocaine or 0.5% prilocaine. More concentrated forms are unnecessary and could lead to toxicity. The volume injected is typically 25–50 ml (sufficient to fill the venous system of an exsanguinated arm) for the upper extremity and 100–120 ml for the lower extremity. Lower extremity techniques are limited by their long onset times and the large total doses of local anesthetic required and are therefore not used as often as upper extremity techniques.

Other local anesthetic agents are not recommended for IVRA due to their potential for cardiotoxicity. Once the local anesthetic is injected into the operative arm, surgical anesthesia will set in within 5 min. Supplemental local anesthetic infiltration at the site of incision may be used in addition. IVRA is a useful technique for upper extremity procedures of short to intermediate duration. It may be supplemented by light sedation based on patient preference.

Disadvantages of IVRA include slow onset, poor muscle relaxation, tourniquet pain (in longer procedures) and short duration of postoperative analgesia. The duration of the block is usually limited to 60–90 min, due to declining effect and increasing tourniquet pain.

- Onset time may be shortened by forcing the injected local anesthetic to distribute peripherally by applying a temporary tight tourniquet around the forearm prior to injection and leaving it on for 10 min.
- Tourniquet pain may be eased by deflating the proximal cuff after inflating the distal cuff in double tourniquet systems.

- For postoperative analgesia, a field block is performed by the surgeon at the end of the procedure.

The tourniquet is usually not deflated until 20 min have elapsed from the time of injection of local anesthetic, thus ensuring that most of the local anesthetic has been taken up by the tissues and avoiding an IV bolus of the local anesthetic with its attendant cardiovascular or neurological effects.

If the tourniquet must be deflated before 20 min, it may be done in cycles of deflation and reinflation. The reinflation should be less than 30 seconds to avoid tissue swelling.

Contraindications to local anesthesia

- Uncooperative patient: this could be mitigated by sedation.
- Infection at the site of infiltration.
- Pre-existing neurological deficit at the site of the block or a systemic progressive neurological condition.
- Anticoagulated patients: this would eliminate certain types of blocks, but these patients could still receive infiltration anesthesia or topical anesthesia if the procedure permits.

Summary

Local anesthetic techniques should be considered in all surgical procedures. They constitute an important adjunct of multimodal analgesia and provide the advantages of faster recovery, improved postoperative pain control, need for less opioids, and decreased incidence of PONV. The appropriate technique should be individualized based on patient and surgeon preference and the requirements of the procedure. The anesthesia provider must pay attention to contraindications and total dose of local anesthetic permissible in each patient to avoid local anesthetic systemic toxicity (LAST). Measures should be taken to prevent, recognize, and promptly treat LAST.[9]

Monitoring

Standard monitoring during anesthesia, as recommended by the ASA,[10] includes the following.

1. The presence of qualified anesthesia personnel in the operating room throughout the procedure.

2. Continual monitoring of the patient's oxygenation via fiO$_2$ monitoring using an in-line oxygen analyzer and pulse oximetry.

3. Ventilation is monitored via capnography and disconnect alarms in the breathing circuit and continual observation.

4. Circulation is monitored by continuous ECG, plethysmography, and heart rate with intermittent measurement of NIBP at least every 5 min.

5. Temperature monitoring is recommended when significant changes in temperature are intended or expected. Core temperature monitoring is recommended by MHAUS (Malignant Hyperthermia Association of United States) in all patients receiving general anesthesia with potential MH triggers for greater than 30 min.[11]

Summary

The anesthetic technique depends on a combination of patient, surgeon, and procedure-related factors. The choice of technique should be in keeping with the goals of ambulatory anesthesia, namely quick recovery and short times to discharge.

MAC is a service and includes a conglomerate of techniques ranging from local anesthesia with monitoring at one end and general anesthesia at the other end.

Every surgical procedure is eligible for local or regional anesthesia, be it topical, infiltration, or a field block. Local anesthesia techniques are an important component of multimodal analgesia and should be used whenever possible.

References

1. Tramèr M, Moore A, McQuay H. Omitting nitrous oxide in general anaesthesia: meta-analysis of intraoperative awareness and postoperative emesis in randomized controlled trials. *Br J Anaesth* 1996;**76**(2):186–93.

2. American Society of Anesthesiologists. Position on Monitored Anesthesia Care 2005, last amended 2013. https://www.asahq.org/For-Members/Standards-Guidelines-and-Statements.aspx (Accessed November 10, 2014).

3. Continuum of Depth of Sedation: Definition of General Anesthesia and Levels of Sedation/Analgesia (2009) http://www.asahq.org/Home/For-Members/Clinical-Information/~/media/For%20Members/Standards%20and%20Guidelines/2012/CONTINUUM%20OF%20DEPTH%20OF%20SEDATION%20442012.ashx (Accessed Feb 23, 2014).

4. Mehta SP, Bhananker SM, Posner KL, Domino KB. Operating room fires: a closed claims analysis. *Anesthesiology* 2013 May;**118**(5):1133–39.

5. Metzner J, Posner KL, Lam MS, Domino KB. Closed claims' analysis. *Best Pract Res Clin Anaesthesiol* 2011 Jun;**25**(2):263–76.

6. Bhananker SM, Posner KL, Cheney FW, Caplan RA, Lee LA, Domino KB. Injury and liability associated with monitored anesthesia care: a closed claims analysis. *Anesthesiology* 2006 Feb;**104**(2):228–34.

7. Aveline C, Le Hetet H, Le Roux A, Vautier P, Cognet F, Vinet E, Tison C, Bonnet F. Comparison between ultrasound-guided transversus abdominis plane and conventional ilioinguinal/iliohypogastric nerve blocks for day-case open inguinal hernia repair. *Br J Anaesth* 2011 Mar;**106**(3):380–86.

8. Brill S, Middleton W, Brill G, Fisher A. Bier's block; 100 years old and still going strong! *Acta Anaesthesiol Scand* 2004 Jan;**48**(1):117–22.

9. Neal JM, Mulroy MF, Weinberg GL; American Society of Regional Anesthesia and Pain Medicine. American Society of Regional Anesthesia and Pain Medicine checklist for managing local anesthetic systemic toxicity: 2012 version. *Reg Anesth Pain Med* 2012 Jan–Feb;**37**(1):16–18.

10. Basic Anesthetic Monitoring, Standards for. http://www.asahq.org/For-Members/~/media/For%20 Members/documents/Standards%20Guidelines%20St mts/Basic%20Anesthetic%20Monitoring%202011.ashx (Accessed Jan 10, 2014).

11. Temperature Monitoring during Surgical Procedures. http://www.mhaus.org/healthcare-professionals/mhaus-recommendations/temperature-monitoring (Accessed Jan 10, 2014).

Chapter

6

Regional anesthesia for ambulatory surgery

Ramprasad Sripada, MD, MMM, CPE, Shuchita Garg, MD, and Johan Raeder, MD, PhD

Introduction

Regional anesthesia techniques (peripheral nerve blocks and neuraxial blocks) offer significant advantages in the ambulatory setting.[1] These not only can provide good surgical conditions for intraoperative anesthesia, but also excellent postoperative analgesia. They may be used as (a) the only anesthetic provided, (b) together with sedation, or (c) as a supplement to general anesthesia. Studies show that regional anesthesia lowers the incidence of nausea and vomiting, improves pain scores, and decreases narcotic use.[2,3] The growth and popularity in regional anesthesia has coincided with dramatically improved intravenous (IV) sedative medications such as propofol,[4] low-dose ketamine,[5,6] and dexmedetomidine. Monitoring "depth" of anesthesia and better titration techniques for IV sedatives have evolved, whereas regional anesthesia-specific technologies have evolved from peripheral nerve stimulation[7] to ultrasound.[8]

Perhaps more than any other specialty, orthopedic surgery lends itself to the practice of regional anesthesia.[9] Nonetheless, general surgery, ophthalmology, and otolaryngology are also leaning towards use of regional anesthesia techniques.

Preoperative preparation

Patient assessment

Patients due for regional anesthesia should basically have the same preoperative assessment and precautions as patients due for general anesthesia. This is both because regional anesthesia has cardiorespiratory risks and complications as well, and also there may be a change of plan intraoperatively, because regional anesthesia may be changed into general anesthesia.

Patients receiving regional anesthesia to extremities should be reminded to avoid using the blocked extremity for at least 24 hours. In addition, patients should be warned that protective reflexes and proprioception for the blocked extremity may be diminished or absent for 24 hours.

Accepted by the surgeon

If the surgeon is unwilling or not cooperative during loco-regional anesthesia, the chance of problems and failure will increase significantly. Sometimes it may simply be a matter of providing the surgeon with better information about the benefits of loco-regional anesthesia or discussing the option of providing adequate sedation in order to let the surgeon work undisturbed. In other cases the surgeon may have valid concerns about muscle relaxation and surgical access, or the surgeon and patient may have made alternative plans in their prior consultations.

Accepted by the patient

Patients who do not consent to loco-regional anesthesia, even after full discussion of the technique, should not be forced into it, unless strong contraindications to general anesthesia are present (see later). Nevertheless, it is wise to spend time with reluctant patients, first stating that their opinions will be heard, then presenting the pros and cons of their treatment options, and ending by stating what method is normally used in cases such as theirs. For both surgeons and patients it is reassuring and positive to know whether the loco-regional technique is used routinely by the team for the specific procedure and type of patient in question; it is also good to remember that "routine" never means "always," and that exceptions will be made from time to time.

Practical Ambulatory Anesthesia, ed. Johan Raeder and Richard D. Urman. Published by Cambridge University Press.
© Cambridge University Press 2015.

Avoid preoperative delay

With some blocks, such as spinal anesthesia, administration and onset take no longer than general anesthesia induction. However, with other blocks, such as epidural anesthesia and brachial plexus blocks, the administration of the block may take time, testing takes time, and failure may occur, especially in inexperienced hands or with obese patients. The use of a separate induction/block room to prepare the blocks may be an advantage, especially in units with anesthetists in training or where operating room (OR) availability creates a bottleneck in the treatment chain. If an induction room is not an option, the block has to be done in the OR. An effective measure, then, is to automatically assume that the block will be effective. The implication of this is that the patient can be immediately placed in position, washed, and draped as soon as the block is done. Usually these procedures are carried out while the plexus block takes effect, and a rapid test of block efficacy may be done using the surgeon's forceps immediately before the start of surgery. In rare cases (a benchmark goal should be less than 1 case out of 10–20) of insufficient block, a very low threshold should be set for immediately starting propofol and opioid, and/or sevoflurane, perhaps with an LMA to induce general anesthesia within 2–3 min, before starting the operation.

Monitoring

As per the ASA standards and recommendations, qualified anesthesia personnel shall be present in the room throughout the conduct of all general anesthetics, regional anesthetics and monitored anesthesia care. During all anesthetics, the patient's oxygenation, ventilation, circulation, and temperature shall be continually evaluated. Standard ASA monitors include continuous EKG; blood pressure every 5 min, pulse oximetry, and end-tidal CO_2 analysis. Respiratory rate and mental status should also be monitored.

Regional anesthesia equipment

1. Regional block carts: a regional anesthesia cart should have all drawers clearly labeled and be portable to enable transport to the patient's bedside. It should have relevant drugs, and equipment available.

    a. Ruler and marking pen for measuring and marking landmarks and injection points.
    b. Alcohol and chlorhexidine swabs.
    c. 25-gauge needle and syringe.
    d. 1% lidocaine to anesthetize the skin for needle puncture.
    e. Chlorhexidine gluconate, antimicrobial skin cleaner.
    f. Syringes for sedation.
    g. Local anesthetic drugs.
    h. Sterile gloves, clear occlusive dressing, lubricating gel, transducer covers.
    i. Suction and airway resuscitation devices.
    j. Standard advanced cardiac life support (ACLS) resuscitation equipment and drugs.
    k. Intralipid lipid emulsion.

2. Stimulating needles of various sizes. Stimulating needles are typically beveled at 45° rather than at 17°, as are more traditional needles, to enhance the tactile sensation of the needle passing through tissue planes and to reduce the possibility of neural trauma. To facilitate the ease of needle visualization, specialized needle designs are being developed that allow greater visibility of the needle when performing ultrasound-guided peripheral nerve blocks (PNBs). Echogenic needle design incorporates echogenic "dimples" at the tip to improve visibility.

3. Continuous epidural and peripheral nerve catheter sets.

4. Ultrasound machines with linear and curved ultrasound probes and a printer.

5. Peripheral nerve stimulators. Peripheral nerve stimulation has greatly aided the practice of regional anesthesia by providing objective evidence of needle proximity to targeted nerves. In the majority of PNBs, stimulation of nerves at a current of 0.5 mA or less suggests accurate needle placement for injection of local anesthetic. Sometimes a combination of peripheral nerve stimulation and ultrasound guidance is used to place PNBs.

6. Injection pressure monitor device. From animal studies, injection pressure has been suggested to be an important and potentially reliable predictor of nerve injury from intraneural injection. Although it has not been proven in humans that there is a relationship between high-pressure intraneural injection and nerve injury, if such relationship does exist then it will be vital for anesthesiologists to have the ability to maintain low injection pressures at all time points during injection for PNBs. Alternatively, the compressed

air injection technique (CAIT) has been studied which involves drawing 10 ml of air into the syringe above the 20 ml saline and compressing this air to 5 ml prior to and during the injection, which could limit the injection pressures generated below 1034 mmHg (25 psig) in an *in vitro* system.[10,11]

Role of ultrasonography (USG) in regional anesthesia

Ultrasound refers to the use of sound waves (typically from 2 to 15 MHz, but in modern probes up to 22 MHz), which are above the frequency of those sound waves that can be heard by the human ear (20–20,000 Hz range). Technological advances in piezoelectric materials, electronics, and software have enabled improved probe design and software capability; this has led to the development of small, portable 2D machines with good resolution and penetration available for bedside "point-of-care" use.

The advantages of the ultrasound technique include the following.

i. Ability to visualize and identify the target nerve(s) and their relationship to surrounding structures (e.g., arteries, veins, lungs, other nerves).

ii. Allow for patient variability (e.g., size, shape, anatomical variations).

iii. Determine depth, angle, and path of the needle to the target nerve.

iv. Real-time visualization of the technique and guidance of the needle to the target.

v. Visualization of the spread of local anesthetic (encircling nerve) and placement of a catheter.

vi. Allow the procedure to be carried out on anesthetized patients safely (e.g., children) and even to be repeated if ineffective.

vii. Portability and safety (no ionizing radiation).

The ultrasound appearance of a nerve is primarily dependent on its size and the amount and make-up of the support tissue (epineurium, perineurium). Axons, or in reality fascicles (collection of axons), appear black (hypoechoic) and the supporting tissue appears bright (hyperechoic).

The most commonly used probe is a high-frequency, linear array probe (5–10 MHz), as this gives good spatial resolution for the nerves and plexuses, which are usually superficial (1–5 cm deep). A low-frequency curvilinear probe (2–5 MHz) can be useful for deeper nerves and plexuses, but it is limited by its poor spatial resolution at increasing depth.[12]

The use of USG in performing blocks has not only increased the success rate of the blocks, but also has proved to be safer and has decreased the rate of complications, especially in high-risk patients. Studies have reported the use of reduced volumes of local anesthetics with USG,[13–15] sufficiently low vascular complications,[16–20] pneumothorax,[21–24] and hemidiaphragmatic paresis.[25] These make it useful in reducing the incidence of local anesthetic induced systemic toxicity (LAST). However, a recent advisory of the American Society of Regional Anesthesia and Pain Medicine concluded that the overall effectiveness of the USG in reducing the frequency of LAST remains to be determined.[26] Speed of performance, learning curve, and availability of the appropriate equipment and logistics still remain as obstacles.

Local anesthetics and adjuvants

Local anesthetics by blocking sodium channels cause reversible neural conduction block. Several local anesthetic agents are available with varying concentrations, onset times, durations, safety profiles, and potencies. Local anesthetic agents are chosen based on desired effects. Profiles of various local anesthetics for infiltration and PNBs are summarized in Table 6.1. Local anesthetic toxicity is always a concern because regional anesthetic techniques involve injection of large volumes of local anesthetics solutions.

Ropivacaine and levobupivacaine have been introduced as less-toxic alternatives to bupivacaine. Levobupivacaine is very similar and equipotent to racemic bupivacaine. Ropivacaine seems to be slightly different and less potent in most applications. Further, ropivacaine seems to have a better separation between motor and sensory block, and has been approved for spinal use and continuous postoperative nerve block infusion. Mepivacaine and preservative-free 2-chloroprocaine have been introduced as short-acting alternatives to lidocaine for spinal anesthesia, with less risk of transient neurologic symptoms (TNS), which are often seen with lidocaine use.

Local anesthetic systemic toxicity (LAST)

Signs and symptoms of LAST include lightheadedness, sight disturbances, tinnitus, perioral paresthesia, drowsiness, confusion, slurred speech, and muscle twitches. With further increasing plasma and CNS

Table 6.1 Local anesthetic agents for infiltration and peripheral nerve blocks (PNBs): Concentration onset, duration, and maximum dose.[a]

Drug	Concentration (mg/ml)	Onset (min)	Duration (hours)	Maximal dose (mg/kg)[b] Infiltration	Maximal dose mg/kg[b] with epinephrine PNBs
Lidocaine	5–20	Fast 10–20	Medium (2–3)	10	7
Mepivacaine	5–20	Fast 10–20	Medium (3–6)	10	7
Bupivacaine	2.5–5	Medium 15–30	Long (6–12)	2.5	3
Levobupivacaine	2.5–5	Medium 15–30	Long (6–12)	4	3
Ropivacaine	2–7.5	Medium 15–30	Long (6–12)	3.5	3.5

[a] Will always depend on the potential for rapid diffusion of a large amount into the circulation, weighed against the potential for side effects with each drug.

[b] The maximum dose may be increased when adrenaline adjunct is used and also when there is infiltration into a large area with a minor risk of the full dose coming into circulation (major vessels) at the same time

concentrations seizures may occur. With even higher concentrations, cardiac arrhythmias and cardio-respiratory arrest are possible. The first signs of minor symptoms of toxicity should always warrant alarm, alert, and preparations for the more serious symptoms of convulsions and cardiac symptoms, which may occur within minutes.

ASRA guidelines

Use incremental injection of local anesthetics. Basically, slow injection of up to 15–20 ml in a healthy, normal adult is considered safe with all commonly used preparations and drugs. When exceeding this amount administer 3–5 ml aliquots, pausing 15–30 s between each injection. When using a fixed needle approach – e.g., landmark, paresthesia-seeking, or electrical stimulation – the time between injections should encompass one circulation time.

When injecting potentially toxic doses of local anesthetic, the use of an intravascular marker is recommended. Although epinephrine is an imperfect marker and its use is open to physician judgment, its benefits likely outweigh its risks in the majority of patients. Ultrasound guidance may reduce the frequency of intravascular injection, but actual reduction of LAST remains unproven in humans.

Treatment of LAST

- Stop injecting local anesthetic; get help.
- Prompt and effective airway management (intubate if needed; i.e., non-fasting patient or failure to control ventilation otherwise), 100% oxygen.

- If seizures occur, halt with benzodiazepines. If benzodiazepines are not readily available, small doses of propofol or thiopental are acceptable. Future data may support the early use of lipid emulsion for treating seizures.
- If cardiac arrest occurs, we recommend standard ACLS with the following modifications:
  - If epinephrine is used, small initial doses. Vasopressin is not recommended.
  - Avoid calcium channel blockers and alpha-adrenergic receptor blockers.
  - If ventricular arrhythmias develop, amiodarone is preferred.
  - Lipid emulsion therapy dosing:
    - 1.5 ml/kg 20% lipid emulsion bolus,
    - 0.25 ml/kg per minute of infusion, continued for at least 10 min after circulatory stability is attained.
    - If circulatory stability is not attained, consider rebolus and increasing infusion to 0.5 ml/kg per minute.
    - 10 ml/kg lipid emulsion for 30 min is recommended as the upper limit for initial dosing.
  - Failure to respond to lipid emulsion and vasopressor therapy should prompt institution of cardiopulmonary bypass (CPB). Because there can be considerable lag in beginning CPB, it is reasonable to notify the closest facility capable of providing it when cardiovascular compromise is first identified during an episode of LAST.[26]

. It should be kept in mind that cardiac arrest from local anesthetic overdose implies sodium channel block in the heart nerves and muscles. Thus, resuscitation may take time for the heart to start again as the sodium channel block needs to be "washed away" first. Thus it is important to prepare for adequate compression and ventilation for some time, and not accept diagnosis of death until at least 45–60 min of non-responsive resuscitation has passed.

Adjuncts

Various agents have been tried as adjuncts to local anesthetics to prolong local anesthetic duration of action and to improve the quality of regional blocks. Except for epinephrine there is a valid controversy if these adjuncts have a true loco-regional effect, or whether the effect sometimes seen is a result of systemic absorption, which could have been achieved with an I.V. dose as well.

- **Epinephrine:** is added to decrease the systemic absorption of local anesthetic and to limit systemic toxicity. There are limited data regarding the efficacy of epinephrine for prolonging the analgesic duration of long-acting local anesthetics. Furthermore, the use of USG and concerns of neurotoxicity may reduce the enthusiasm of its use for some physicians. Brummett and Williams recommend the use of epinephrine for nerve blocks done without ultrasound guidance or blocks in which the needle tip and local anesthetic spread is not adequately visualized, as a safety measure to detect intravascular injection.[27]
- **Buprenorphine, opioids:** Buprenorphine is an opioid receptor, mu agonist, and kappa antagonist. While earlier studies have shown efficacy from the addition of buprenorphine to combinations of mepivacaine, tetracaine, and epinephrine,[28] the results from more recent studies[29] were not very impressive. The rationale for adding opioids to local anesthetic infiltration has been the demonstration of opioid receptors in peripheral tissue. While these are evident in tissues after some period of inflammation, their presence is disputed in native tissue.[30] It remains unclear whether the co-administration of adjuvants such as an opioid, a α_2-agonist, or ketamine is beneficial. Further studies are needed to elucidate this controversial topic. The question of dosage and volume is another interesting area of investigations.

- **Clonidine:** Meta analyses and systematic reviews clearly show an analgesic benefit from the addition of clonidine to the local anesthetics.[31,32] Most studies used between 100 and 150 μg with higher doses causing sedation, bradycardia, and hypotension.[31]
- **Bicarbonate:** This does not seem to have any effect on block duration, although some studies report a shortening time to block onset[33] and less aching during induction, especially with acid local anesthetic solutions such as lidocaine- and epinephrine-containing drugs.
- **Dexamethasone:** Further research is needed to better delineate the impact of dexamethasone with long-acting local anesthetics both with and without other adjuvants.
- **Dexmedetomidine** is currently not approved for use in peripheral nerve blockade in the United States.

Neuraxial anesthesia

Anatomy

The spinal cord in adults extends from the base of the skull up to L1/L2 in adults and L3 vertebral level in infants. The dural sac extends from the base of the skull up to sacral (S2) vertebral in adults. In adults, it is generally safe to place a spinal needle below L2, unless there is a known anatomical variation.

A few landmarks that are worth a look and are relevant in day-to-day clinical practice would be:

- The C7 spinous process – most prominent in the cervical region when the neck is flexed.
- A line drawn at the level of the prominent spinous process passes through the T4 vertebra.
- A line drawn at the level of the tip of the scapulae passes through the T7 vertebra.
- A line drawn between the iliac crests passes though the L4 vertebra.
- The sacral cornu is at the level of the S5 vertebra.

Spinal anesthesia (subarachnoid block)

Spinal anesthesia remains one of the oldest regional techniques and involves injection of local anesthetic in the subarachnoid space. Its rapid onset, minimal expense, and easy administration are key advantages in outpatient procedures. Spinal anesthesia can be used for lower extremity, lower abdominal, and urogenital surgeries. However, limitations include pain with regression, urinary retention, and the inability to ambulate resulting from weak lower extremities.[34]

Limitations and arguments against the use of spinal anesthesia for day-case surgery are problems in ambulation due to motor weakness and disturbed proprioception, immediate onset of pain at home when it wears off, urinary retention, and insufficient monitoring of side effects such as PDPH (post-dural puncture headache) and TNS and severe neurologic disturbances such as spinal hematoma.[35] Salinas and Liu reviewed some of the major controversies.[36]

As ambulatory patients are mobilized and are prone to feel symptoms of a spinal headache, a thin needle (i.e., 27G) of pencil point design should be used and the incidence of mild headache is expected to be less than 1–2% and even lower in the elderly or obese patients. Theoretically 29 G needles should be even better in this respect, but in clinical use they are more difficult to direct even with an introducer, and spinal flow is so low that there is a risk of multiple dural punctures and also failure.

The occurrence of TNS has been associated particularly with ambulatory surgery (rapid mobilization), the lithotomy position, or manipulation of the hip joint during knee arthroscopy, and almost exclusively with lidocaine.[36] TNS is a benign and self-limiting condition, but in a study by Tong et al. the patients with TNS had more pain during the first 72 h after surgery and reduced activities of daily living for 24 h compared with the patients without TNS.[37] Variation of the lidocaine concentration or hyperbaricity seems to have little influence on the incidence,[37] but there seems to be a lower incidence when the lidocaine dose is reduced.[36] In a study of 36 patients with 25 mg lidocaine spinally, no TNS was observed.[38] However, in order for lidocaine doses of less than 40 mg to be effective, an opioid adjunct is usually needed.[36] In the study of Buckenmaier et al., 20 μg fentanyl was added to 25 mg lidocaine for anorectal procedures,[39] whereas Lennox et al. added sufentanil 10 μg to only 10 mg lidocaine for gynecologic laparoscopy.[40] In the latter study it seems as though anesthesia was on the lower threshold for acceptance, as 30% of the patients reported perioperative discomfort. However, motor recovery and discharge readiness were even faster than in a comparator group receiving desflurane anesthesia.[40] A mixture of lidocaine (20 mg) with fentanyl (20 μg) was sufficient for knee arthroscopy in the study of Ben-David et al.[41] Another approach to avoid TNS is to use ropivacaine

or bupivacaine. In studies of identical doses of these two drugs, either 12 mg[42] or 15 mg,[43] there was no TNS. A conclusion in favor of ropivacaine was made, as motor block was less prominent and recovery faster compared with bupivacaine. This may be due to non-equipotency in dosing, as bupivacaine should probably be dosed lower than ropivacaine for equal effect.[44] Future studies are needed to clarify whether a clinical issue of less motor block and shorter recovery with ropivacaine at the minimal effective dose remains.

Bupivacaine for ambulatory spinal anesthesia is usually combined with an opioid to reduce the dose needed and the duration of motor block. With a combination of bupivacaine 15 mg + fentanyl 10 μg, 50–75% of patients had impairment of walking and standing for more than 90 min. This was in spite of a low incidence of motor block: fewer than 25% of the patients had measurable perioperative weakness in the leg musculature.[45] Urinary retention delayed average discharge by 30 min when spinal levobupivacaine (10 mg) or ropivacaine (15 mg) was compared with lidocaine.[5,44] In a study of hernia repair, Gupta et al. used fentanyl (25 μg) together with bupivacaine (either 6 mg or 7.5 mg).[46] The 6 mg dose necessitated supplemental I.V. analgesia in some cases, and average discharge time was in the range of 5–6 h in both groups. In this study, 17% of the patients needed catheterization, resulting in 5% being admitted overnight.[46] In a study of bupivacaine (10 mg) spinally for hysteroscopy, recovery and discharge were significantly longer than with remifentanil + propofol anesthesia.[47]

It is debatable whether patients undergoing ambulatory surgery with spinal anesthesia can be discharged before voiding. Mulroy et al. claim that otherwise healthy patients less than 70 years old, with no history of voiding problems, and who are not undergoing surgery in the perianal or perineal region or having hernia repair may be discharged safely 2 h after bupivacaine (6 mg) spinally, even if they not have voided.[38]

An approach for further bupivacaine dose reduction is to administer hyperbaric bupivacaine and then place the patient in the lateral decubitus position for 10–15 min to achieve unilateral spinal block. This was used successfully by Korhonen et al., who compared 4 mg bupivacaine with a mixture of 3 mg bupivacaine + 10 μg fentanyl for knee arthroscopy.[48] Of the two, the latter group had a higher rate of fast-tracking and their recovery unit stay was shorter, but discharge-readiness was similar in both groups, with a mean value of 3 h.[47] A major problem with opioid adjunct to spinal anesthesia is the high frequency of pruritus, at an incidence of 25–75%.[41,47] With a combination of I.V. droperidol[41] and nalbuphine, Ben-David et al. were able to reduce significantly the incidence of both pruritus and nausea, without provoking any more pain.[41] Another interesting adjunct is clonidine, which was optimally dosed at 15 μg with better block quality and no delay in recovery (i.e., about 2 h) when added to 8 mg ropivacaine.[49] Merivirta and co-workers added clonidine 15 μg to 5 mg unilateral bupivacaine, and found an increased need for initial vasopressors with clonidine, but a better block quality, and no delay in discharge-readiness.[50]

A simpler and promising development in ambulatory spinal anesthesia is the launch of new, safe, short-acting local anesthetic agents. Articaine 50 mg was shown to provide discharge-readiness within 3 h, significantly faster than prilocaine,[51] and 40–50 mg of 2-chloroprocaine seems even faster with ambulation and discharge-readiness within 2 h.[52]

The 2-chloroprocaine (introduced in 1952) fell into disgrace in the 1980s after reports of neurotoxicity following an unintentional intrathecal injection of large doses of 2-chloroprocaine with sodium bisulphite during intended epidural anesthesia. There is growing evidence that this problem originated from the antioxidant sodium bisulphite rather than from the local anesthetic itself. Several encouraging volunteer studies and clinical studies were carried out during the last few years. Therefore, it is worthwhile considering new data gained with a preservative-free solution of 2-chloroprocaine.[53]

Choice of adjuncts

For outpatients, lipophilic opioids and low-dose clonidine can be used as intrathecal adjuncts, whereas several other agents studied (adrenaline, neostigmine, morphine) are not suitable because they cause delayed home discharge and/or side effects.

Low doses of lipophilic intrathecal opioids improve the quality of anesthesia[54] without delaying home discharge significantly.[40,55–57] Compared with morphine, small doses of lipophilic opioids have a shorter duration of action and a low risk of respiratory depression.[58] Fentanyl (10–25 μg) or sufentanil (10 μg) have been used together successfully with different local anesthetics.

Clonidine 15 μg combined with ropivacaine or 2-chloroprocaine (2 CP) improves the quality of spinal anesthesia with a recovery time suitable for day surgery. Hypotension, bradycardia, or sedation developed after higher doses of clonidine (45–75 μg), whereas with a 15-μg dose these systemic side effects were avoided.[49,59]

Epidurals

There are few recent reports in the literature on epidural anesthesia for ambulatory care. Epidural anesthesia is usually regarded as more time-consuming compared with other techniques. Our data on epidural anesthesia with mepivacaine showed discharge readiness after 2 h, whereas that after a lidocaine spinal was about 30 min less.[60] A study by Mulroy and co-workers actually showed a faster discharge, namely about 2 h after surgery, with epidural block with either lidocaine or 2-chloroprocaine when compared with spinal lidocaine or low-dose bupivacaine.[38] In another study of 256 hemorrhoidectomy patients, either 20 ml lidocaine 1% or bupivacaine 0.5% epidurally was used, but the observation time in hospital was a minimum of 5 h and 2% of the patients were admitted due to urinary retention.[61] In a study of lower body surgery, epidural administration of 16 ml lidocaine 1.6% was used, but all the patients were observed for 6 h in the hospital.[62] Although epidural needles are thick and some outpatients used NSAIDs or had a history of bruising, epidural steroid injections caused no hematoma in a mixed population of 1035 patients.[63] However, a recent case report describes a 35-year-old woman with no risk factors, apart from perioperative ketorolac administration, who developed an epidural hematoma after discharge from an ambulatory arthroscopy under epidural anesthesia.[64] More recently, studies have concluded that epidural washout (epidural bolus of 30 ml saline at the end of surgery) facilitates the regression of both motor and sensory block following epidural anesthesia without reducing the postoperative analgesic benefit.[65]

Caudal anesthesia

Caudal epidural block involves injection of a drug into the epidural space through the sacral hiatus.

Caudal block is applicable widely in pediatric day surgery, providing excellent analgesia for most day-case procedures below the umbilicus. Using weaker local anesthetic solutions can minimize the potential for lower limb weakness delaying discharge with caudal block (e.g. 0.125% bupivacaine).[66] Several studies have failed to demonstrate that urinary retention is a significant problem after day-case caudal block.[67,68]

One of the main drawbacks with single-shot local anesthetic caudal block is that effective analgesia lasts for only a few hours. Recently, addition of NMDA antagonists and alpha-2 antagonists has been shown to significantly prolong caudal analgesia initiated by local anesthetics. Thus, clonidine 1–2 µg/kg doubles and ketamine 0.5 mg kg quadruples the duration of analgesia.[69] These drugs are suitable for day-case practice as their use is not associated with significant cardiorespiratory, sedative, or untoward psychological effects.

Combined spinal epidural anesthesia

Combined spinal epidural (CSE) anesthesia is well established for inpatient surgery and obstetrics but is still in its infancy in day-case surgery.[70] It combines the rapidity, density, and reliability of subarachnoid block with the flexibility of continuous epidural block. Although, at first sight, CSE techniques appear to be more complicated than epidural or spinal block alone, intrathecal drug administration and siting of the epidural catheter are both enhanced by the combined, single space, needle-through-needle method. CSE is an effective way to reduce the total drug dosage required for anesthesia and analgesia, thus making a truly selective blockade possible.[71] The security of an epidural catheter allows minimal dosing of local anesthetic and therefore more precise predictability of day-surgery spinal anesthesia.[70] In contrast with epidural anesthesia, the other leading central neuraxial technique, CSE has a lower failure rate and a faster onset time.[72] For ambulatory knee surgery, CSE allowed Urmey and colleagues to reduce the dose of spinal lidocaine from 80 mg to 40 mg.[73] Similarly, Pawlowski and others used CSE to identify appropriate doses of spinal mepivacaine in order to eliminate the risk of TNS.[74]

Truncal peripheral nerve blocks

Paravertebral blocks

Paravertebral anesthesia is a unilateral alternative to epidural anesthesia with prolonged postoperative pain relief. It has been used successfully for ambulatory breast surgery[75] and inguinal hernia repair.[76]

In a study using paravertebral ropivacaine for hernia repair, the average time for block administration was 12 min and analgesia was provided for 15 h, which was significantly better than with local infiltration block with ropivacaine.[77] However, in a series of 30 patients, there were two cases of block failure and two cases of prolonged recovery due to epidural effects.[76]

Unilateral paravertebral anesthesia may be a good choice alone or as an adjunct to sedation for breast cancer surgery. In one study the data actually indicated a lower incidence of cancer relapse after this block, although some confounders could be present from the nonrandomized retrospective design.[78] In any case, there seems to be better initial pain relief after this block and minor side effects, at least after moderate or more extensive procedures.[79]

Transversus abdominis plane (TAP) block

A recent review of seven randomized controlled studies of TAP blocks for postoperative pain showed that there is a substantial reduction in postoperative opioid consumption and improved pain scores after surgeries involving the anterior abdominal wall.[80] When used regularly, the landmark approach is effective, reliable, and relatively easy to perform. The key to a successful block is proper identification of the triangle of Petit and directing the needle in a slightly anterior direction. There is also a general agreement that reliable spread of the drug occurs between the T10 and L1 dermatomes with an ultrasound-guided approach. In particular, adequate volume is more important than a high concentration of local anesthetic. With either technique 20–40 ml of the local anesthetic is injected. The block is gaining popularity because of the easy technique and favorable risk profile. Its use is limited by the need for bilateral blocks when incisions cross the midline and the limitation to analgesia for somatic pain, sparing visceral coverage.[81] Recently, ultrasound-guided TAP catheters with ambulatory perineural infusions have been used successfully in patients undergoing inguinal hernia repair.[82]

Ilioinguinal field block for inguinal hernia repair

Aasbo et al. compared preoperative inguinal field block plus perioperative sedation with general anesthesia and wound infiltration for inguinal hernia repair.[83] They found that patients anesthetized with an inguinal field block had a shorter recovery time, less pain, better mobilization, and greater satisfaction than patients who received general anesthesia and wound infiltration. These differences lasted for the whole 1-week observation period. Even though there are reports of transient femoral nerve palsy following this technique,[84] the use of inguinal field block seems to be highly recommended for inguinal hernia repair in day-case surgery as an alternative to skilled surgeons doing the local anesthesia infiltration themselves.

Rectus sheath block (RSB)

First described by Schleich in 1899, for providing muscle relaxation and analgesia, interest has been renewed for abdominal wall analgesia in laparotomies and hernia procedures.[81] RSB is performed bilaterally with large volumes of local anesthetic. It provides excellent analgesia for laparoscopy, resulting in significantly lower pain scores and opioid administration.[85] It also provides superior analgesia after laparotomy than intraperitoneal or intraincisional local anesthesia.[86]

Peripheral nerve blocks

Painful stimuli are initiated by tissue injury and transmitted by A-delta and C fiber nociceptors to the dorsal horn neurons in the spinal cord. In this response to injury, a variety of neurotransmitters such as prostaglandin, bradykinin, serotonin, and substance P are released which leads to increased activity of the dorsal horn neurons. Local anesthesia/regional blocks inhibit the transmission of the noxious afferent stimuli from the operative site to the spinal cord and brain, and it is desirable to maintain this effect well into the postoperative period. This sustained postoperative analgesia decreases the risks of hyperalgesia, allodynia, and increased pain.[9] Ultrasound guidance enables the imaging of peripheral nerves and vessels and the possibility of guiding the block needle with real-time imaging, thus reducing the risk of nerve damage.

Upper extremity peripheral nerve blocks: Brachial plexus can be blocked using ultrasound guidance right from the level of the roots till distal nerves. Upper extremity blocks have many advantages over general anesthesia with systemic opioids. Advantages include effective postoperative analgesia, decreased requirements for opioids and the potential complications associated with their use, and an ability to avoid instrumenting the airway. These blocks can provide successful surgical anesthesia in a high majority of cases, with a very low complication rate.

Table 6.2 Peripheral nerve block techniques, surgeries, and risks.[87]

Regional technique	Surgery, notes/risks
Upper extremity peripheral nerve blocks	
Interscalene brachial plexus (BP) block	Surgeries over the lateral two-thirds of the clavicle, proximal humerus, and shoulder joint. Shoulder arthroscopy, rotator cuff repair, total shoulder arthroplasty. Performed using paresthesia, nerve stimulation (NS), ultrasound guidance (USG), or a combination (NS+USG). Ulnar-sparing common, Horner syndrome, ipsilateral paresis of phrenic and laryngeal nerves, spinal cord damages, epidural spread. Hadzic *et al.* showed that none of the patients treated with Interscalene BP required additional analgesics as compared to the general anesthesia (GA) group in which 8% patients required pain management despite wound infiltration and single injection IA instillation of local anesthetic.[88]
Supraclavicular BP block	Surgery on upper arm, elbow, forearm, wrist, and fingers. Superficial location. Fast-onset, dense blockade. Single/double injection technique. Pneumothorax, ulnar-sparing, hemidiaphragmatic paresis.
Axillary BP block	Surgery on hand, forearm. Superficial and compressible, wide variation of the positioning of the four main nerves. Low risk profile, multiple injections required.

Table 6.2 (cont.)

Regional technique	Surgery, notes/risks
Infraclavicular BP block	Surgical procedures below the midhumeral level. Deeper in location, USG helps to visualize better. Single posterior cord injection is more effective than single medial/lateral cords. Pneumothorax.
Suprascapular nerve block	Shoulder surgery. Used when interscalene approach to BP contraindicated. Often combined with axillary nerve block.
Lower extremity peripheral nerve blocks	
Femoral nerve block	Knee arthroscopy, total knee arthroscopy (TKA) and anterior cruciate ligament (ACL) repair, ankle surgery. Superficial and compressible location. Risk of fall with quadriceps weakness. Usually performed in conjunction with sciatic nerve block.
Adductor canal block	Knee surgery. Decreased risk of fall (motor weakness) as compared with femoral block.
Saphenous nerve block	Performed in conjunction with sciatic nerve block. Surgeries on knee, ankle, and medial and lower leg. No fall concerns as they do not affect quadriceps.
Sciatic nerve block – approaches: classic, sub-gluteal	Combined with femoral nerve block for ACL and TKA surgery. Surgery of lower leg, ankle, and foot in conjunction with femoral or saphenous nerve block. Foot drop with high concentration blocks.
Lumbar plexus block Psoas compartment block	Hip arthroscopy, total hip arthroplasty, surgeries on thigh and knee. Retroperitoneal hematoma is a possible complication.
Popliteal approach for sciatic nerve	Surgical procedures below the knee, foot/ankle surgery, Achilles tendon surgery, sural nerve biopsy, short saphenous vein stripping. This block provides great analgesia for a calf tourniquet as well. Medial aspect of the leg missed, needs to be supplemented with saphenous nerve block. Popliteal fossa is amenable to both single injections and catheter placement.
Ankle block	Surgery of the foot and toes especially those patients who cannot hemodynamically tolerate the depressant effects of GA or neuraxial blockade. Three superficial and two deep nerves: posterior tibial, sural, deep peroneal, superficial peroneal (terminal branches of sciatic nerve) and saphenous nerves (extension of the femoral nerve) can all be blocked utilizing ultrasound guidance resulting in anesthesia of the entire foot (ankle block).

Lower extremity peripheral nerve blocks: For single lower extremity surgery there are several choices of regional technique. The choice for all kinds of foot surgery (including those with an ankle tourniquet) remains the ankle block. Although simple and efficacious for foot surgery, the ankle block technique is somewhat unreliable. Combined with a saphenous or femoral nerve block, posterior popliteal sciatic nerve block seems a more reliable alternative. The use of long-acting local anesthetics is advocated and it seems safe to discharge the patients before the block has worn off.[89,90] For unilateral knee surgery spinal can be an option with a request to the surgeon to provide appropriate cover with local anesthetic.

The use of regional foot blocks in conjunction with general anesthesia is thought to prolong the period of postoperative pain relief and thus be beneficial for patients undergoing day-case surgery. In one study by Clough and colleagues of outpatient bony forefoot surgery, however, supplemental foot block did not alter the consumption of postoperative analgesic tablets or overall patient satisfaction.[91] The authors concluded that although the foot block prolonged the time until postoperative pain was first perceived, it was not a major benefit when used as an analgesic in the outpatient setting.

Continuous ambulatory peripheral nerve blocks (CPNB)

Although single-injection nerve blocks (sPNB) provide excellent analgesia, they usually provide postoperative analgesia for a shorter duration of 12–16 h or less. CPNB increases both duration and density of local anesthetic effects. CPNB are performed by placement of a percutaneous perineural catheter that helps with continuous infusion of local anesthetics to extend the duration of postoperative analgesia. They are placed with the help of either nerve stimulation and/or ultrasound guidance. This technique may now be used in the ambulatory patients in the outpatient setting[92,93] and may be continued outside of the hospital setting for eligible patients.

Continuous wound catheters are placed (usually by surgeons) to infuse local anesthetics (LA), directly into a surgical site, providing improved pain relief while reducing the need for analgesics. One must be aware of the signs of LA toxicity including agitation, confusion, tachycardia, arrhythmias, hypotension and convulsions.

Peripheral nerves blocks with a catheter suitable for continuous LA infusions include: interscalene catheters which are commonly placed for shoulder surgeries, such as total shoulder arthroplasty, hemiarthroplasty, etc. In patients with severe respiratory problems, an ultrasound-guided suprascapular nerve block catheter can be placed. Supraclavicular and infraclavicular catheters are placed for arm, elbow, wrist, and hand surgeries. Femoral catheters are placed commonly for knee surgeries including total knee arthroplasty, etc. Popliteal catheters are placed in combination with saphenous catheters for ankle and foot surgeries including total ankle fusion, ankle arthroplasty, etc. Single/bilateral paravertebral catheters are placed for breast surgeries including mastectomies.

Indwelling catheter placement requires strict adherence to sterile procedure. The American Society of Regional Anesthesia and Pain Medicine (ASRA) recommends sterile precautions, including antiseptic hand-washing, sterile gloves, surgical hats and masks, and the use of alcohol-based chlorhexidine antiseptic solution.[94] A sterile drape is applied to isolate the area of skin preparation. When using an ultrasound-guided technique, the transducer must either be covered with a sterile sleeve or be positioned outside of the sterile field. The Tuohy needle remains

a popular choice for many practitioners when transitioning from sPNB to CPNB placement. A significant advantage of CPNB placed for postoperative analgesia is that it does not require the injection of a large, concentrated dose of LA. Interscalene catheters, for example, provide excellent analgesia after initial injection of only 20 ml of 0.125% bupivacaine.[95] This total dose of bupivacaine (25 mg) is considerably lower than doses typically used for sPNB (100–150 mg). As with many aspects of CPNB placement, there is variability among institutions regarding how to secure the catheter. Catheter dressing focuses on preventing leakage, dislodgement, and infection. Liquid adhesives are commonly applied to the skin before the dressing. Sterile adhesive strips and other fixation devices can also be used at the catheter insertion site to prevent dislodgement. Catheter tunneling is practiced at many institutions in hopes of minimizing infection and dislodgement.

The optimal combination of local anesthetic concentration and volume to be infused through a perineural catheter remains to be determined. One trend that seems to be consistent is that analgesia can be achieved at most locations using low concentrations of long-acting local anesthetics (ropivacaine 0.2%, bupivacaine 0.125%) infused at rates from 5 to 12 ml per hour.[95]

The benefits of CPNBs[93] include:

- facilitate same-day discharge
- decrease the time to achieve discharge criteria
- reduce analgesic requirements
- decrease in postoperative joint inflammation and inflammatory markers
- reduce sleep disturbances and opioid-related side effects
- decrease baseline/dynamic pain
- increase patient satisfaction
- increase ambulation and help with functioning improvement
- early resumption of passive range of motion of joints
- potential reduction of the incidence of postsurgical chronic pain and reduction of costs.

Intravenous regional anesthesia

This is a simple method that may sometimes be used by experienced surgeons without involving the anesthesiologist (also see Chapter 5, Anesthetic Techniques). This practice may be controversial; at the very least, the surgeon should have fast and adequate backup in case of cuff failure, systemic toxicity, and convulsions. The method is most reliable when carried out on the upper extremities, although anesthesia of deeper bone/joint structures may be inadequate. Also, the surgical procedure should be limited to about 1 hour, because the anesthesia will wear off, tissue hypoxia will evolve, and the discomfort caused by the cuff may become significant. The method is to establish an intravenous cannula on the dorsum of the hand and then to elevate the extremity and wrap the whole arm tightly in elastic wrapping, starting with the fingers, in order to "empty" out the venous blood. Then the proximal part of a double cuff is inflated to 150 mmHg above systolic blood pressure, and the wrapping is released. Then 40–50 ml of lidocaine (5 mg/ml) is injected via the intravenous cannula. After 5–10 min the distal part of the cuff may be filled and then the proximal part deflated, and surgery may start. The cuff should not be released before at least 20–30 min has elapsed (risk of free lidocaine and convulsions). The method is good for superficial surgery, tendon surgery, and soft tissue procedures.

Head and neck nerve blocks

Ophthalmology

Retrobulbar blocks confer sensory blockade to the contents of the orbit from the first (ophthalmic) division of the trigeminal nerve. The ophthalmologists in the day care setting for cataract surgery frequently perform these along with supratrochlear nerve blocks. Minimal if any I.V. sedation is required for routine cataract surgery.

Superficial cervical plexus block

This block involves injection of LA near the superficial cervical plexus posterior to the lateral border of the sternocleidomastoid muscle at the midpoint of the muscle. It provides sensory block to the anterolateral neck, and may be useful for breast surgery in conjunction with paravertebral blocks.

How to make a final choice of anesthetic technique in the individual case

There is no conclusive evidence to highlight any technique as being superior in terms of safety, i.e., a close to zero incidence of mortality or permanent disability.

The choice must be made according to total quality for the patient and their experience as well as the cost-effectiveness for the unit. Quality for individual patients varies and depends upon personal preferences, such as being awake, fear of needles, risk, and tolerance of side effects such as postoperative nausea and pain. Cost-effectiveness will also vary with the surgical unit in question: acquisition costs of drugs, staffing, out-of-theater induction or regional block facilities, postoperative recovery facilities, and so on. However, the following are some general approaches to consider.

1. For superficial surgery or cases with minor surgical invasiveness, LA with individually tailored and minimized sedation may be preferred.
2. For surgery of middling duration, in areas suitable for regional anesthesia, with an anticipated medium or high intensity of postoperative pain, a regional nerve block or neuraxial block may be recommended. The same may be valid for patients with a definite preference for regional techniques or for patients with a high risk of nausea or vomiting.
3. For other procedures general anesthesia is usually chosen, mostly due to the decreased time required for preparation and the ease of administration. With general anesthesia care must be taken to ensure optimal prophylaxis against pain and nausea in the postoperative period.

Conflicts/controversies with the regional anesthesia techniques

What are the contraindications to loco-regional anesthesia?

- Patients who do not consent.
- For patients with nerve injury or neurologic deficit in the area of planned block, it is a good general rule to avoid loco-regional techniques. Although loco-regional anesthesia has not been shown to worsen any neurologic deficit, it may be wise to avoid the potential for speculation and discussion with the patient afterwards about these issues. This means that if there is a good indication for loco-regional anesthesia, if general anesthesia presents problems, or if the patient is otherwise motivated to have such an approach, it may well be done. In any case, it is wise to assess neurologic function before applying the anesthesia, and also

to document the discussion with the patient and the decision made before going ahead.

- Uncooperative patients may be poor subjects for loco-regional anesthesia. Again, the contraindication is relative and must be weighed against the alternatives. Using ultrasound may be a tool to decrease the risk of major nerve damage in such patients.

- Infection at the site of the block is an absolute contraindication. Also a tattoo may be a relative contraindication if the needle has to go directly through a pigmented skin area. Such pigments may be drawn in with the needle tip and become neurotoxic. This concern is most valid with spinal anesthesia and the problem can usually be managed by moving the needle a few millimeters to a skin spot without pigmentation.

- Anticoagulated patients should be evaluated more strictly for neuraxial blocks in the outpatient setting than as inpatients. A postoperative hematoma developing after discharge is more dangerous in terms of diagnosis and delays from pressure ischemia or nerve tissue injury than it is in a carefully observed inpatient.

Anticoagulation: ASRA guidelines[96]

Unfractionated (UFH) SQ heparin: No contraindication on regional anesthesia with twice-daily dosing and total daily dose < 10,000 U. The safety of neuraxial blockade in patients receiving doses greater than 10,000 U of UFH daily, or more than twice-daily dosing of UFH, has not been established. Heparinize 1 hour after neuraxial technique, remove catheter 2–4 hours after last heparin dose.

UFH IV heparin: Delay needle/catheter placement 2–4 hours after last dose, document normal aPTT. Heparin may be restarted 1 hour following procedure. Heparinization with an indwelling neuraxial catheter is associated with increased risk; monitor neurologic status.

LWMH: With twice-daily dosing delay procedure at least 12 hours from the last dose of LMWH. For "treatment" dosing of LMWH, at least 24 hours should elapse prior to procedure. LMWH should not be administered within 24 hours after the procedure. Remove neuraxial catheter *4 hrs before first LMWH dose.*

Warfarin: Normal INR (before neuraxial technique); remove catheter when INR ≤ 1.5 (initiation of therapy). Warfarin therapy should be discontinued 4–5 days prior to neuraxial procedure. INR should be within the normal range at time of procedure. Remove catheter when INR ≤ 1.5.

Antiplatelet medications: Aspirin or other NSAIDs present no contraindication to block placement. Clopidogrel should be discontinued 7 days, ticlopidine 14 days, and GP II b/IIIa inhibitors 8–48 hours in advance (8 hours for tirofiban and eptifibatide, 24–48 hours for abciximab).

Dabigatran: Discontinue 7 days prior to procedure; for shorter time periods, document normal TT. First postoperative dose: 24 h after needle placement and 2 h post catheter removal (whichever is later).

Rivaroxaban: Needle placement 22–26 h after discontinuation. No neuraxial or deep/plexus catheters during rivaroxaban therapy. First dose 6 h postoperatively.

Thrombolytics and fibrinolytics: Absolute contraindication. There are no data available to suggest a safe interval between procedure and initiation or discontinuation of these medications. Follow fibrinogen levels and observe for signs of neural compression.

Herbal therapy: No evidence for mandatory discontinuation before neuraxial technique; be aware of potential drug interactions.

What are the prerequisites for successful loco-regional use in ambulatory care?

Ensure a low block failure rate

This comes with training and experience, but may be challenged by time constraints and a stressful working environment. Induction rooms may lower the failure rate, as does the use of good equipment such as nerve stimulators and, in particular, appropriate ultrasound imaging and experience in its use.

Avoid prolonged block

A prolonged neuraxial block may delay recovery and discharge due to prolonged leg paralysis and occasionally complications such as urinary retention, but it will also ensure prolonged analgesia. For ambulatory surgery these neuraxial blocks should be done with short-lasting drugs, unless a prolonged surgical procedure is anticipated. A better strategy for potentially prolonged procedures is to use short-acting drugs, but insert a catheter in case repeated dosing becomes necessary.

For nerve blocks with a limited area of paralysis it may be totally advantageous to have a prolonged block, because pain protection is better and longer-lasting. If the patient has been given appropriate information it is usually acceptable to discharge a patient with a paralyzed arm in a sling or a paralyzed foot within a bandage or plaster.

Early discharge with long-acting peripheral nerve blockade: is it safe?

Whether one should discharge patients before a peripheral block has worn off is controversial. Concerns about possible nerve damage and the risk of accidental harm to an anesthetized limb remain arguments against early discharge. In a prospective study involving 2382 peripheral nerve blocks of both the upper and lower extremities with early discharge, the incidence of complications was very low, and most patients (98%) were highly satisfied with the choice of anesthesia.[97] Only 6 patients (0.25%) had a persistent paresthesia after 7 days (which later resolved) that might have been associated with the nerve block. The authors concluded that even longer-acting local anesthetics would be beneficial in order to reduce the frequent incidence of persistent pain at 7 days.[97]

Summary

The success of day-case surgery depends, to a large extent, on both effective control of postoperative pain and minimization of side effects such as sedation, nausea, and vomiting. Regional anesthesia assumes a significant position in the outpatient setting by fulfilling the above requirements. Careful patient selection and ultrasound-guided regional anesthesia techniques have made it all the more popular and acceptable over the last couple of decades. Newer local anesthetics and adjuncts make the duration of the technique very malleable. It is very likely that the growth in ambulatory surgery heralds a promising future in terms of role and demand of regional anesthesia.

Clinicians must consider several factors when choosing a specific block. These include the preferences of the surgeon and patient, the duration of surgery, and the surgical and postoperative requirement for motor examination. The location of block performance largely depends on the anesthesiologist's performance and local environment. Variables include OR turnover, available resources, and practice conditions.

References

1. M. F. Mulroy, S. B. McDonald. Regional anesthesia for outpatient surgery. *Anesthesiol Clin North Am.* 2003;**21**(2):289–303.

2. S. M. Klein, A. Bergh, S. M. Steele, G. S. Georgiade, R. A. Greengrass. Thoracic paravertebral block for breast surgery. *Anesth Analg.* 2000;**90**(6):1402–05.

3. S. Larsson, D. Lundberg. A prospective survey of postoperative nausea and vomiting with special regard to incidence and relations to patient characteristics, anesthetic routines and surgical procedures. *Acta Anaesthesiol Scand.* 1995;**39**(4):539–45.

4. T. Tan, R. Bhinder, M. Carey, L. Briggs. Day-surgery patients anesthetized with propofol have less postoperative pain than those anesthetized with sevoflurane. *Anesth Analg.* 2010;**111**(1):83–85.

5. S. Badrinath, M. N. Avramov, M. Shadrick, T. R. Witt, A. D. Ivankovich. The use of a ketamine–propofol combination during monitored anesthesia care. *Anesth Analg.* 2000;**90**(4):858–62.

6. S. Himmelseher, M. E. Durieux. Ketamine for perioperative pain management. *Anesthesiology.* 2005;**102**(1):211–20.

7. B. A. Williams, S. L. Orebaugh, B. Ben-David, P. E. Bigeleisen. Electrical stimulation: An important force behind the growth of regional anesthesia. *Can J Anaesth.* 2007;**54**(7):585–86; author reply 586–87.

8. S. L. Orebaugh, B. A. Williams, M. L. Kentor. Ultrasound guidance with nerve stimulation reduces the time necessary for resident peripheral nerve blockade. *Reg Anesth Pain Med.* 2007;**32**(5):448–54.

9. A. K. Jacob, M. T. Walsh, J. A. Dilger. Role of regional anesthesia in the ambulatory environment. *Anesth Clinics.* 2010;**28**(2):251–66.

10. B. C. Tsui, M. P. Knezevich, J. J. Pillay. Reduced injection pressures using a compressed air injection technique (CAIT): An in vitro study. *Reg Anesth Pain Med.* 2008;**33**(2):168–73.

11. B. C. Tsui, L. X. Li, J. J. Pillay. Compressed air injection technique to standardize block injection pressures. *Can J Anaesth.* 2006;**53**(11):1098–102.

12. B. N. S. Carty. Ultrasound-guided regional anaesthesia. *BJA: CEACCP Contin Educ Anaesth Crit Care Pain.* 2007;**7**(Issue 1):20–24.

13. B. D. O'Donnell, G. Iohom. An estimation of the minimum effective anesthetic volume of 2% lidocaine in ultrasound-guided axillary brachial plexus block. *Anesthesiology.* 2009;**111**(1):25–29.

14. U. Eichenberger, S. Stockli, P. Marhofer, *et al.* Minimal local anesthetic volume for peripheral nerve block: A new ultrasound-guided, nerve dimension-based method. *Reg Anesth Pain Med.* 2009;**34**(3):242–46.

15. B. O'Donnell, J. Riordan, I. Ahmad, G. Iohom. Brief reports: A clinical evaluation of block characteristics using one milliliter 2% lidocaine in ultrasound-guided axillary brachial plexus block. *Anesth Analg.* 2010;**111** (3):808–10.

16. M. S. Abrahams, M. F. Aziz, R. F. Fu, J. L. Horn. Ultrasound guidance compared with electrical neurostimulation for peripheral nerve block: A systematic review and meta-analysis of randomized controlled trials. *Br J Anaesth.* 2009;**102**(3):408–17.

17. P. Marhofer, K. Schrogendorfer, H. Koinig, S. Kapral, C. Weinstabl, N. Mayer. Ultrasonographic guidance improves sensory block and onset time of three-in-one blocks. *Anesth Analg.* 1997;**85**(4):854–57.

18. P. Marhofer, K. Schrogendorfer, T. Wallner, H. Koinig, N. Mayer, S. Kapral. Ultrasonographic guidance reduces the amount of local anesthetic for 3-in-1 blocks. *Reg Anesth Pain Med.* 1998;**23**(6):584–88.

19. F. C. Liu, J. T. Liou, Y. F. Tsai, *et al.* Efficacy of ultrasound-guided axillary brachial plexus block: A comparative study with nerve stimulator-guided method. *Chang Gung Med J.* 2005;**28**(6):396–402.

20. A. R. Sauter, M. S. Dodgson, A. Stubhaug, A. M. Halstensen, O. Klaastad. Electrical nerve stimulation or ultrasound guidance for lateral sagittal infraclavicular blocks: A randomized, controlled, observer-blinded, comparative study. *Anesth Analg.* 2008;**106**(6):1910–15.

21. N. A. Bryan, J. D. Swenson, P. E. Greis, R. T. Burks. Indwelling interscalene catheter use in an outpatient setting for shoulder surgery: Technique, efficacy, and complications. *J Shoulder Elbow Surg.* 2007;**16** (4):388–95.

22. Z. J. Koscielniak-Nielsen, H. Rasmussen, L. Hesselbjerg. Pneumothorax after an ultrasound-guided lateral sagittal infraclavicular block. *Acta Anaesthesiol Scand.* 2008;**52**(8):1176–77.

23. J. M. Neal. Ultrasound-guided regional anesthesia and patient safety: An evidence-based analysis. *Reg Anesth Pain Med.* 2010;**35**(2 Suppl):S59–67.

24. A. Bhatia, J. Lai, V. W. Chan, R. Brull. Case report: pneumothorax as a complication of the ultrasound-guided supraclavicular approach for brachial plexus block. *Anesth Analg.* 2010;**111**(3):817–19.

25. A. T. Gray, J. J. Laur. Regional anesthesia for ambulatory surgery: Where ultrasound has made a difference. *Int Anesthesiol Clin.* 2011;**49**(4):13–21.

26. J. M. Neal, C. M. Bernards, J. F. T. Butterworth, *et al.* ASRA practice advisory on local anesthetic systemic toxicity. *Reg Anesth Pain Med.* 2010;**35** (2):152–61.

27. C. M. Brummett, B. A. Williams. Additives to local anesthetics for peripheral nerve blockade. *Int Anesthesiol Clin.* 2011;**49**(4):104–16.

28. K. D. Candido, A. P. Winnie, A. H. Ghaleb, M. W. Fattouh, C. D. Franco. Buprenorphine added to the local anesthetic for axillary brachial plexus block prolongs postoperative analgesia. *Reg Anesth Pain Med.* 2002;**27**(2):162–67.

29. K. D. Candido, J. Hennes, S. Gonzalez, *et al.* Buprenorphine enhances and prolongs the postoperative analgesic effect of bupivacaine in patients receiving infragluteal sciatic nerve block. *Anesthesiology.* 2010;**113**(6):1419–26.

30. C. Stein. Targeting pain and inflammation by peripherally acting opioids. *Front Pharmacol.* 2013;**4**:123.

31. D. M. Popping, N. Elia, E. Marret, M. Wenk, M. R. Tramer. Clonidine as an adjuvant to local anesthetics for peripheral nerve and plexus blocks: A meta-analysis of randomized trials. *Anesthesiology.* 2009;**111**(2):406–15.

32. C. J. McCartney, E. Duggan, E. Apatu. Should we add clonidine to local anesthetic for peripheral nerve blockade? A qualitative systematic review of the literature. *Reg Anesth Pain Med.* 2007;**32**(4):330–38.

33. J. E. Tetzlaff, H. J. Yoon, J. Brems, T. Javorsky. Alkalinization of mepivacaine improves the quality of motor block associated with interscalene brachial plexus anesthesia for shoulder surgery. *Reg Anesth.* 1995;**20**(2):128–32.

34. S. H. Wilson, C. Rest, B. Pearce-Smith, M. E. Hudson, J. E. Chelly. Regional anesthesia for ambulatory surgery: The ideal technique for a growing practice. *Anesthesiology News.* 2013;Sect. 1.

35. H. Wulf. New perspectives for day-case spinals! Old drugs for an ancient technique? *Acta Anaesthesiol Scand.* 2011;**55**(3):257–58.

36. F. V. Salinas, S. S. Liu. Spinal anaesthesia: Local anaesthetics and adjuncts in the ambulatory setting. *Best Pract Res Clin Anaesthesiol.* 2002;**16** (2):195–210.

37. D. Tong, J. Wong, F. Chung, *et al.* Prospective study on incidence and functional impact of transient neurologic symptoms associated with 1% versus 5% hyperbaric lidocaine in short urologic procedures. *Anesthesiology.* 2003;**98**(2):485–94.

38. M. F. Mulroy, F. V. Salinas, K. L. Larkin, N. L. Polissar. Ambulatory surgery patients may be discharged before voiding after short-acting spinal and epidural anesthesia. *Anesthesiology.* 2002;**97**(2):315–19.

39. C. C. Buckenmaier, 3rd, K. C. Nielsen, R. Pietrobon, *et al.* Small-dose intrathecal lidocaine versus ropivacaine for anorectal surgery in an ambulatory setting. *Anesth Analg.* 2002;**95** (5):1253–57, table of contents.

40. P. H. Lennox, H. Vaghadia, C. Henderson, L. Martin, G. W. Mitchell. Small-dose selective spinal anesthesia for short-duration outpatient laparoscopy: Recovery

characteristics compared with desflurane anesthesia. *Anesth Analg.* 2002;**94**(2):346–50, table of contents.

41. B. Ben-David, P. J. DeMeo, C. Lucyk, D. Solosko. Minidose lidocaine–fentanyl spinal anesthesia in ambulatory surgery: Prophylactic nalbuphine versus nalbuphine plus droperidol. *Anesth Analg.* 2002;**95**(6):1596–600, table of contents.

42. F. Lopez-Soriano, B. Lajarin, F. Rivas, J. M. Verdu, J. Lopez-Robles. [Hyperbaric subarachnoid ropivacaine in ambulatory surgery: comparative study with hyperbaric bupivacaine]. *Rev Esp Anestesiol Reanim.* 2002;**49**(2):71–75.

43. J. B. Whiteside, D. Burke, J. A. Wildsmith. Comparison of ropivacaine 0.5% (in glucose 5%) with bupivacaine 0.5% (in glucose 8%) for spinal anaesthesia for elective surgery. *Br J Anaesth.* 2003;**90**(3):304–08.

44. M. B. Breebaart, M. P. Vercauteren, V. L. Hoffmann, H. A. Adriaensen. Urinary bladder scanning after day-case arthroscopy under spinal anaesthesia: Comparison between lidocaine, ropivacaine, and levobupivacaine. *Br J Anaesth.* 2003;**90**(3):309–13.

45. C. O. Imarengiaye, D. Song, A. J. Prabhu, F. Chung. Spinal anesthesia: Functional balance is impaired after clinical recovery. *Anesthesiology.* 2003;**98**(2):511–15.

46. A. Gupta, K. Axelsson, S. E. Thorn, *et al.* Low-dose bupivacaine plus fentanyl for spinal anesthesia during ambulatory inguinal herniorrhaphy: A comparison between 6 mg and 7.5 mg of bupivacaine. *Acta Anaesthesiol Scand.* 2003;**47**(1):13–19.

47. G. Danelli, M. Berti, A. Casati, *et al.* Spinal block or total intravenous anaesthesia with propofol and remifentanil for gynaecological outpatient procedures. *Eur J Anaesthesiol.* 2002;**19**(8):594–99.

48. A. M. Korhonen, J. V. Valanne, R. M. Jokela, P. Ravaska, K. Korttila. Intrathecal hyperbaric bupivacaine 3 mg + fentanyl 10 microg for outpatient knee arthroscopy with tourniquet. *Acta Anaesthesiol Scand.* 2003;**47**(3):342–46.

49. M. De Kock, P. Gautier, L. Fanard, J. L. Hody, P. Lavand'homme. Intrathecal ropivacaine and clonidine for ambulatory knee arthroscopy: A dose–response study. *Anesthesiology.* 2001;**94**(4):574–78.

50. R. Merivirta, K. Kuusniemi, P. Jaakkola, K. Pihlajamaki, M. Pitkanen. Unilateral spinal anaesthesia for outpatient surgery: A comparison between hyperbaric bupivacaine and bupivacaine–clonidine combination. *Acta Anaesthesiol Scand.* 2009;**53**(6):788–93.

51. M. P. Hendriks, C. J. de Weert, M. M. Snoeck, H. P. Hu, M. A. Pluim, M. J. Gielen. Plain articaine or prilocaine for spinal anaesthesia in day-case knee arthroscopy: A double-blind randomized trial. *Br J Anaesth.* 2009;**102**(2):259–63.

52. A. Sell, T. Tein, M. Pitkanen. Spinal 2-chloroprocaine: Effective dose for ambulatory surgery. *Acta Anaesthesiol Scand.* 2008;**52**(5):695–99.

53. M. R. Hejtmanek, J. E. Pollock. Chloroprocaine for spinal anesthesia: A retrospective analysis. *Acta Anaesthesiol Scand.* 2011;**55**(3):267–72.

54. B. Ben-David, E. Solomon, H. Levin, H. Admoni, Z. Goldik. Intrathecal fentanyl with small-dose dilute bupivacaine: Better anesthesia without prolonging recovery. *Anesth Analg.* 1997;**85**(3):560–65.

55. H. Vaghadia, D. Viskari, G. W. Mitchell, A. Berrill. Selective spinal anesthesia for outpatient laparoscopy. I: Characteristics of three hypobaric solutions. *Can J Anaesth.* 2001;**48**(3):256–60.

56. B. Ben-David, M. Maryanovsky, A. Gurevitch, *et al.* A comparison of minidose lidocaine–fentanyl and conventional-dose lidocaine spinal anesthesia. *Anesth Analg.* 2000;**91**(4):865–70.

57. C. J. Jankowski, J. R. Hebl, M. J. Stuart, *et al.* A comparison of psoas compartment block and spinal and general anesthesia for outpatient knee arthroscopy. *Anesth Analg.* 2003;**97**(4):1003–09, table of contents.

58. S. S. Liu, S. B. McDonald. Current issues in spinal anesthesia. *Anesthesiology.* 2001;**94**(5):888–906.

59. B. R. Davis, D. J. Kopacz. Spinal 2-chloroprocaine: the effect of added clonidine. *Anesth Analg.* 2005;**100**(2):559–65.

60. V. Dahl, C. Gierloff, E. Omland, J. C. Raeder. Spinal, epidural or propofol anaesthesia for out-patient knee arthroscopy? *Acta Anaesthesiol Scand.* 1997;**41**(10):1341–45.

61. P. Labas, B. Ohradka, M. Cambal, J. Olejnik, J. Fillo. Haemorrhoidectomy in outpatient practice. *Eur J Surg.* 2002;**168**(11):619–20.

62. A. A. Weinbroum, G. Lalayev, T. Yashar, R. Ben-Abraham, D. Niv, R. Flaishon. Combined pre-incisional oral dextromethorphan and epidural lidocaine for postoperative pain reduction and morphine sparing: A randomised double-blind study on day-surgery patients. *Anaesthesia.* 2001;**56**(7):616–22.

63. T. T. Horlocker, Z. H. Bajwa, Z. Ashraf, *et al.* Risk assessment of hemorrhagic complications associated with nonsteroidal antiinflammatory medications in ambulatory pain clinic patients undergoing epidural steroid injection. *Anesth Analg.* 2002;**95**(6):1691–97, table of contents.

64. A. Gilbert, B. D. Owens, M. F. Mulroy. Epidural hematoma after outpatient epidural anesthesia. *Anesth Analg.* 2002;**94**(1):77–78, table of contents.

65. E. Y. Park, H. K. Kil, W. S. Park, N. H. Lee, J. Y. Hong. Effect of epidural saline washout on regression of sensory and motor block after epidural anaesthesia

with 2% lidocaine and fentanyl in elderly patients. *Anaesthesia.* 2009;**64**(3):273–76.

66. A. R. Wolf, R. D. Valley, D. W. Fear, W. L. Roy, J. Lerman. Bupivacaine for caudal analgesia in infants and children: The optimal effective concentration. *Anesthesiology.* 1988;**69**(1):102–06.

67. L. M. Broadman, R. S. Hannallah, A. B. Belman, P. T. Elder, U. Ruttimann, B. S. Epstein. Post-circumcision analgesia – A prospective evaluation of subcutaneous ring block of the penis. *Anesthesiology.* 1987;**67**(3):399–402.

68. Q. A. Fisher, C. M. McComiskey, J. L. Hill, *et al.* Postoperative voiding interval and duration of analgesia following peripheral or caudal nerve blocks in children. *Anesth Analg.* 1993;**76**(1):173–77.

69. B. Cook, E. Doyle. The use of additives to local anaesthetic solutions for caudal epidural blockade. *Paediatr Anaesth.* 1996;**6**(5):353–59.

70. N. Rawal. Analgesia for day-case surgery. *Br J Anaesth.* 2001;**87**(1):73–87.

71. N. Rawal, B. Holmstrom, J. A. Crowhurst, A. Van Zundert. The combined spinal–epidural technique. *Anesth Clin North Am.* 2000;**18**(2):267–95.

72. B. Holmstrom, K. Laugaland, N. Rawal, S. Hallberg. Combined spinal epidural block versus spinal and epidural block for orthopaedic surgery. *Can J Anaesth.* 1993;**40**(7):601–06.

73. W. F. Urmey, J. Stanton, M. Peterson, N. E. Sharrock. Combined spinal–epidural anesthesia for outpatient surgery. Dose–response characteristics of intrathecal isobaric lidocaine using a 27-gauge Whitacre spinal needle. *Anesthesiology.* 1995;**83**(3):528–34.

74. J. Pawlowski, R. Sukhani, A. L. Pappas, *et al.* The anesthetic and recovery profile of two doses (60 and 80 mg) of plain mepivacaine for ambulatory spinal anesthesia. *Anesth Analg.* 2000;**91**(3):580–84.

75. C. C. Buckenmaier, 3rd, S. M. Steele, K. C. Nielsen, A. H. Martin, S. M. Klein. Bilateral continuous paravertebral catheters for reduction mammoplasty. *Acta Anaesthesiol Scand.* 2002;**46**(8):1042–45.

76. C. R. Weltz, S. M. Klein, J. E. Arbo, R. A. Greengrass. Paravertebral block anesthesia for inguinal hernia repair. *World J Surg.* 2003;**27**(4):425–29.

77. S. M. Klein, R. Pietrobon, K. C. Nielsen, *et al.* Paravertebral somatic nerve block compared with peripheral nerve blocks for outpatient inguinal herniorrhaphy. *Reg Anesth Pain Med.* 2002;**27**(5):476–80.

78. A. K. Exadaktylos, D. J. Buggy, D. C. Moriarty, E. Mascha, D. I. Sessler. Can anesthetic technique for primary breast cancer surgery affect recurrence or metastasis? *Anesthesiology.* 2006;**105**(4):660–64.

79. J. F. Moller, L. Nikolajsen, S. A. Rodt, H. Ronning, P. S. Carlsson. Thoracic paravertebral block for breast cancer surgery: A randomized double-blind study. *Anesth Analg.* 2007;**105**(6):1848–51, table of contents.

80. P. L. Petersen, O. Mathiesen, H. Torup, J. B. Dahl. The transversus abdominis plane block: A valuable option for postoperative analgesia? A topical review. *Acta Anaesthesiol Scand.* 2010;**54**(5):529–35.

81. H. P. Sviggum, A. D. Niesen, B. D. Sites, J. A. Dilger. Trunk blocks 101: Transversus abdominis plane, ilioinguinal–iliohypogastric, and rectus sheath blocks. *Int Anesthesiol Clin.* 2012;**50**(1):74–92.

82. J. W. Heil, B. M. Ilfeld, V. J. Loland, N. S. Sandhu, E. R. Mariano. Ultrasound-guided transversus abdominis plane catheters and ambulatory perineural infusions for outpatient inguinal hernia repair. *Reg Anesth Pain Med.* 2010;**35**(6):556–58.

83. V. Aasbo, A. Thuen, J. Raeder. Improved long-lasting postoperative analgesia, recovery function and patient satisfaction after inguinal hernia repair with inguinal field block compared with general anesthesia. *Acta Anaesthesiol Scand.* 2002;**46**(6):674–78.

84. K. R. Ghani, R. McMillan, S. Paterson-Brown. Transient femoral nerve palsy following ilio-inguinal nerve blockade for day case inguinal hernia repair. *J R Coll Surg Edinb.* 2002;**47**(4):626–29.

85. S. Azemati, M. B. Khosravi. An assessment of the value of rectus sheath block for postlaparoscopic pain in gynecologic surgery. *J Minim Invasive Gynecol.* 2005;**12**(1):12–15.

86. H. Willschke, A. Bosenberg, P. Marhofer, *et al.* Ultrasonography-guided rectus sheath block in paediatric anaesthesia – A new approach to an old technique. *Br J Anaesth.* 2006;**97**(2):244–49.

87. S. H. Wilson, C. Rest, B. Pearce-Smith, M. E. Hudson, J. E. Chelly. Regional anesthesia for ambulatory surgery: The ideal technique for a growing practice. *Anesthesiology News.* 2013;**39**(4)(April 2013):1–11.

88. A. Hadzic, B. A. Williams, P. E. Karaca, *et al.* For outpatient rotator cuff surgery, nerve block anesthesia provides superior same-day recovery over general anesthesia. *Anesthesiology.* 2005;**102**(5):1001–07.

89. A. Casati, B. Borgi, G. Fanelli, *et al.* A double-blinded, randomized comparison of either 0.5% levobupivacaine or 0.5% ropivacaine for sciatic nerve block. *Anesth Analg.* 2002;**94**:987–90.

90. F. J. Singelyn. Single-injection applications for foot and ankle surgery. *Best Pract Res Clin Anaesthesiol.* 2002;**16**:247–54.

91. T. M. Clough, D. Sander, R. S. Bale, A. S. Laurence. The use of a local anesthetic foot block in patients undergoing outpatient bony forefoot surgery: A prospective randomized controlled trial. *J Foot Ankle Surg.* 2003;**42**:24–29.

92. B. M. Ilfeld, F. K. Enneking. Continuous peripheral nerve blocks at home: A review. *Anesth Analg.* 2005;**100**:1822–33.

93. J. Aguirre, A. Del Moral, I. Cobo, A. Borgeat, S. Blumenthal. The role of continuous peripheral nerve blocks. *Anesth Res Pract.* 2012;**2012**:560879.

94. J. R. Hebl. The importance and implications of aseptic techniques during regional anesthesia. *Reg Anesth Pain Med.* 2006;**31**:311–23.

95. J. D. Swenson, G. S. Cheng, D. A. Axelrod, J. J. Davis. Ambulatory anesthesia and regional catheters: When and how. *Anesth Clin.* 2010;**28**(2):267–80.

96. T. T. Horlocker, D. J. Wedel, J. C. Rowlingson, *et al.* Regional anesthesia in the patient receiving antithrombotic or thrombolytic therapy: American Society of Regional Anesthesia and Pain Medicine Evidence-Based Guidelines (Third Edition). *Reg Anesth Pain Med.* 2010;**35**(1):64–101.

97. S. M. Klein, K. C. Nielsen, R. A. Greengrass, D. S. Warner, A. Martin, S. M. Steele. Ambulatory discharge after long-acting peripheral nerve blockade: 2382 blocks with ropivacaine. *Anesth Analg.* 2002;**94** (1):65–70, table of contents.

Multimodal management of pain and postoperative nausea and vomiting (PONV) in ambulatory surgery

Dawn Schell, MD, and Jaspreet Somal, MD

A. Introduction

As ambulatory surgery evolves to include increasingly complex procedures and patients, the prevention and management of postoperative pain and nausea/vomiting (PONV) becomes even more important. Uncontrolled PONV can cause patient distress and dissatisfaction, a delay in discharge, and increase the economic burden on the healthcare system.[1]

Increasing evidence supports a multimodal approach to the management of acute PONV. A multimodal approach utilizes both pharmacological and non-pharmacological techniques and ideally produces an additive or synergistic increase in therapeutic efficacy but avoids a similar increase in side effects.[2] These techniques frequently include not only postoperative treatment strategies but preoperative and intraoperative prevention strategies as well. Ultimately, the goal is the management of patients' pain and nausea/vomiting without untoward side effects, thus improving the recovery process and postoperative course.[3] In ambulatory settings, the ideal analgesic/anti-emetic would not produce sedation, confusion, or postoperative nausea and vomiting, and have minimal effects on ventilation and hemodynamics.

Multimodal treatments can be broadly grouped into three categories.

1. Pharmacological agents administered systemically that act on various central and peripheral receptors/pathways.
2. Regional techniques which act through central neuraxial blockade, peripheral nerve blocks, or local infiltration and field blocks.
3. Miscellaneous non-pharmacological techniques such as TENS, acupuncture, acustimulation, hypnosis, etc.

B. Multimodal management of postoperative pain

The goals of treating pain in the ambulatory setting are multiple: (1) to improve patient comfort and satisfaction, (2) to produce earlier mobilization and thereby decrease risks due to immobility (DVT, pneumonia), (3) to minimize respiratory and cardiac complications, (4) to decrease the likelihood of the development of chronic pain, and (5) to reduce the overall cost of care. The Joint Commission (TJC) issued pain treatment standards that apply to all TJC-accredited hospitals and ambulatory centers in the United States, thus emphasizing the importance of pain management for patients, health care providers, and institutions. The hallmark of most guidelines and recommendations of various regulatory agencies is to provide effective pain control and treat pain as a "fifth vital sign." Additionally, all discharge criteria require adequate pain management; therefore, the continuing success of ambulatory surgery will depend on the successful implementation of postoperative pain management strategies.

The physiology of pain transmission is a complex and evolving science that is too complicated to be discussed extensively here. However, the goal of multimodal analgesia is to target different receptors and pathways, thereby providing improved analgesia without the associated side effects of higher doses of each drug/technique individually. With evolving understanding, acute postoperative pain is now recognized to have two components: an earlier inflammatory component and a later neuropathic component. Just alleviating the inflammatory component in susceptible patients might not be sufficient; addressing the neuropathic pain component can be equally important in the prevention of chronic pain.[4] Observed advantages of

Practical Ambulatory Anesthesia, ed. Johan Raeder and Richard D. Urman. Published by Cambridge University Press.
© Cambridge University Press 2015.

the use of non-opioid pharmacologic agents include diminished allodynia and hyperalgesia that result from central spinal cord wind-up and sensitization caused by the surgical insult.[2] Based on the available evidence, the ASA Task Force on Acute Pain Management recommends a multimodal, around-the-clock regimen of non-steroidal anti-inflammatory drugs (NSAIDs), acetaminophen, and cyclooxygenase (COX)-2 inhibitors to treat surgical pain and limit the use of opioids.

C. Pharmacologic management of pain

1. NSAIDS

Non-steroidal anti-inflammatory drugs are commonly used in the perioperative period due to their favorable side-effect profile. They do not cause sedation or respiratory depression, PONV, itching, or the other unfavorable adverse effects of opioids. They are broadly classified into non-specific COX inhibitors and selective COX-2 inhibitors.

a. Non-specific COX inhibitors

This class of drugs inhibits COX-1 and often also COX-2 enzymes. Commonly used non-specific COX inhibitors include ibuprofen, ketorolac, naproxen, and diclofenac and can be given preoperatively (PO ibuprofen), intraoperatively (IV ketorolac), or postoperatively as an oral, rectal, or topical medication.

The use of NSAIDS in combination with other analgesics has been shown to significantly decrease the need for rescue analgesic medication in the early post-discharge period, leading to an improvement in the quality of recovery and patient satisfaction with their pain management after outpatient surgery.[5]

Mechanism of action

NSAIDs inhibit cyclooxygenase (prostaglandin synthase), decreasing the conversion of arachidonic acid to prostaglandins, prostacyclin, and thromboxanes. The extent of enzyme inhibition varies among the different NSAIDS, although there are no studies relating the degree of cyclooxygenase inhibition with anti-inflammatory efficacy in individual patients.

Side effects

NSAIDs have a range of side effects that can limit their use in susceptible patient populations. The most common side effects of NSAIDS are related to the inhibition of prostaglandin synthesis and include renal injury, GI bleeding, platelet inhibition/increased risk of surgical bleeding, bronchospasm in asthmatics and an increased risk of adverse cardiovascular thrombotic events (MI, stroke) in patients with chronic use or pre-existing cardiovascular disease.[6]

The judicious short-term use of NSAIDS with careful patient selection can minimize these side effects and provide an effective substitute for opioid-based analgesics, especially when used in combination with other drugs.

b. Selective COX-2 inhibitors

The principal benefit of the selective COX-2 inhibitors is the production of comparable analgesia and anti-inflammatory effects to the non-selective NSAIDs, but without many of the accompanying side effects. They decrease postoperative pain, opioid use, PONV, and recovery room length of stay.[7] Celecoxcib, the only FDA-approved COX-2 inhibitor still available in the United States, provides very good analgesia in ambulatory patients.[7]

Mechanism of action

The selective COX-2 inhibitors demonstrate at least a 200- to 300-fold selectivity for inhibition of COX-2 over COX-1.

Side effects

When compared with non-selective NSAIDs, COX-2 inhibitors cause less gastroduodenal toxicity,[8,9] no risk of bleeding due to platelet inhibition and lack of bronchoconstriction.

However, significant side effects include a dose-dependent increase in ischemic cardiovascular disease risk with prolonged use, worsening of heart failure, an increase in blood pressure, and possible atrial fibrillation. COX-2 inhibitors carry an FDA "black-box" warning regarding cardiovascular risk, although this risk appears to be related to long-term use. To date, there is no evidence of increased cardiovascular risk when treating short-term postoperative pain. Nevertheless, it is recommended to avoid these drugs during the perioperative period in patients with unstable cardiovascular disease.

2. Acetaminophen

Acetaminophen is a widely available analgesic that is used in combination with other analgesics like NSAIDs and opioids for the management of postoperative pain during ambulatory surgery. It is a relatively weak analgesic as compared to NSAIDs, but has better tolerance and side-effect profile.

The combination of acetaminophen and an NSAID may offer superior analgesia compared with either drug alone. It can be used as an oral premedication (15–25 mg/kg, maximum 2g) or as part of a postoperative pain regimen either alone or as a combination therapy.[10–12] It is also available as a rectal suppository, although with slower and less predictable bioavailability than oral use. Intravenous preparations can be administered intraoperatively, although in the US, they still cost significantly more than oral preparations. The lack of side effects like respiratory depression, sedation, PONV, and itching make it a favorable drug for ambulatory settings, obese patients, and patients with respiratory disease.

Mechanism of action

Despite the similarities to NSAIDs, the mode of action of acetaminophen has been uncertain, but it is now generally accepted that it inhibits COX-1 and COX-2 through metabolism by the peroxidase function of these isoenzymes.[13]

Side effects

The most significant side effect of acetaminophen is hepatotoxicity with overdose. Acetaminophen-induced hepatitis is acute in onset, progresses rapidly, is characterized by marked elevation of plasma aminotransferases (> 3000 IU/l), and is associated with a rising prothrombin time. Risk factors for hepatotoxicity include excessive dosing and chronic alcoholism. In general, toxicity is likely to occur with single ingestions greater than 250 mg/kg or 12 g over a 24-hour period;[14] however, more recent evidence suggests that hepatotoxicity can occur with substantially lower doses over a 24-hour period. Because of this, the FDA has recommended against prescribing more than 4 g acetaminophen in a 24-hour period.[15]

3. Opioids

Historically, opioids have been a mainstay of perioperative analgesia; however, their attendant side effects limit their usefulness in the ambulatory setting. Unfortunately, even at therapeutic dosages, opioids can produce pruritus, nausea/vomiting, constipation, sedation, sleep disturbances and, most seriously, respiratory depression. As a result, there has been an increased emphasis on the utilization of non-opioid pharmacologic therapies in preference to opioids.

Ideally, one should utilize opioids in conjunction with non-opioid therapies[16] to minimize their side effects.

Although the types of opioids utilized in ambulatory settings do not differ from the inpatient setting, there is a greater emphasis on the early administration of oral opioids to ensure adequate analgesia in the home going patient. The most commonly used opioids are the short-acting ones: hydrocodone, oxycodone and codeine. There is little evidence to recommend one oral opioid over another with the exception of codeine. Codeine is a pro-drug and is metabolized to its active metabolite, morphine, by a hepatic P450 isoenzyme. Unfortunately, there is substantial variability in the rate of metabolism of codeine due to individual variations in this P450 isoenzyme activity. This leads to unpredictable metabolism, with some individuals being slower metabolizers and others ultra-rapid metabolizers. Drugs that inhibit this isoenzyme lead to reduced analgesic efficacy of codeine. Alternatively, the ultra-rapid metabolizers produce morphine at a much higher rate leading to respiratory depression and overdose with normal dosages in those individuals. Between 1969 and 2012, the FDA received 13 reports of deaths in children who were prescribed codeine. Due to this, the FDA has placed a black-box warning on the use of codeine in children undergoing tonsillectomy and adenoidectomy.[17] In lieu of this, given the other available alternatives, codeine cannot be recommended for routine use in ambulatory surgery.

Some ambulatory units have successfully added sustained release oxycodone (Oxycontin™) to their home-going analgesic regimen in procedures more likely to cause prolonged pain. This can be especially useful for supplementing analgesia after regional blocks have worn off and can be dosed at convenient 12-hour intervals.

Tramadol, a combined mu agonist and serotonin and norepinephrine reuptake inhibitor, can also be used for short-term analgesia, although the evidence for its superiority over other analgesics is mixed. It seems to have found wider acceptance in Europe than the US.

4. Miscellaneous drugs

IV lidocaine has been studied extensively and several studies have reported lower postoperative pain values and less opioid administration in lidocaine groups in comparison with control groups. The effects of systemic lidocaine can be explained by inhibition of NF-k B, protein kinase C, and NMDA receptors.[18]

A review by McCarthy *et al.* showed that in open and laparoscopic abdominal surgery, as well as in ambulatory surgery patients, intravenous perioperative infusion of lidocaine resulted in significant reductions in postoperative pain intensity and opioid consumption.[19] Pain scores were reduced at rest and with cough or movement for up to 48 hours postoperatively. Opioid consumption was reduced by up to 85% in lidocaine-treated patients when compared with controls. Infusion of lidocaine also resulted in earlier return of bowel function, allowing for earlier rehabilitation and shorter duration of hospital stay.[19] Subsequent studies have not uniformly supported these findings so additional studies are needed to establish any firm recommendations for the use of IV lidocaine infusions in ambulatory settings. In the author's experience, however, they are quite useful to prevent coughing during emergence in intubated patients in whom you prefer to avoid opioids.

Ketamine is an IV anesthetic agent that exerts its clinical effects by non-competitive antagonism at the *N*-methyl-D-aspartate and certain opioid receptors. Ketamine has direct analgesic properties at plasma concentrations significantly lower than those producing loss of consciousness[20] and can be administered at low doses as a continuous infusion to produce a significant opioid-sparing effect. The addition of ketamine to propofol infusions may attenuate propofol-induced hypoventilation and provide earlier recovery of cognition.[21] Adjunctive use of ketamine during propofol sedation provides significant analgesia and minimizes the need for supplemental opioids when given at subhypnotic doses.[22] Given before the end of surgery in ambulatory procedures, ketamine allows a reduction of approximately 40% in morphine requirements without altering the recovery profile.[23] Whereas anesthetic doses of ketamine are associated with unpleasant psychomimetic side effects, many studies have reported improved postoperative mood and function after perioperative administration of subanesthetic doses of ketamine.[21]

Gabapentinoid compounds have also been used as part of multimodal analgesia in the postoperative period. Gabapentin in combination with other analgesics seems to be an effective adjunct to improve pain control in the early stages of recovery in children and adolescents undergoing spine surgery and has a significant 24-hour opioid-sparing effect and improves pain score for both abdominal hysterectomy and spinal surgery. Nausea may be reduced in abdominal hysterectomy.[24,25] Most favorable data on gabapentin came from the single 1200-mg dose in the preoperative period, with a significant reduction in morphine use and minimal side effects, when used in mastectomy patients.[26] A single dose, however, has been associated with sedation and confusion and may limit its use in ambulatory settings.

Glucocorticoid steroids have an adjuvant role in the multimodal analgesic regimen in the perioperative setting, and help to reduce pain and to prolong analgesic effects from 24 to 72 hours after breast surgery when used in combination with NSAIDs and local anesthetic infiltration.[12] A typical single dose of dexamethasone is 4–8 mg in an adult for PONV prophylaxis, although high doses are needed (8–16 mg) to achieve analgesic effect in adults. Although some have raised concerns about an increased incidence of wound complications, to date there is no evidence to support this. Also, experimental animal data on fracture non-union does not seem to be confirmed in human studies so far.

α-2 agonists dexmedetomidine and clonidine have been studied as part of a multimodal regimen. Different mechanisms have been proposed, such as central action via the agonism of α-2-receptors in the dorsal horn of the spinal cord and inhibition of substance P. The peripheral action is thought to be due to cross tolerance with opioid mu-receptors and blockade of peripheral nerve fibers, especially C-fibers.[27]

Dexmedetomidine, as part of a perioperative analgesic regimen, decreases opioid requirements, PONV, and postoperative stay.[28] It can also be especially useful in patients with pulmonary compromise because it does not cause respiratory depression. Low doses of clonidine have been shown to be a useful analgesic adjunct when administered neuraxially or in combination with peripheral nerve blocks. The addition of low doses of clonidine to either intrathecal or peripheral bupivacaine has been found to prolong analgesia without increasing side effects.[27] Additionally, in open cholecystectomy patients, clonidine administered IV or via wound infiltration with bupivacaine provided effective postoperative analgesia and reduced morphine requirements. In this study, however, the incidence of complications was less with wound infiltration.[29]

One should be mindful of the potential adverse effects of these drugs such as sedation, hypotension, and bradycardia, especially when administered neuraxially. Overall, the value of these drugs in ambulatory settings is sufficiently unclear to make any recommendations for their routine use.

A summary of all non-opioid analgesics, including some less commonly used drugs, is listed in Table 7.1.

Table 7.1 Summary of commonly used non-opioid drugs for acute postoperative pain.

Drug	Mechanism of action	Dose and route of administration (adult)	Advantages	Limitations and side effects
Acetaminophen	Cyclooxygenase enzyme inhibition	Premedication: 15–25 mg/kg PO, IV, PR (max 2 g) 10–15 mg/kg every 6 hours, not to exceed 4 g/24 hours	Opioid-sparing Cost-effective No respiratory/CNS depression Premedication compatible	Low potency High doses (> 4 g/24 h) may lead to liver toxicity
NSAID	Non-selective COX inhibitor	Adults: ketorolac 30 mg IV ibuprofen 200–600 mg PO q 6 h naproxen sodium 220–440 mg PO q 12 h Children: ketorolac 0.1 mg/kg IV ibuprofen 10 mg/kg PO q 6 h	Opioid-sparing Cost-effective No respiratory/CNS depression Premedication compatible	Prostaglandin inhibitor. Can result in renal, GI, or platelet dysfunction in susceptible population
Selective COX-2 inhibitors	COX-2 inhibition	Celecoxib 200–400 mg PO preoperatively 100 mg PO q 12 h	Less theoretical risk of bleeding All advantages associated with NSAIDs	Increased risk of thrombotic events and GI side effects
Gabapentin	Inhibits alpha-2-delta-1 subunit of Ca^{2+} channels and inhibits neuronal Ca^{2+} influx and decrease in release of excitatory neurotransmitters	Variable dose PO use	Opioid-sparing Decrease in opioid-related side effects Can be given as premedication, has pre-emptive analgesic effect Synergistic analgesic effect with epidural	Sedation Dizziness Dosage regimen not fully established Knowledge still evolving but side effects limit use
Pregabalin	Inhibits alpha-2-delta-1 subunit of Ca^{2+} channels and inhibits neuronal Ca^{2+} influx and decrease in release of excitatory neurotransmitters	Variable dose 150–300 mg PO	Opioid-sparing Useful preventive analgesic effect	Sedation Dizziness Vomiting Headache Confusion Side effects limit usefulness in ambulatory settings
Ketamine	NMDA receptor antagonist	Intraoperative IV infusion Dose is variable (1–5 µg/kg/min)	Opioid-sparing and extended analgesic effect especially in chronic pain patients Useful in opioid-resistant pain	Dose-dependent psychomimetic effects such as hallucinations, nightmares, sedation, nausea, and vomiting

Table 7.1 (cont.)

Drug	Mechanism of action	Dose and route of administration (adult)	Advantages	Limitations and side effects
Dexamethasone	Unknown but likely anti-inflammatory and reduces the inhibition of impulse generated from injured nerve fibers	IV 4–16 mg perioperative PO 8–16 mg premedication	Reduce the pain Anti-emetic Useful as adjuvant	Steroid side effects in high doses No solo analgesic effect
IV lidocaine		Perioperative 1–2 mg/kg load and 2–3 mg/kg/h continuous infusion	Reduces pain and opioid requirements, nausea, vomiting, duration of ileus, earlier intake of enteral food, rehabilitation, and discharge	Questionable benefit in non-abdominal and non-breast surgery Potential for local anesthetic toxicity if other routes of LA used simultaneously
Dexmedetomidine	Membrane hyperpolarization via G1 – protein-gated K channels	Perioperative 0.1–1 μg/kg hour	Moderate analgesic effect, opioid-sparing Potential for good sedative for sedation and MAC procedures to avoid opioids	Bradycardia Hypotension
Miscellaneous Magnesium, Beta-blockers	Membrane stabilization effect (although exact mechanism and effectiveness debatable)			Not much literature available so dosing and indications not clear but anecdotal reports claim benefit

+ The dosing information is recommended for adults.

D. Role of regional anesthesia in multimodal pain management

Regional anesthetic techniques provide benefit in ambulatory surgery settings by reducing the need for opioids and providing analgesia for many hours after surgery. Other potential benefits include reducing the incidence of PONV, greater patient satisfaction, early mobilization, and decrease in the time spent in PACU and readmission rates.[30] Regional techniques include neuraxial blocks (spinal, epidural, and combined spinal epidural), peripheral nerve blocks, field blocks (TAP block), and local infiltration of the wound with local anesthetic solution. It is very important to take into account the preoperative, intraoperative, and postoperative effects of the block being considered and whether it will be used as the primary anesthetic (surgical block) or as an adjuvant. Factors like patient and surgeon preference, type and duration of the surgery, and impact of postoperative motor block on local discharge policies all must be taken into consideration before committing to a particular technique. Table 7.2 briefly summarizes the different regional blocks commonly used in the ambulatory setting along with their advantages and limitations.

Local anesthetic infiltration in the wound has been shown to be effective in reducing the immediate postoperative pain and opioid consumption. Recently,

Table 7.2 Summary of commonly used regional anesthetic techniques in ambulatory settings

Technique	Advantages	Disadvantages/ limitations	Recommendations
Neuraxial anesthesia	• Very good intraoperative analgesia, better postoperative analgesia • Minimizes intraoperative opioids	• Prolonged block and urinary retention can delay discharge and interfere with discharge criteria	• Use short-acting local anesthetic and lowest possible dose
Upper extremity blocks: interscalene, suprascapular, axillary, specific peripheral nerve blocks, etc.	• Provide excellent perioperative analgesia • Opioid-sparing • Improve anesthesia workflow	• Potential complications can occur with individual blocks • Adequate time management and block • Can utilize catheter for prolonged analgesia	• Expertise and timing of blocks should be optimized by training and developing protocols
Lower extremity blocks: lumbar plexus, femoral, sciatic nerve or distal nerve blocks, intra-articular LA/opioid	• Provide excellent intraoperative analgesia • Provide extended postoperative analgesia and can expedite mobilization and discharge	• Primary or secondary block failure • Resulting motor weakness can result in fall risk • Can utilize catheter for prolonged analgesia	• Use these blocks in carefully selected patient population in expert hands
Transversus abdominis plane block and trunk blocks[53]	• Decreased opioid consumption, improved pain scores • May facilitate early discharge	• High failure rate • Is not effective for visceral pain	• Trunk blocks work better when combined with multimodal techniques

FDA-approved liposomal bupivacaine (Exparel™), which is an extended release bupivicaine, has shown some promising results in reducing opioid requirements and providing extended analgesia for up to four days post-infiltration.[31] However, caution must be exercised, as the manufacturer has warned against simultaneous administration of other local anesthetics due to concerns about potential toxicity.[32] Currently, it is only approved for local wound infiltration and not for regional blocks.

Improved technology now permits the discharge of patients with infusion pumps connected to indwelling peripheral nerve catheters or subcutaneous catheters that deliver low-dose local anesthetics continuously for several days postoperatively.[33,34] These pumps have allowed procedures to be performed as outpatients that previously required several day inpatient admissions.

E. Non-pharmacologic management of pain

Many unconventional analgesia techniques such as acupuncture, electro acupuncture (electric current is applied to the acupuncture needles), acupressure (pressure is applied with fingers or band to acupuncture points), transcutaneous electrical nerve stimulation (TENS), transcutaneous electrical acupoint stimulation (TAES), and Capsicum plaster have shown promising results in isolated clinical trials; however, their incorporation in routine clinical practice is limited due to the lack of practitioner expertise and lack of high-quality randomized controlled trials.[35,36]

However, these techniques do offer many advantages. They are noninvasive, inexpensive, easy to perform, and produce minimal adverse effects. They have also demonstrated some efficacy in the prevention and treatment of postoperative nausea and vomiting, emergence delirium, shivering, and hypothermia-related distress. However, until larger randomized, controlled studies support their routine use, it is unlikely that they will enjoy routine use in an ambulatory surgery setting.

The authors' approach in ambulatory settings for the adult patient is as follows.

- Identify any special issues and contraindications (chronic pain, organ impairment) that may pose challenges to the pain management or preclude the use of any drug.
- Administer 1.5–2 g acetaminophen and 200–400 mg celecoxib orally preoperatively.
- Utilize regional blocks or local anesthetic infiltration when possible.
- If not administered preoperatively, administer 1 g IV acetaminophen (maximum single dose) intraoperatively.
- Administer 30 mg of IV ketorolac if not contraindicated due to concerns about bleeding, unless celecoxib can be used (orally) instead. Some practitioners administer both a preoperative dose of celecoxib and an intraoperative dose of ketorolac, although safety data related to administering these NSAIDs together is lacking.
- Consider administering dexamethasone IV just after induction, in order to reduce the risk of both nausea and pain. While dexamethasone is an effective anti-emetic in smaller doses (4–8 mg), larger doses may be needed to achieve an analgesic effect (8–16 mg).
- Minimize/avoid the use of intraoperative opioids. Administer postoperative opioids only as dictated by the patient's pain levels postoperatively.
- Manage post-discharge pain with the prescription of NSAIDs, continuous local anesthetic peripheral blockade when possible, and short-acting opioids for rescue.

The considerations for special patient populations can be found elsewhere in this book.

F. Multimodal management of PONV in the ambulatory surgery

The management of PONV in ambulatory settings can also present significant challenges to the practitioner. Patient discomfort, increased morbidity, a delay in hospital discharge, and unplanned admission can all result from uncontrolled PONV.

Like pain pathways, the various receptors and pathways (chemoreceptor trigger zone) that contribute to nausea and vomiting are complicated and poorly understood and their discussion is beyond the scope of this chapter. However, it is well documented that effective management of PONV in high-risk patients involves targeting different receptors and pathways through the use of various pharmacological and non-pharmacological strategies. Even then, the response may vary in different patients and a perfect recipe for prevention and management of PONV does not exist.[37] Figure 7.1 illustrates the complexity involved with evaluating and treating patients at risk for PONV.

G. Preventive strategies and pharmacotherapy

Prevention of PONV is paramount in the management of PONV and the benefit of pharmacological prophylaxis in moderate and high-risk patients is without dispute. However, the benefit is less clear in low-risk patients. Authorities like the Society for Ambulatory Anesthesia (USA) and the Royal College of Anaesthetists (UK) recommend against the routine use of anti-emetic medication in low-risk patients in ambulatory settings.[38] Therefore, prophylaxis must be selected by weighing the risks and benefits of each drug in any given scenario.

Prevention of PONV starts with the identification of moderate and high-risk patients utilizing various scoring systems (Apfel) that identify patient and surgical characteristics to define risk (Table 7.3). Once identified, the provider can then take measures to decrease the risk of PONV in patients at risk. These measures may include pharmacologic prophylaxis with dexamethasone and/or 5-HT3 antagonist, scopolamine transdermal patch, avoidance/minimization of conventional pharmacological triggers (e.g., inhalational agents, opioids, nitrous oxide, neostigmine), maximization of regional anesthetic techniques, and utilization of non-pharmacological strategies when possible. The intraoperative administration of ultrashort-acting remifentanil may not be as problematic as other opioids in causing PONV. However, it must be remembered that remifentanil can cause hyperalgesia and an increased need for analgesic agents postoperatively.

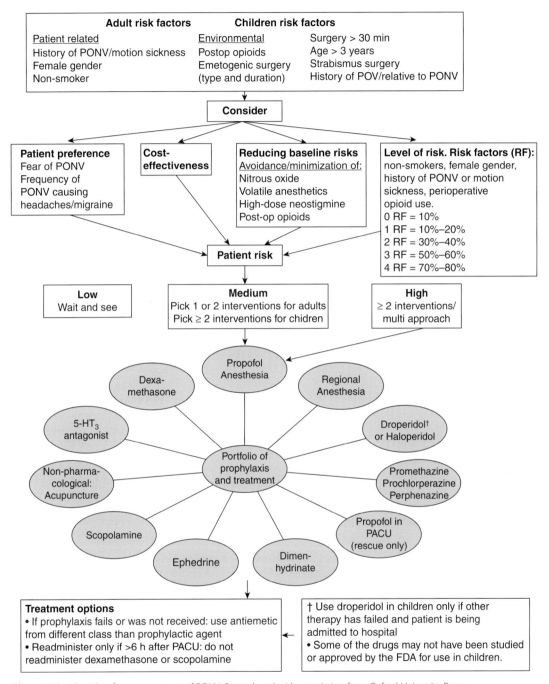

Figure 7.1. Algorithm for management of PONV. Reproduced with permission from Oxford University Press.

Utilization of a total intravenous anesthetic (TIVA) technique with aggressive pharmacologic prophylaxis has also been demonstrated to eliminate vomiting and significantly decrease nausea in a group of high-risk patients.[39]

H. Treatment strategies for breakthrough PONV

For treatment of a failed prophylactic anti-emetic for PONV occurring in the PACU, an anti-emetic from a

Table 7.3 Risk factors for postoperative nausea and vomiting

Patient-related	• History of PONV or motion sickness • Female gender • Non-smoker • Age: younger patients have more PONV
Anesthesia-related	• Volatile anesthetic agents use • Nitrous oxide use • Opioid use • Neostigmine use
Surgery-related	• Duration of surgery • Type of surgery • High-risk procedures include ENT surgery, gynecologic surgery, strabismus surgery, breast surgery, shoulder surgery
Miscellaneous	• Pain • Hypotension • Anxiety

different drug class not previously given should be administered. Additionally, evidence proves that combination therapy is more efficacious than single agent therapy.[37,38,40] For example, if the patient received ondansetron prior to emergence, another dose of ondansetron is unlikely to be effective. Instead, an anti-histamine or phenothizine would be a better option. Due to the relatively short half-life of most anti-emetic medications, however, prophylactic anti-emetics from the same drug class may need to be repeated after 12–24 hours.

If no prior anti-emetic prophylaxis was given, a 5-HT$_3$ antagonist should be the initial treatment. Second-line treatment of breakthrough PONV should utilize droperidol, promethazine, small doses of propofol, dimenhydrinate, or dexamethasone.[37,41–43] All anti-emetic therapies and their dosing are found in Table 7.4.

It must be noted, however, that in 2001, the FDA placed a "black-box warning" on droperidol after the discovery that some patients had experienced episodes of ventricular dysrhythmias after receiving droperidol – some of which were fatal. Although the dosages these patients received were far greater than commonly used anti-emetic dosages, this has significantly reduced the popularity of droperidol as an anti-emetic. The authors agree with many experts that this

"black-box warning" should not preclude the use of droperidol for PONV in anti-emetic dosages (0.5–0.75 mg). We do, however, typically administer it at the beginning of the case because by doing so, we have monitored the patient for the requisite "2–3 hours" recommended by the FDA prior to discharge.

In patients with known congenital or acquired prolonged QT syndrome and in pediatric patients who may have undiagnosed long QT syndrome, one should be especially cautious with the use of any anti-emetic that may prolong the QT interval (droperidol, 5-HT$_3$ antagonists, phenothiazines). At the authors' institution, the electrophysiologists prefer the use of scopolamine, dexamethasone, and anti-histamines such as dimenhydrinate in patients with known QT prolongation. If PONV persists despite these therapies, they recommend the use of other anti-emetics (e.g., ondansetron) only with inpatient ECG monitoring.

The treatment of recognized PONV should also include the treatment of conditions which may exacerbate PONV, such as anxiety, pain, hypotension, hypoxia, and inadequate hydration. Commonly used drugs for the prevention and treatment of PONV are listed in Table 7.4. These drugs are also discussed below along with their mechanisms of action, common adverse effects, and cautions prior to use.

HT$_3$ antagonists: ondansetron, granisetron, dolasetron, palonosetron

- Act through antagonism of 5-HT$_3$ receptors.
- Adverse effects: dose-dependent QT interval prolongation, headache, dizziness.
- Caution: avoid in patients with congenital or prolonged QT.

Antidopaminergics:

Phenothiazines: chlorpromazine, prochlorperazine, promethazine

- Act through antagonism of dopaminergic (D2) receptors in the central nervous system.
- Adverse effects include sedation and extrapyramidal side effects such as dystonia and akathisia.
- Caution: avoid in patients with Parkinson's disease.

Butyrophenones: droperidol, haloperidol

- Act through antagonism of central D2 receptors, mild alpha receptor antagonism.
- Adverse effects include sedation, QT interval prolongation, hypotension, rare extrapyramidal side effects, neurolepsis.

Table 7.4 Commonly used pharmacological anti-emetic agents: mechanism of action and dosing (for adults)

Class	Examples	Advantages	Recommend dosing
5-HT$_3$ antagonist	Ondansetron Granisetron Dolasetron Palonosetron	Highly efficacious in prevention of nausea and vomiting	Ondansetron: IV 4 mg PO 8 mg Granisetron: IV 1 mg
Anti-dopaminergic	Butyrophenones (droperidol, haloperidol) Phenothiazines (prochlorperazine, promethazine)	Highly efficacious in prevention and treatment of nausea and vomiting	Droperidol: IV 0.625–1.25 mg Haloperidol: IV 0.5–2 mg Prochlorperazine: IV 5–10 mg PO 5–10 mg 3–4 times/day
Anti-histamines	Diphenhydramine Dimenhydrinate promethazine	Effective pre- or postoperatively	Diphenhydramine: PO, IM, IV 25–100 mg Dimenhydrinate: PO, IV 25–50 mg Promethazine: PO, IM, IV 12.5–50 mg
Anticholinergic	Scopolamine	Effective alone or as a combination prophylactic therapy agent with other anti-emetics	Transdermal patch 1.5 mg ideally 4–12 h before the induction of anesthesia
Steroids	Dexamethasone	Useful in prevention of PONV	Dexamethasone: IV 4–16 mg administered at the beginning of anesthesia
NK-1 receptor antagonists	Aprepitant Fosaprepitant	Prevention or treatment of PONV	Aprepitant: PO 40 mg before induction Fosaprepitant IV

- Avoid in patients with congenital or prolonged QT. Benzamide: metoclopramide
- Act through antagonism of dopamine (D2) receptor antagonism, some 5-HT$_3$ receptor antagonism.
- Adverse effects include extrapyramidal side effects, agitation, sedation.
- Short duration, low efficacy.

Antihistamines: diphenhydramine, dimenhydrinate, promethazine (also antidopaminergic)

- Act through H1-receptor antagonism, some antidopaminergic (promethazine) antimuscarinic (diphenhydramine) and anti-alpha adrenergic effects and antiserotonergic effects (promethazine).
- Adverse effects include sedation, anticholinergic side effects, QT interval prolongation in overdose.
- Caution: sedative action.

Anticholinergics: atropine, scopolamine, hyoscine

- Act through antagonism of CNS muscarinic receptors.
- Adverse effects include antimuscarinic side effects such as dry mouth, sedation, blurred vision, tachycardia, inhibition of sweating, urinary retention, etc., agitation in elderly patients.

Steroids: dexamethasone, methylprednisolone

- Exact mechanism of action still unknown.
- Adverse effects include hyperglycemia in susceptible population, potential for immune suppression, delayed wound healing, etc.
- Caution: can cause hyperglycemia,[44] the clinical significance of which is not known, and increased incidence of postoperative infection.[45,46]

NK-1 antagonists: aprepitant, fos aprepitant

- Acts through antagonism of NK 1 receptor in the central and peripheral nervous system and inhibition of action of substance P47.

- Long-term therapy can cause GI upset, hypotension, alopecia, anorexia, fatigue.
- Few studies evaluating efficacy in PONV but may have significant benefit as a prophylactic anti-emetic.

Cannabinoid receptor agonists: nabilone, dronabinol

- Acts on cannabinoid receptors (CB1 and CB2 receptors) in the peripheral nervous system, CNS and immune cells.
- Can cause drowsiness, confusion, administration can precipitate psychosis and panic attacks.
- Efficacy is not documented for PONV.

Miscellaneous: ephedrine, midazolam

- Precise mechanism of action of ephedrine is unknown, although several studies have confirmed positive effect on PONV. Midazolam most likely works by decreasing dopamine's input at the chemoreceptor trigger zone; it is effective when given after induction,[48] rather than as a premedication.
- Adverse effects of midazolam include sedation, agitation, confusion, amnesia, respiratory depression; ephedrine can cause cardiovascular stimulation.

I. Non-pharmacological strategies for prevention of nausea and vomiting

Adequate hydration with fluids helps to prevent PONV as the NPO patient may be dehydrated which may be exacerbated by intraoperative fluid losses. In addition, acupuncture and acupressure have been shown to decrease the incidence of PONV by both a direct and opioid-sparing effect. Acustimulation at the P6 acupoint also has demonstrated efficacy in the prevention of PONV. Uncontrolled pain may contribute to PONV, although this may be a result of increased perioperative opioid administration. Perioperative anxiolysis and hypnosis may also have a beneficial effect on prevention of the PONV.[34]

J. Management of PONV after ambulatory center discharge

Approximately 30–60% patients may experience PONV after discharge to home and this is commonly termed post-discharge nausea and vomiting (PDNV), which may lead to readmission or emergency department visit.[49,50] PDNV may persist many days beyond surgery. Commonly recognized risk factors for PDNV include: (i) female gender; (ii) age < 50 years; (iii) history of PONV; (iv) PACU opioids; and (v) nausea in the PACU.[37] Possible useful approaches to help decrease the incidence of PDNV include: (i) prophylactic combination anti-emetic therapy; (ii) TIVA substituting propofol for inhalation anesthesia; (iii) P6 acupoint stimulation; and (iv) use of home anti-emetics.[37] The management of PDNV should extend into the postoperative and post-discharge period and include prescription of oral anti-emetics such as ondansetron or dolasetron, more expensive options such as aprepitant and additional non-opioid-based analgesics (NSAIDs, acetaminophen). Continuous pump infusions of local anesthetics for nerve catheters should be utilized for opioid-sensitive patients.[51,52]

The authors' preference for prevention and management of PONV in a high-risk patient receiving GA:

- Preoperative reassurance and/or anti-anxiety medication.
- Application of scopolamine patch in patients < 65 years with history of PDNV.
- Administration of 4–16 mg IV dexamethasone and 0.625 mg droperidol after induction.
- Avoidance of nitrous oxide, minimize or avoid opioids.
- Consider utilization of TIVA techniques and avoidance of the anesthesia gases.[20]
- Administration of 4 mg ondansetron prior to emergence.

References

1. Shnaider I, Chung F. Outcomes in day surgery. *Curr Opin Anaesthesiol.* Dec 2006;**19**(6):622–29.
2. Elvir-Lazo OL, White PF. The role of multimodal analgesia in pain management after ambulatory surgery. *Curr Opin Anaesthesiol.* Dec 2010;**23**(6):697–703.
3. Habib AS, White WD, Eubanks S, Pappas TN, Gan TJ. A randomized comparison of a multimodal management strategy versus combination antiemetics for the prevention of postoperative nausea and vomiting. *Anesth Analg.* Jul 2004;**99**(1):77–81.
4. Kehlet H, Jensen TS, Woolf CJ. Persistent postsurgical pain: risk factors and prevention. *Lancet.* May 13 2006;**367**(9522):1618–25.

5. White PF, Tang J, Wender RH, *et al.* The effects of oral ibuprofen and celecoxib in preventing pain, improving recovery outcomes and patient satisfaction after ambulatory surgery. *Anesth Analg.* Feb 2011;**112**(2):323–29.

6. Bhala N, Emberson J, Merhi A, *et al.* Vascular and upper gastrointestinal effects of non-steroidal anti-inflammatory drugs: meta-analyses of individual participant data from randomised trials. *Lancet.* Aug 31 2013;**382**(9894):769–79.

7. White PF, Sacan O, Tufanogullari B, Eng M, Nuangchamnong N, Ogunnaike B. Effect of short-term postoperative celecoxib administration on patient outcome after outpatient laparoscopic surgery. *Can J Anaesth.* May 2007;**54**(5):342–48.

8. Emery P, Zeidler H, Kvien TK, *et al.* Celecoxib versus diclofenac in long-term management of rheumatoid arthritis: randomised double-blind comparison. *Lancet.* Dec 18–25 1999;**354**(9196):2106–11.

9. Simon LS, Weaver AL, Graham DY, *et al.* Anti-inflammatory and upper gastrointestinal effects of celecoxib in rheumatoid arthritis: a randomized controlled trial. *JAMA.* Nov 24 1999;**282**(20):1921–28.

10. Derry CJ, Derry S, Moore RA. Single dose oral ibuprofen plus paracetamol (acetaminophen) for acute postoperative pain. *Cochrane Database Syst Rev.* 2013;**6**:CD010210.

11. Hong JY, Won Han S, Kim WO, Kil HK. Fentanyl sparing effects of combined ketorolac and acetaminophen for outpatient inguinal hernia repair in children. *J Urol.* Apr 2010;**183**(4):1551–55.

12. Hval K, Thagaard KS, Schlichting E, Raeder J. The prolonged postoperative analgesic effect when dexamethasone is added to a nonsteroidal antiinflammatory drug (rofecoxib) before breast surgery. *Anesth Analg.* Aug 2007;**105**(2):481–86.

13. Graham GG, Scott KF. Mechanism of action of paracetamol. *Am J Ther.* Jan–Feb 2005;**12**(1):46–55.

14. Makin AJ, Wendon J, Williams R. A 7-year experience of severe acetaminophen-induced hepatotoxicity (1987–1993). *Gastroenterology.* Dec 1995;**109**(6):1907–16.

15. Krenzelok EP. The FDA Acetaminophen Advisory Committee Meeting – what is the future of acetaminophen in the United States? The perspective of a committee member. *Clin Toxicol (Phila).* Sep 2009;**47**(8):784–89.

16. Day case and short stay surgery: 2. *Anaesthesia.* May 2011;**66**(5):417–34.

17. Kuehn BM. FDA: No codeine after tonsillectomy for children. *JAMA.* Mar 20 2013;**309**(11):1100.

18. Brinkrolf P, Hahnenkamp K. Systemic lidocaine in surgical procedures: effects beyond sodium channel blockade. *Curr Opin Anaesthesiol.* Aug 2014;**27**(4):420–25.

19. McCarthy GC, Megalla SA, Habib AS. Impact of intravenous lidocaine infusion on postoperative analgesia and recovery from surgery: a systematic review of randomized controlled trials. *Drugs.* Jun 18 2010;**70**(9):1149–63.

20. Sneyd JR, Carr A, Byrom WD, Bilski AJ. A meta-analysis of nausea and vomiting following maintenance of anaesthesia with propofol or inhalational agents. *Eur J Anaesthesiol.* Jul 1998;**15**(4):433–45.

21. Mortero RF, Clark LD, Tolan MM, Metz RJ, Tsueda K, Sheppard RA. The effects of small-dose ketamine on propofol sedation: respiration, postoperative mood, perception, cognition, and pain. *Anesth Analg.* Jun 2001;**92**(6):1465–69.

22. Badrinath S, Avramov MN, Shadrick M, Witt TR, Ivankovich AD. The use of a ketamine–propofol combination during monitored anesthesia care. *Anesth Analg.* Apr 2000;**90**(4):858–62.

23. Suzuki M, Tsueda K, Lansing PS, *et al.* Small-dose ketamine enhances morphine-induced analgesia after outpatient surgery. *Anesth Analg.* Jul 1999;**89**(1):98–103.

24. Chang CY, Challa CK, Shah J, Eloy JD. Gabapentin in acute postoperative pain management. *Biomed Res Int.* 2014;**2014**:631756.

25. Mathiesen O, Moiniche S, Dahl JB. Gabapentin and postoperative pain: a qualitative and quantitative systematic review, with focus on procedure. *BMC Anesthesiol.* 2007;**7**:6.

26. Dirks J, Fredensborg BB, Christensen D, Fomsgaard JS, Flyger H, Dahl JB. A randomized study of the effects of single-dose gabapentin versus placebo on postoperative pain and morphine consumption after mastectomy. *Anesthesiology.* Sep 2002;**97**(3):560–64.

27. Chan AK, Cheung CW, Chong YK. Alpha-2 agonists in acute pain management. *Expert Opin Pharmacother.* Dec 2010;**11**(17):2849–68.

28. Tufanogullari B, White PF, Peixoto MP, *et al.* Dexmedetomidine infusion during laparoscopic bariatric surgery: the effect on recovery outcome variables. *Anesth Analg.* Jun 2008;**106**(6):1741–48.

29. Bharti N, Dontukurthy S, Bala I, Singh G. Postoperative analgesic effect of intravenous (i.v.) clonidine compared with clonidine administration in wound infiltration for open cholecystectomy. *Br J Anaesth.* Oct 2013;**111**(4):656–61.

30. Mears DC, Mears SC, Chelly JE, Dai F, Vulakovich KL. THA with a minimally invasive technique, multi-modal anesthesia, and home rehabilitation: factors associated with early discharge? *Clin Orthop Relat Res.* Jun 2009;**467**(6):1412–17.

31. Candiotti K. Liposomal bupivacaine: an innovative nonopioid local analgesic for the management of postsurgical pain. *Pharmacotherapy.* Sep 2012;**32**(9 Suppl):19S–26S.

32. Pacira Pharmaceuticals Inc. Exparel (Bupivacaine Liposome Injectable Suspension) Product Monograph. In: Inc. PP, ed. http://www.exparel.com/pdf/Exparel_Monograph.pdf. New Jersey: Pacira Pharmaceuticals, Inc; 2012.

33. Boezaart AP, Davis G, Le-Wendling L. Recovery after orthopedic surgery: techniques to increase duration of pain control. *Curr Opin Anaesthesiol.* Dec 2012;**25**(6):665–72.

34. Moore JG, Ross SM, Williams BA. Regional anesthesia and ambulatory surgery. *Curr Opin Anaesthesiol.* Dec 2013;**26**(6):652–60.

35. Liodden I, Norheim AJ. Acupuncture and related techniques in ambulatory anesthesia. *Curr Opin Anaesthesiol.* Dec 2013;**26**(6):661–68.

36. Wang SM, Harris RE, Lin YC, Gan TJ. Acupuncture in 21st century anesthesia: is there a needle in the haystack? *Anesth Analg.* Jun 2013;**116**(6):1356–59.

37. Kovac AL. Update on the management of postoperative nausea and vomiting. *Drugs.* Sep 2013;**73**(14):1525–47.

38. Gan TJ, Meyer TA, Apfel CC, *et al.* Society for Ambulatory Anesthesia guidelines for the management of postoperative nausea and vomiting. *Anesth Analg.* Dec 2007;**105**(6):1615–28, table of contents.

39. Scuderi PE, James RL, Harris L, Mims GR, 3rd. Multimodal antiemetic management prevents early postoperative vomiting after outpatient laparoscopy. *Anesth Analg.* Dec 2000;**91**(6):1408–14.

40. Chandrakantan A, Glass PS. Multimodal therapies for postoperative nausea and vomiting, and pain. *Br J Anaesth.* Dec 2011;**107** Suppl 1:i27–40.

41. Kazemi-Kjellberg F, Henzi I, Tramer MR. Treatment of established postoperative nausea and vomiting: a quantitative systematic review. *BMC Anesthesiol.* 2001;**1**(1):2.

42. Kovac AL, O'Connor TA, Pearman MH, *et al.* Efficacy of repeat intravenous dosing of ondansetron in controlling postoperative nausea and vomiting: a randomized, double-blind, placebo-controlled multicenter trial. *J Clin Anesth.* Sep 1999;**11**(6):453–59.

43. Scuderi PE, James RL, Harris L, Mims GR, 3rd. Antiemetic prophylaxis does not improve outcomes after outpatient surgery when compared to symptomatic treatment. *Anesthesiology.* Feb 1999;**90**(2):360–71.

44. Lukins MB, Manninen PH. Hyperglycemia in patients administered dexamethasone for craniotomy. *Anesth Analg.* Apr 2005;**100**(4):1129–33.

45. Hans P, Vanthuyne A, Dewandre PY, Brichant JF, Bonhomme V. Blood glucose concentration profile after 10 mg dexamethasone in non-diabetic and type 2 diabetic patients undergoing abdominal surgery. *Br J Anaesth.* Aug 2006;**97**(2):164–70.

46. Nazar CE, Lacassie HJ, Lopez RA, Munoz HR. Dexamethasone for postoperative nausea and vomiting prophylaxis: effect on glycaemia in obese patients with impaired glucose tolerance. *Eur J Anaesthesiol.* Apr 2009;**26**(4):318–21.

47. Diemunsch P, Joshi GP, Brichant JF. Neurokinin-1 receptor antagonists in the prevention of postoperative nausea and vomiting. *Br J Anaesth.* Jul 2009;**103**(1):7–13.

48. Lee Y, Wang JJ, Yang YL, Chen A, Lai HY. Midazolam vs ondansetron for preventing postoperative nausea and vomiting: a randomised controlled trial. *Anaesthesia.* Jan 2007; **62**(1):18–22.

49. Gold BS, Kitz DS, Lecky JH, Neuhaus JM. Unanticipated admission to the hospital following ambulatory surgery. *JAMA.* Dec 1 1989;**262**(21):3008–10.

50. Gupta A, Wu CL, Elkassabany N, Krug CE, Parker SD, Fleisher LA. Does the routine prophylactic use of antiemetics affect the incidence of postdischarge nausea and vomiting following ambulatory surgery? A systematic review of randomized controlled trials. *Anesthesiology.* Aug 2003;**99**(2):488–95.

51. Chinnappa V, Chung F. Post-discharge nausea and vomiting: an overlooked aspect of ambulatory anesthesia? *Can J Anaesth.* Sep 2008;**55**(9):565–71.

52. Coloma M, White PF, Ogunnaike BO, *et al.* Comparison of acustimulation and ondansetron for the treatment of established postoperative nausea and vomiting. *Anesthesiology.* Dec 2002;**97** (6):1387–92.

53. Petersen PL, Stjernholm P, Kristiansen VB, *et al.* The beneficial effect of transversus abdominis plane block after laparoscopic cholecystectomy in day-case surgery: a randomized clinical trial. *Anesth Analg.* Sep 2012;**115**(3):527–33.

Chapter

8

Practical recipes from start (preop) to finish (post-discharge)

Niraja Rajan, MBBS, Srikantha Rao, MD, MS, and Johan Raeder, MD, PhD

Preoperative logistics

This chapter primarily describes the typical adult patient undergoing intermediate extensive surgery under general anesthesia at an Ambulatory Surgery Center (ASC). It also provides basic principles for creating a successful ambulatory anesthetic.

Most ASCs have different methods of obtaining preoperative information and providing instructions to their patients. To provide a safe anesthetic the following information is required:

1. Preoperative health information including a past medical history (coexisting medical illnesses, concurrent medical problems), relevant surgical history, and history of problems in the perioperative period.
2. Some ASCs have criteria to exclude patients based on their state requirements and their individual capabilities; for example, some ASCs have a BMI limit due to equipment and safety constraints. Other ASCs have limitations on the duration of the surgical procedure or length of recovery room stay depending on their state requirements.
3. Any language barriers and need for interpreter services.
4. Whether the patient will have a responsible adult with them on the day of surgery, to transport them to their residence, receive postoperative instructions, and take care of them for at least the first 24 hours following surgery, when the residual effects of the anesthetic drugs may still be present.
5. Any required preoperative testing is ordered and its results reported to the anesthesiologists prior to surgery.

All of the above information can be collected prior to the day of surgery (DOS) either via a phone interview or filled out by the patient on the internet via a questionnaire (secure patient portal) or on the DOS (in person upon arrival to the ASC). A disadvantage of collecting the information on the DOS is the potential for last-minute cancellations.

Collecting all of the above information will help exclude patients who are not suitable candidates for ambulatory surgery.

Pre-admission testing (PAT)

Most ambulatory surgical procedures tend to be low to intermediate risk. Patients are usually ASA 1–2 with some exceptions. Preoperative testing is therefore unnecessary in the vast majority of patients and procedures.[1] An otherwise healthy patient undergoing an intermediate-risk procedure requires no preoperative testing. Women in the reproductive age group (who have not had a tubal ligation or hysterectomy) would require a urine pregnancy test on the day of surgery.

Patients with diabetes mellitus should have their blood glucose checked in the preoperative area and, depending on the length of surgery, again intraoperatively and subsequently in the recovery room.[2] ECG should only be performed when indicated, such as in patients with history of cardiovascular disease or significant arrhythmias (see Chapter 3).

Preoperative instructions

These instructions are given to patients in the following manner:

1. Over the telephone at the time of collection of information prior to DOS.
2. Through the patient portal website.
3. Written instructions at the surgeon's office.

Practical Ambulatory Anesthesia, ed. Johan Raeder and Richard D. Urman. Published by Cambridge University Press.
© Cambridge University Press 2015.

Typical preoperative instructions include the following:

1. Time of arrival at the ASC (on the DOS);
2. NPO instructions which usually follow the ASA NPO guidelines;
3. Removal of non-essential precious items such as jewelry prior to arrival at the facility;
4. Details of attire including make-up;
5. Details of removable prosthetic devices, contact lenses, glasses, hearing aids, dentures, etc.;
6. Details of the caretaker/responsible adult accompanying them following/after surgery;
7. Medications that may be withheld on the day of surgery (DOS):
   - Angiotensin-converting enzyme inhibitors and angiotensin receptor-blocking agents to avoid serious intraoperative hypotension due to vasoplegia;
   - oral hypoglycemics and long-acting insulin;[2]
   - antiplatelet agents and anticoagulants: depending on the type of surgery, warfarin and clopidogrel are held for 5–7 days prior to surgery;
   - herbal medications; should preferably be withheld 5–7 days prior to surgery;
   - most other medications are continued.
8. New medications, including deep venous thrombosis (DVT) prophylaxis, prescribed to be taken on the DOS.
9. Prophylactic anti-emetics to be taken on the DOS, in high-risk patients.
10. Oral non-opioid pain prophylaxis (acetaminophen, NSAID) according to individual facility's practice guidelines.

Preoperative evaluation

Patients should be screened ahead of time for their suitability to be treated at an ASC, their need for anti-emetic and analgesic prophylaxis, and their need for DVT prophylaxis. In most ASCs, the preoperative evaluation is done on the day of surgery by the anesthesiologist. After a review of the patient's history and performing a directed and focused physical exam-including an airway exam, the anesthetic plan is formulated.

Premedications

Premedications may include the following.

- Anxiolytics: if needed, a short-acting benzodiazepine (midazolam 1–2 mg) is given intravenously just prior to transport to the operating room (OR). For severely anxious patients, an oral benzodiazepine may be prescribed (to be taken) the night before and/or the morning of surgery. Typical examples include lorazepam 0.5–1 mg or diazepam 5–10 mg orally the night before and the morning of surgery.
- Antiemetics: patients identified on the screening questionnaire as at high risk for postoperative nausea and vomiting (PONV), or who report a prior history of severe PONV may be prescribed transdermal scopolamine patch applied preferably 12 hours prior to surgery, or aprepitant 40 mg or ondansetron 8 mg by mouth 2–3 hours prior to scheduled surgery.[3]
- Antibiotics: prophylaxis against surgical site infections should be administered intravenously within the hour before incision (within 2 hours before incision for vancomycin and ciprofloxacin).
- DVT prophylaxis: sequential compression devices, subcutaneous heparin or low molecular weight heparin.
- Analgesics: (see also postoperative pain/analgesia section). It may be practical to administer oral non-opioid analgesics such as acetaminophen or NSAIDs (ibuprofen or naproxen or COX-2 inhibitors) as premedication.

Anesthetic plan

For a successful ambulatory anesthetic, the recipe should be planned at in advance, keeping discharge criteria in mind. The outcome of an ideal ambulatory anesthetic is a patient who meets discharge criteria in the shortest possible time after surgery. To this end (patient is awake and oriented or at baseline, with all his protective reflexes intact, minimal or controlled pain, nausea and bleeding, and ambulatory), short-acting anesthetic agents (without prolonged effects that may delay emergence) should be used.

Anesthetic technique

While surgeries could be performed under local, regional or general anesthesia, this chapter will focus on general anesthesia using a suitable combination of different drugs and techniques.

Anesthesia technique

For general anesthesia (GA), the standard technique would involve using IV induction and maintenance with a potent volatile anesthetic agent, possibly with an addition of nitrous oxide (see below). A total intravenous anesthesia (TIVA) technique could also be used. Intraoperative and postoperative analgesia is provided by a multimodal technique using short-acting IV opioids with IV NSAIDs (ketorolac or parecoxib) and/or acetaminophen, supplemented by infiltration of local anesthetic into the wound by the surgeon or a field block or regional anesthetic by the anesthesiologist.

General anesthesia with IV induction and maintenance with an inhalational anesthetic

IV induction: the patient is induced using IV propofol, titrated to hypnosis. A dose of 1.5–2.5 mg/kg of ideal body weight provides a rough estimate to the dose required to achieve hypnosis. In patients older than 65 years of age, pretreatment with ephedrine 10 mg IV may prevent the hypotension that occurs when a larger dose than necessary is given in these patients due to their longer circulation times.[4,5]

Maintenance of anesthesia is by inhalation of a mixture of air, oxygen, and sevoflurane or desflurane (at 1–2 MAC concentration). The use of nitrous oxide is controversial. The advantages of using nitrous oxide are that it is non-irritating, reduces the amount of halogenated agent required for maintenance, and due to reduced solubility, allows for quicker emergence. The disadvantages to using nitrous oxide are an increased incidence of PONV and relative contraindications in patients undergoing certain surgeries (tympanomastoidectomy) or coexisting medical illnesses such as pulmonary hypertension or pernicious anemia (secondary to vitamin B12 cyanocobalamin deficiency).

For a healthy individual undergoing intermediate extensive surgery at a low risk for PONV, nitrous oxide could be a useful adjunct in the maintenance of general anesthesia.[6]

General anesthesia with IV induction and maintenance with an IV and inhalational anesthetic combination

IV induction with propofol is followed by maintenance of GA using either air–oxygen with inhaled agent (sevoflurane or desflurane) or with nitrous oxide–oxygen with an inhaled agent at half a MAC plus a propofol infusion at 75–100 µg/kg/min. The advantage of a combination of using half a MAC of each agent is one of smooth onset during induction, PONV prophylaxis, and a smooth emergence.

General anesthesia with IV induction and maintenance using a TIVA technique

TIVA with propofol alone: IV induction is achieved with propofol 1.5–2 mg/kg, followed by maintenance of GA with air–oxygen and an IV propofol infusion at a dose of 150–200 µg/kg/min for the first 10 min, and then reduced to surgical anesthesia, typically 100–150 µg/kg/min (based on patient characteristics and procedure specifics). This technique completely avoids inhalational anesthetics and is useful in patients at high risk for PONV or patients who are susceptible to malignant hyperthermia (MH). Analgesia is provided by IV acetaminophen or ketorolac or loco-regional techniques. This technique is chosen when you wish to avoid the use of opioids.

TIVA with propofol combined with other drugs: best and most logical is to provide one syringe with propofol for stable level of hypnosis (see above, maintenance at 80–100 µg/kg/min) and another syringe with opioid analgesic to be adjusted according to surgical need.

> Alfentanil: 1 µg/kg/min as an infusion
> Remifentanil: 0.05–0.2 µg/kg/min infusion
> Other analgesics:
> Ketamine: 1 mg/kg for the entire surgery, not to exceed to 100 mg.
>
> Dexmedetomidine: 1 µg/kg for the entire case, not to exceed to 100 µg.
>
> Alfentanil (1 mg to 200 mg propofol), remifentanil (1 mg to 500 mg propofol) or ketamine can also be added to the same syringe as propofol and the infusion titrated to surgical anesthesia. One must be careful of the total dose of these drugs added to the propofol.

Remember that if postoperative pain is anticipated, non-opioids and loco-regional techniques should be given before the end of surgery. With remifentanil infusions, it is wise to administer a dose of fentanyl 1–2 µg/kg 10 min before the end of surgery, and then additional opioids, if needed after the emergence from anesthesia.

TCI refers to target controlled infusion, where a microprocessor-controlled syringe pump controls and varies automatically the rate of infusion of a drug, to attain a target level (set by the operator) in the patient's blood. However, these devices are not FDA-approved in the United States.

General anesthesia with inhalational induction

For the needle-phobic or the difficult IV access patient, inhalational induction is an alternative. The patient breathes a 30/70 mixture of oxygen and nitrous oxide and the inhalational agent sevoflurane is slowly added to the mixture until unresponsiveness, at which point IV access is established. The patient's ventilation is assisted, if required. Alternatively, sevoflurane (with the vaporizer dial set to 8%) may be given in high-flow oxygen by mask, without nitrous oxide to achieve unresponsiveness. After insertion of an IV catheter, the patient may be given IV propofol (1 mg/kg) to achieve an adequate depth of anesthetic for insertion of a laryngeal mask airway (LMA).

Airway management

The LMA is the mainstay of airway devices commonly used for GA and will be discussed in detail in this chapter. There are several other supraglottic airway devices available that could be used as alternatives. These will not be discussed in this chapter.

The LMA is available in disposable (plastic) or reusable (silicone) varieties from several manufacturers. There are several types of LMAs available with advantages to each type.

The LMA is ideal in the ambulatory setting for airway management for several reasons:

- LMAs can be inserted after IV induction or inhalational induction at a lighter depth than required for endotracheal intubation.
- LMA insertion does not require the use of muscle relaxants.
- The procedure length in ambulatory settings is usually optimal for LMA use.
- These are elective cases and patients tend to be fasting (are at low risk for pulmonary aspiration of gastric contents).
- Both spontaneous ventilation and controlled ventilation are possible with an LMA, depending on the requirements of the procedure.
- Many procedures performed at ASCs do not require profound/deep skeletal muscle relaxation, making the LMA an ideal alternative to endotracheal intubation. Additionally, procedures that were previously done with patients breathing spontaneously with a facemask could also be maintained using an LMA, freeing up the operator's hands.
- It is important to maintain an adequate depth of anesthesia to avoid coughing and laryngospasm that may occur in lighter planes of anesthesia or with varying depth of surgical stimulation.

Table 8.1 Examples of the types of LMAs.

Name	Description	Comments
Classic LMA	Original reusable LMA	
Flexible™ LMA	Wire-reinforced, flexible airway tubing that allows it to be positioned away from the surgical field	Useful in head and neck procedures or prone position
Proseal™ LMA	Consists of a separate channel for gastric suctioning, has a built in bite-block	Allows for 50% higher ventilation pressures
LMA Supreme™	Similar to the Proseal, but is disposable	
Fastrach™ LMA	Consists of a short inserting handle, rigid shaft, and an epiglottic elevating bar	Facilitates tracheal intubation
LMA CTrach™	Similar to the Fastrach, but has a video screen and fiber-optics built in for viewing the larynx	

Table 8.2 Suggested LMA size and maximum cuff volume based on the patient's weight.

Patient weight in kg	LMA size	Maximum cuff volume in ml
< 5	1	4
5–10	1.5	7
10–20	2	10
20–30	2.5	14
30–50	3	20
50–70	4	30
70–100	5	40
> 100	6	50

Table 8.3 Commonly used neuromuscular blocking agents.

Drug	Intubating dose	Duration of action
Depolarizing agents		
Succinylcholine	0.3–1.1 mg/kg	6 minutes
Non-depolarizing agents		
Vecuronium	0.05–0.1 mg/kg	25–40 minutes
Rocuronium	0.6–1.2 mg/kg	31–67 minutes
Cis-atracurium	0.15–0.20 mg/kg	44–77 minutes

- When controlled ventilation is desired, a Proseal/Supreme™ LMA is probably a better choice as they allow for a 50% greater ventilation pressure without a leak.
- The size of the LMA inserted is based on the patient's weight as recommended by the manufacturer.

It is advisable to use the largest size LMA permissible by patient weight. Under-sizing the LMA can lead to improper seating, partial airway obstruction, inadequate ventilation, easy dislodgement, and a tendency to over-inflate the cuff to compensate for the leak. Insertion of a smaller LMA and cuff overinflation in turn can lead to dislodgement, sore throat, and, in some cases, nerve palsies.[7]

Do not exceed the recommended cuff inflation volumes, and the use of a cuff pressure measurement device is recommended when in doubt. The incidence of sore throat following LMA use is 13% and is mostly mild in severity.

Keep in mind that the LMA is a supraglottic airway device and therefore does not completely isolate the upper airway tract. An endotracheal tube may be preferred in patients where there is a potential risk for aspiration, such as patients with severe untreated/symptomatic gastro-esophageal reflux disease, massive trauma, pregnancy, and other conditions associated with delayed gastric emptying. The incidence of aspiration with an LMA is very low (0.012%) if general rules are followed.[7] The commonest reason for regurgitation and aspiration with an LMA is inadequate depth of anesthesia and improper patient selection. An alternative to conventional LMA is the Proseal™ type LMA with a gastric tube to empty stomach contents and decrease the

risk of gastric contents passing upwards through the esophagus, increasing the risk of aspiration. Providers should follow the manufacturer's recommendations for cleaning and sterilizing the LMA when using reusable LMAs.

For procedures requiring skeletal muscle relaxation to improve surgical exposure, or procedures in need of 100% patient immobility (middle ear surgery, eye surgery, and microsurgery) or procedures requiring isolation of the upper respiratory tract, endotracheal intubation is usually the preferred technique of airway management, although the use of LMAs may be feasible in carefully selected patients.

Endotracheal tubes come in different varieties and are sized based on the patient's age and gender. The size of the endotracheal tube is the internal diameter of the tube in mm. Adult women are intubated with 7.0 endotracheal tubes and men with 8.0 endotracheal tubes. Different types of tubes (micro laryngoscopy, reinforced, laser, RAE oral and nasal) are available for different procedures. The endotracheal tube has a low-pressure, high-volume cuff, which when inflated just enough to prevent a leak allows for positive pressure ventilation and protects the airway from aspiration.

Endotracheal intubation may be facilitated by muscle relaxation, which is preferred in the elderly or the ASA 3–4 patient to avoid the hypotension that often occurs when high-dose remifentanil (with propofol) is used to facilitate tracheal intubation. The choice of muscle relaxant depends on the type and duration of the procedure. For a short procedure, where continuous muscle relaxation is not required, the lowest effective dose of a short-acting agent should be used. The degree of muscle relaxation and adequacy of reversal should be monitored with a neuromuscular monitor that records muscle response to a peripheral nerve using acceleromyography. Muscle relaxation should be completely reversed using neostigmine at the end of the procedure, before extubation. If the extent of spontaneous recovery of muscle function is greater than 90%, neostigmine need not be given. Due to the mixed evidence of the effect of neostigmine on PONV, reversal of residual skeletal muscle paralysis using neostigmine should take precedence over the potential risk of PONV associated with its use. With vecuronium or rocuronium, sugammadex (currently not FDA-approved in the US) is a very efficient and rapid alternative for paralytic reversal.

Succinylcholine is a depolarizing muscle relaxant and does not need to be reversed, but its use is associated with postoperative myalgia and infrequent anaphylactic reactions.

Monitoring

For the typical healthy adult undergoing intermediate-risk surgery as an outpatient, standard monitoring as recommended by the ASA should suffice.[8] This includes the following.

1. The presence of qualified anesthesia personnel in the operating room throughout the procedure.
2. Continual monitoring of the patient's oxygenation via FiO_2 monitoring using an in-line oxygen analyzer and pulse oximetry.
3. Ventilation is monitored via capnography and disconnect alarms in the breathing circuit and continual observation.
4. Circulation is monitored by continuous ECG, plethysmography and heart rate with intermittent measurement of NIBP at least every 5 minutes.
5. Temperature monitoring is recommended when significant changes in temperature are intended or expected. Core temperature monitoring is recommended by MHAUS (Malignant Hyperthermia Association of United States) in all patients receiving general anesthesia for greater than 30 min.[9]

Maintaining normothermia is an important goal of a well-planned anesthetic. For intermediate extensive procedures, it is advisable to use a forced air-warming device for this purpose. A helpful measure is to ensure that the patient does not become hypothermic before entering the OR by keeping them in a warm environment and if necessary prewarm the patient before

admitting to the OR, by warm blankets or actively using forced air gowns.

Next, when the patient is positioned for surgery, all pressure points are checked and padded if necessary, with the intent to prevent potential nerve injuries.

The desired intravenous crystalloid is infused to replace any deficit based on fasting time and for maintenance of normovolemia during the procedure. Pre- and intraoperative IV fluid loading (15–20 ml/kg) could prevent PONV especially for procedures scheduled later in the day.[10,11]

Analgesia (see also Chapter 4 on Pharmacology)

A multimodal approach is used to manage intraoperative and postoperative pain. The goal is to use different pharmacological types of analgesics with different routes of administration to provide surgical analgesia with minimal adverse effects.

Multimodal analgesia decreases the risk of PONV and PDNV, by decreasing the need for both intraoperative and postoperative opioids. To produce a meaningful reduction in opioid-induced side effects, a multimodal analgesia regimen should reduce opioid requirements by at least 30%.

Opioids, although effective analgesics, have significant adverse effects, particularly in ambulatory anesthesia, which delay discharge and may even result in a transfer or admission to a hospital. It is therefore prudent to use opioid-sparing techniques first and then use opioids for severe pain or breakthrough pain. Administer analgesics keeping in mind their pharmacokinetics so that their peak effects occur prior to emergence.

Our recipe consists of the following.

1. The use of regional anesthesia (single-shot or continuous infusions) whenever possible (various techniques available for different procedures are discussed in detail in Chapter 6 on Regional Anesthesia).
2. Field blocks or infiltration of local anesthetics into the wound (or intra-articular) by the surgeon.
3. Supplemental preoperative oral analgesics such as acetaminophen, NSAIDS, and gabapentin when indicated.
4. Supplemental preoperative intravenous analgesics such as acetaminophen or ketorolac.
5. Intraoperative narcotics, generally the shorter-acting agents are preferred. In our center typically

fentanyl or alfentanil in combination with other analgesic techniques are used.

6. Acetaminophen is a weak analgesic and suitable for mild pain. Although its potency is low, its favorable side-effect profile makes it suitable for combining with other analgesics.[12,13] It is available in both oral and injectable forms. It lacks the adverse effects of NSAIDs, such as inhibition of platelet aggregation, gastric bleeding, and renal effects.[14,15] When IV acetaminophen is administered, it is important to warn patients not to exceed the total daily recommended dosing for acetaminophen. This is especially important because many of the oral analgesics the patient will be taking post-discharge contain acetaminophen in combination with an opioid.

7. Non-selective NSAIDs are available in oral and parenteral formulations. They decrease opioid requirements and attenuate inflammatory pain response, providing excellent pain relief. Due to their side-effect profile, they are to be used with caution in the elderly, patients with bleeding disorders, hepatic or renal disease, cardiac failure, hypovolemia or sepsis, and following certain surgical procedures (i.e. plastic-reconstructive surgery and tonsillectomy).[16–18]

8. Selective cyclooxygenase (COX-2) inhibitors do not affect platelet function or increase the risk of GI bleeding.[19] Rofecoxib was removed from the market over concerns about increased risk of adverse cardiovascular events, but this does not seem to be a problem with present COX-2 inhibitors when used for a short period of 3–10 days.[20] Celecoxib and parecoxib are contraindicated in patients with sulfonamide allergy and patients with cardiac and renal disease.

9. The NMDA antagonist ketamine has analgesic properties due to its effect on the NMDA receptor. In a low dose via infusion (0.25–0.5 mg/kg/h), ketamine can reduce opioid consumption.[21] However, due to its hemodynamic and psychomimetic side-effect profile, it is not commonly used for relief of mild to moderate pain, especially in the ambulatory setting. It is an option in severe pain, unresponsive to conventional analgesic or opioid-tolerant patients.

10. Centrally acting alpha-2 receptor agonists clonidine and dexmedetomidine also provide analgesia through their effects on the dorsal horn of the spinal cord. Clonidine is limited by its side effects of bradycardia, hypotension, and excessive sedation. It is used as an additive to local anesthetics to prolong the duration of neuraxial and peripheral nerve blocks.[22] As dexmedetomidine has opioid-sparing effects,[23] without respiratory depression, it may be useful in patients at risk for respiratory depression or airway obstruction (patients with OSA).

11. Gabapentin and pregabalin are analogs of GABA and useful in the treatment of neuropathic pain. Their use in the perioperative period has not been studied extensively. They are useful adjuncts in patients at risk for developing neuropathic pain postoperatively.[24] They can cause dizziness and somnolence, another limiting factor in their use in the ambulatory setting.

12. Glucocorticoids reduce inflammatory response to surgical stress and can thus have analgesic properties. Dexamethasone preoperatively in a dose of 8–16 mg IV has been shown to have analgesic effects (as well as an anti-emetic effect) but does have the potential to increase serum glucose[25] and delay wound healing. It is also a useful additive to local anesthetics in the dose of 8 mg to prolong the duration of peripheral nerve blocks.

In summary, our recipe for analgesia consists of regional anesthesia whenever possible, infiltration of local anesthetic when possible, acetaminophen and NSAIDs (either IV or oral) administered preoperatively if no contraindications exist, and a short-acting IV opioid intraoperatively.

PONV

Postoperative nausea and vomiting is a highly distressing complication of general anesthesia and is especially bothersome in the ambulatory setting, where it is one of the important causes of delayed discharge from PACU or even leads to hospital admission. The ideal ambulatory anesthetic is planned keeping PONV prophylaxis in mind.

The first step is to identify patients at risk for PONV.[26] Risk factors for PONV include the following.

1. Patient factors: female gender, age < 50 years, history of PONV or motion sickness and non-smoking.

Table 8.4 Common anti-emetic drugs and doses used at our center.

Drug	Dose and route	Timing	Common adverse effects
Aprepitant	40 mg orally	1–3 hours before induction	
Dexamethasone	4 mg IV	After induction of GA	Interference with wound healing and hyperglycemia with higher doses
Diphenhydramine	25–50 mg IV	After induction of GA or in the PACU	Dry mouth, sedation
Ondansetron	4 mg IV	End of surgery	Headache, QT prolongation with higher doses
Promethazine	6.25–12.5 mg IV	After induction of GA or in the PACU	Sedation
Promethazine	25–50 mg per rectum	In the PACU	Sedation
Metoclopramide	10 mg IV	After induction of GA	Extrapyramidal side effects
Scopolamine	Transdermal	2–24 hours before induction of GA	Visual disturbances, dry mouth, dizziness

2. Anesthetic factors: use of volatile anesthetics, duration of anesthesia, use of nitrous oxide, postoperative opioid use.
3. Surgical factors: duration of surgery and certain types of surgeries, i.e., cholecystectomy, gynecological surgery, eye surgery, and laparoscopic surgeries.

Patients are then scored based on the number of risk factors using the Apfel[27] or Koivuranta[28] scoring systems. The greater the number of risk factors, the higher the risk of PONV. The risk scores have a sensitivity and specificity between 65% and 70%.[3] Both volatile anesthetics and postoperative opioids cause a dose-dependent increase in PONV. The effect of volatile anesthetics is usually prominent up to 6 hours postoperatively and the effect of postoperative opioids lasts as long as the opioids are used. It is uncertain, based on current evidence, if the use of intraoperative neostigmine contributes to PONV.[29]

The following strategies can be used to reduce the risk for PONV.

1. Avoidance of GA whenever possible.
2. When GA is required, use propofol for induction and maintenance, avoid nitrous oxide and volatile agents, minimize opioids.
3. Supplemental oxygen has no effect and is not recommended for PONV prophylaxis.
4. IV fluids in doses of 20–30 ml/kg preoperatively.

Based on whether the patient is at low, moderate, or high risk for PONV, administer prophylactic or rescue anti-emetics.[3] These include 5-HT$_3$ antagonists (ondansetron 4 mg IV), neuroleptics (droperidol or haloperidol 1.25 mg IV), dexamethasone (a dose of 4–8 mg will do for anti-emesis; giving 8–16 mg provides analgesia, too).

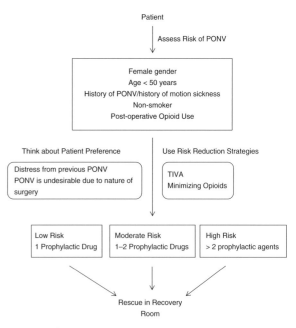

Principles of PONV Management

A multimodal approach to reduce PONV includes strategies to reduce risk of PONV combined with one or more prophylactic agents. Rescue anti-emetic therapy is indicated in patients complaining of nausea or vomiting in the PACU. First, the patient should be evaluated for treatable causes of nausea or vomiting, such as hypotension or hypoxia.

Then, the rescue drugs are basically the same as the prophylactic drugs, but should be from a different pharmacologic class than the prophylactic drugs previously given to the patient. Also metoclopramide and/or ephedrine may be used for treatment of emesis.

PDNV (post-discharge nausea/vomiting) is particularly important to prevent because these patients are at home and do not have access to intravenous, fast-acting rescue anti-emetics. Among ambulatory surgery patients, the incidence of PONV is 33–50%.[26,30]

The prevention of PDNV involves excellent multimodal analgesia strategies, which would reduce postoperative opioid consumption. Combination therapy with long-acting IV and oral anti-emetic in PACU would also reduce PDNV. In some ambulatory practices, patients at high risk for PDNV are often given a prescription for ondansetron tablets to be taken as long as they are taking opioids for pain control. If identified early in the preoperative interview, patients are given a prescription for a transdermal scopolamine patch to be applied the night before surgery.[31]

Recovery: the post anesthesia care unit (PACU)

After emergence, tracheal extubation or LMA removal, the patient is transported to the PACU. The goal of a successful ambulatory anesthetic is to have the patient ready for discharge in the shortest possible time. The advantages to this approach are better patient comfort, reduced hospital-acquired infections, and reduced costs.

A patient is ready to be discharged home when certain predetermined discharge criteria are met. These criteria vary among institutions and are patient-dependent. The patient can then continue with Phase III/late recovery in their home environment.

The Aldrete Scoring System[32] is widely used across institutions and is a modification of the APGAR scoring system. It assesses if a patient can transition from Phase I recovery to Phase II recovery.

Table 8.5 Discharge criteria from Phase 1 recovery to Phase 2 recovery.

Patient sign	Criterion	Score
Activity	Able to move 4 extremities*	2
	Able to move 2 extremities	1
	Able to move 0 extremities	0
Respiration	Able to breathe and cough	2
	Dyspnea	1
	Apneic or obstructed airway	0
Circulation	BP ± 20% of pre-anesthesia level	2
	BP ± 20–49% of pre-anesthesia level	1
	BP ± 50% of pre-anesthesia level	0
Consciousness	Fully awake	2
	Arousable (by name)	1
	Non-responsive	0
Oxygen saturation	$SPO_2 > 92\%$ on room air	2
	Requires supplemental O_2 to maintain $SPO_2 > 90\%$	1
	$SPO_2 < 90\%$ with supplemental O_2	0

* Or at baseline.

Most institutions use an updated or modified Aldrete Scoring system. Assessment of patient readiness for discharge to home from Phase II recovery is by the Post Anesthesia Discharge Scoring System, PADSS.[33]

Recovery then continues at home under the care of a responsible adult who has received discharge instructions in the PACU.

Although there are other scoring systems to assess patient recovery, they each have limitations and will not be further elaborated here. Many ambulatory practices use a combination of the Aldrete scoring system and the PADSS.

The patient must score 8 or higher with no zeroes in any category to be discharged to Phase II recovery.

The patient must score 8 or higher with no zeroes in any category to be discharged home.

Table 8.6 Discharge criteria from Phase 2 recovery to home.

Patient sign	Criterion	Score
Dressing	Dry and clean	2
	Wet and stationary	1
	Growing area of wetness	0
Pain	Pain-free	2
	Mild pain controlled with oral analgesics	1
	Severe pain requiring IV analgesics	0
Ambulation	Can stand and walk straight	2
	Dizzy when upright	1
	Dizzy when supine	0
Nausea	None	2
	Mild nausea	1
	Nausea and vomiting	0
Vital Signs	BP and pulse ± 20% of pre-anesthesia level	2
	BP and pulse ± 20–40% of pre-anesthesia level	1
	BP and pulse > 40% of pre-anesthesia level	0

It is not necessary to require patients to void before discharge. This practice has been shown to cause delayed discharge. If a patient is at high risk for urinary retention, they are observed for an extra hour and residual urine in the bladder is measured via ultrasound (bladder scan). If it is in excess of 400 ml they are catheterized to empty the bladder and then discharged home with clear instruction about when to seek medical assistance (if they do not void further).

It is also not necessary to insist that patients drink and retain fluids prior to discharge. The ASA task force on post-anesthetic care practice guidelines recommends that oral fluid intake not be part of a discharge protocol. Forcing oral intake of fluids may actually increase the incidence of PONV.

Fast-tracking is a process whereby patients bypass Phase I recovery and go directly to Phase II from the OR.[34] Not all patients are suitable for fast-tracking.

Scoring systems are tools to assist the practitioner, not a substitute for clinical judgment or common sense. They should therefore be individualized based on comorbidities and social factors.

Discharge from the facility is a physician responsibility. For all patients receiving GA, regional anesthesia, or sedation, an anesthesiologist must be present in the building until the patient is discharged. For patients receiving no sedation and only local anesthesia by the surgeon, it is the surgeon's responsibility to discharge the patient.

The patient must be discharged into the care of a responsible adult who will remain with the patient overnight. They must be provided with written instructions regarding diet, activity, medications, and follow-up appointments. Circumstances which would require them to seek medical attention should also be clearly outlined, along with the emergency contact information for the surgeon or his/her designee.

Post-discharge follow up

Most ambulatory care practices have a system of follow up where the patient receives a phone call on POD 1 or 2. This is important to ensure patient safety during the late recovery phase. During this call, they are asked about how much pain they experienced, if the pain was relieved or made tolerable by their current dose of oral analgesics, nausea or vomiting episodes if any, and oral intake. They are also asked about how long the regional/local anesthetic lasted, ambulation and the ability to carry out permitted daily activities, fever, and unusual pain or bleeding. Any early postoperative complications are identified and either treated or the patient is directed to seek medical attention. Compliance with postoperative instructions is verified and clarifications are provided.

> Give two cooks the same ingredients and the same recipe; it is fascinating to observe how, like handwriting, their results differ. After you cook a dish repeatedly, you begin to understand it. Then you can reinvent it a bit and make it yours. A written recipe can be useful, but sometimes the notes scribbled in the margin are the key to a superlative rendition. Each new version may inspire improvisation based on fresh understanding (David Tanis, *Heart of the Artichoke: and Other Kitchen Journeys*)

Typical patient flow through an ASC – a step-by-step checklist

Obtain health information
  Suitable for ASC?
  Special needs?
  PAT required?

Scheduling
  NPO instructions
  Medications to be withheld or taken
  (anti-emetics or DVT prophylaxis)

Arrival at the ASC
  Pre-anesthetic evaluation
  Pre-medications (anxiolytics, analgesics,
    anti-emetics, antibiotics, DVT prophylaxis)
  Regional anesthesia?

To the operating room
  MAC-local/regional anesthesia or general anesthesia
    (induction, maintenance & emergence)
  Risk reduction for PONV
  PONV prophylaxis
  Multimodal analgesia

Recovery in PACU (Phase 1 and/or 2)
  Discharge scoring
  Transition to oral analgesics
  Rescue anti-emetics
  Discharge instructions given to responsible adult
  Discharged by physician

Patient's home (late recovery phase)
  Adequate hydration
  Analgesia
  Anti-emetics
  Follow-up appointment

Post-discharge phone call on POD # 1 or 2
  Record outcome measures in patient's chart
    Response to analgesics
    Duration of nerve blocks
    PDNV, if any
    Adherence with post-discharge instructions
Level of activity

Special considerations

In this section, we will deal with specific groups and their anesthetic management in the ambulatory setting.

Obesity

Obesity is defined as having a Body Mass Index (BMI) of ≥ 30 kg/m^2. It is further classified into Class I (BMI 30–34.9 kg/m^2), Class II (BMI 35–39.9 kg/m^2), and Class III (BMI ≥ 40 kg/m^2). Class III obesity is further subdivided into super-obesity (BMI 50–59 kg/m^2) and super-super obesity (BMI ≥ 60 kg/m^2).[35] Obesity is a worldwide epidemic and in 2009–2010, the prevalence of obesity was 35.5% among adult men and 35.8% among adult women in the US.[36] Obese patients may present for a wide variety of surgical procedures, which may or may not be linked to their obesity, ranging from outpatient bariatric surgery to cataract surgery.

Preoperative preparation by systems

Respiratory

Check for associated obstructive sleep apnea (OSA). Some patients may already be diagnosed with OSA and using CPAP. Instruct them to bring their CPAP device on the day of surgery and use it in the post-operative period not just at night but also for daytime sleeping.

For patients who are undiagnosed but high risk for OSA (based on the STOP-BANG screening questionnaire),[37] the type of surgery will determine whether they need a sleep study preoperatively. Procedures that are low to intermediate risk, and not likely to be associated with severe postoperative pain, are amenable to loco-regional techniques or non-opioid analgesics for pain management and can be safely performed on obese patients in the ambulatory setting without the need for a sleep study.

Check for the potential for difficult intubation and obtain previous anesthesia records. The neck circumference appears to be the biggest predictor of difficult intubation in morbidly obese patients.[38] These patients are also difficult to mask ventilate. Whether a patient with a known difficult airway should be anesthetized at a free-standing ASC is debatable. This decision should take into account availability of skilled back up to assist the anesthesiologist if necessary and the availability of difficult airway equipment.[39]

These patients tend to have perioperative hypoxemia and require close monitoring. They are also sensitive to the respiratory depressant effects of anxiolytics such as midazolam, which should be administered with caution, in titrated doses.

Cardiovascular

Obese patients tend to have coexisting arterial hypertension and left ventricular diastolic dysfunction. Many of these patients have restricted mobility, making it difficult to assess their functional capacity. They may therefore have undiagnosed coronary artery disease. The need for preoperative cardiac testing depends on the surgical procedure and presence of comorbidities. Most low- to intermediate-risk ambulatory procedures can be carried out without further cardiac testing.

Patients with suspected obesity hypoventilation syndrome are not candidates for outpatient surgery.

Obese patients are at high risk for thromboembolic events and should receive deep venous thrombosis (DVT) prophylaxis perioperatively, and early ambulation must be encouraged after surgery. They may sometimes require DVT prophylaxis for up to 3 weeks postoperatively.[40]

Gastrointestinal

Obesity is frequently associated with gastroesophageal reflux and patients may already be on medications to treat it. These drugs should be continued on the day of surgery. For patients who are not on anti-reflux medications, consider preoperative famotidine or ranitidine to decrease gastric volumes and increase gastric pH. Current fasting guidelines (6 hours for solids, 2 hours for clear liquids) are acceptable in obese patients.[41]

Endocrine

Many of these patients have insulin resistance and diabetes. They should be given appropriate instructions for managing their anti-diabetic regimen on the day of surgery. Blood glucose levels should be checked and managed in the perioperative period.

Miscellaneous

Ensure that these patients have a responsible caregiver to bring them to their surgery, receive discharge instructions, and take them home after surgery. Ensure that the surgery center has the appropriate equipment (stretchers, OR tables) to accommodate the girth and weight of these patients. It can be difficult to obtain IV access in these patients. Ultrasound guidance can be used to locate and cannulate peripheral veins in these situations.

Intraoperative

Loco-regional techniques of anesthesia, accompanied by minimal sedation, are preferred whenever possible in these patients. For patients in whom GA is indicated, the following tips may be useful. Before induction of GA, position these patients head-up or ramped up to raise the head and shoulders. Avoid the supine position. The head-up position improves functional residual capacity (FRC) and allows for a longer period of apnea before desaturation.[39]

Preoxygenate with 100% oxygen with a tight mask with PEEP of 5–10 cm, and have the patient take at least four vital capacity breaths of 100% oxygen before induction of GA. Have difficult airway equipment available in the room. Sedated, topicalized fiber-optic intubation may be indicated in patients who appear difficult to mask ventilate on the preoperative examination. A videolaryngoscope may be used in other patients to facilitate tracheal intubation. Optimal positioning ultimately is the key to successful atraumatic intubation in these patients.[42,43]

Rapid sequence induction may be indicated in patients at risk for aspiration. In these cases, the decision should be made on an individual basis after airway assessment.

Maintenance of anesthesia can be achieved by any of the techniques mentioned earlier in the chapter.

Pay close attention to positioning to avoid nerve injuries in these patients.

Pay attention to the following dose adjustments.

1. Propofol: induction (bolus) dose should be based on ideal body weight and maintenance (infusion) dose should be based on total body weight.
2. Succinylcholine: dose should be based on total body weight due to increased pseudocholinesterase activity with increasing weight and larger extracellular fluid volume.
3. Rocuronium: dose based on ideal body weight. If dosed according to total body weight, expect a longer duration of action.
4. Benzodiazepines: dose according to ideal body weight. They are highly lipophilic and therefore distribute in the fat compartment resulting in prolonged duration of action if dosed according to total body weight.
5. Fentanyl: dose according to ideal body weight.
6. Remifentanil: dose according to ideal body weight. Pharmacokinetics of remifentanil are similar in

obese and non-obese patients making this a useful adjunct for TIVA in the obese patient.

7. Dexmedetomidine: dose according to total body weight. In doses of 0.2–0.7 µg/kg/h, it produces effective sedation, analgesia, and minimal respiratory depression making it ideal in these situations.

8. Neostigmine: dose according to total body weight for prompt early reversal.

9. Sugammadex: currently not FDA-approved in the US, but may be useful in obese patients.[44]

The goals of fluid management are maintaining normovolemia and avoiding rapid fluid boluses.

Some tips for effective mechanical ventilation of the lungs in these patients are as follows.

10. Do not exceed tidal volumes of 10 ml/kg,[45,46] based on ideal weight.

11. No specific ventilatory (volume control or pressure control) mode is better in these patients.

12. Moderate PEEP (5–10 cm H_2O) with recruitment measures prevents atelectasis.[47]

13. Higher levels of PEEP could impair venous return and cause hypotension.

14. Titrate FiO_2 to maintain acceptable oxygen saturations, avoid 100% oxygen as it could lead to absorption atelectasis.

Emergence

Ensure adequate reversal of neuromuscular blockade. Extubate in the semi-recumbent or semi-sitting or propped-up position to maximize FRC. Administer supplemental oxygen and observe the patient for a few minutes before transporting out of the operating room.

Postoperative

1. Consider using BIPAP or CPAP in the recovery room until the patient is fully awake.

2. Ensure adequate analgesia as stated earlier in the chapter using opioid-sparing techniques.

3. Encourage early ambulation.

4. Patients who are unable to maintain oxygen saturation greater than 95% without supplemental oxygen or non-invasive ventilation should be monitored in the hospital and not discharged home.

5. Patients who are likely to require a significant amount of opioids for pain management are also not candidates for discharge.

6. Both the patient and their caregiver should be given explicit instructions on using CPAP not just at night but anytime the patient is sleeping.

To summarize, perioperative outcomes in obese patients are influenced by the invasiveness of the surgery, the anesthetic technique, the presence of comorbidities, and the BMI (> 50 kg/m²). Ambulatory surgery appears to be safe in patients with BMI < 40 kg/m² when comorbid conditions are well managed. Patients with BMI between 40 and 50 kg/m² require thorough preoperative assessment and screening to rule out obesity-related comorbidities (obesity-related hypoventilation, OSA, CAD, pulmonary hypertension, CHF) which would preclude them from ambulatory surgery.[48]

The child (see also Chapter 11, Pediatrics)

Anesthetic care in children usually begins with local anesthesia pads on both hands (i.e., EMLA® cream) to prepare for painless venous access. If the child accepts oral tablets or mixture, an appropriate dose of acetaminophen and/or an NSAID should be administered orally 1 hour or more before surgery for pain prophylaxis. If this is not possible due to the child's resistance, these drugs may be given IV or rectally after the start of anesthesia. Usually sedative premedication is not needed in a well-assured child accompanied by a close relative. The use of preoperative sedatives may prolong the postoperative recovery and discharge, and also disturb the normal diurnal sleep pattern. Still, in an agitated child, midazolam oral mixture 0.5 mg/kg may be a reasonable option to control the preoperative situation when needed. An alternative may be rectally diazepam suspension, 0.5–1.0 mg/kg.

A quiet and familiar atmosphere around the child can be very helpful for facilitating an uneventful preparation. Clear fluids (except milk products) until 2 hours before the start of anesthesia should be permitted. If surgery is planned after lunch, an early morning light breakfast, up to 6 hours prior to surgery, should be allowed. The child should preferably wait as little as possible in the general waiting area, and preferably with his/her parents surrounded with toys, books, or video screens available in a room furnished with regular rather than hospital-type furniture. It is usually wise to avoid mixing children waiting for surgery with discharge ready children, unless the latter are happy and fully recovered.

For routine inductions, it may be wise to keep the child as normally dressed as possible (including shoes), sitting on a parent's knee with some toys available and/ or a computer screen with cartoons running close by. Although an IV induction may be preferred because it is safer and faster, it may not be possible in smaller children. IV induction can help decrease the chance of aspiration and enable better management of laryngospasm and bradycardia. Even though children undergoing elective ambulatory surgery may be appropriately fasting, they do sometimes have stomach content anyway either because they don't tell their parents about recent food intake or parents do not tell the provider from fear of surgery cancellation.

If IV placement is planned prior to induction, consider removing the EMLA patch a few minutes prior to IV placement to minimize skin pallor and vasoconstriction, although this is not critical. One can usually show the child, with a gentle squeeze (do it gently, but say that you are squeezing hard!) that the topical anesthesia works. After vein cannulation, a Lactated Ringers or 0.9% normal saline solution should be started, and a pulse oximeter placed. Then, intravenous induction with opioid plus propofol can be performed.

Alternatively, an inhalational induction can be performed, usually with sevoflurane (8% in oxygen until deep sleep), followed by venous access. This technique may be preferred in these cases:

- the child or parent insists (i.e., gentle persuasion does not make them change their minds, for instance due to a good previous experience) on inhalational induction;
- cannulation in the EMLA treated area is unsuccessful, and there are no good veins outside the EMLA-applied area;
- unsuccessful cannulation after two attempts inside the EMLA-applied area or one attempt outside the EMLA-applied area.

In children who did not have EMLA or if the EMLA-applied area does not have a good vein for cannulation, it is reasonable to make one quick attempt. One can tell the child that just before skin penetration they will feel pain briefly, but then they will feel no more pain.

For very short procedures (5–10 min), one can just ventilate the child manually through the anesthesia mask; longer cases may warrant an LMA, if appropriate. For some procedures such as tonsillectomies, adenoidectomies and dental surgery the child will likely need to be intubated. This is because the surgeon will be working in the mouth and may dislodge the LMA, and also, as in the case of tonsillectomy, an endotracheal tube will allow for better control of the airway in case of profuse bleeding. However, in cases where there are experienced surgeon-anesthesiologist teams and in the presence of good communication, an LMA can be used for adeno-tonsillectomies.

There are special considerations in children when propofol is used. Children will require about 50–100% more than adults during induction, and 25–50% more during maintenance, mostly due to pharmacokinetic differences, such as small initial distribution volume and higher clearance (see chapter 4, Pharmacology). For opioids and muscle relaxants the dose will be about the same (per kg) as in adults, although slightly more remifentanil may be needed due to higher drug clearance.

For volatile anesthetics, the MAC values are generally 25–50% higher in children compared to adults, and vary according to the child's age. If nitrous oxide is available, it may be a useful adjunct in 50% (small children) to 66% concentration in oxygen, in addition to either intravenous or inhalational anesthesia. Nitrous oxide is not a cardiorespiratory depressant in healthy outpatients and has a very rapid on–off effect, and can help reduce the dose of other agents. This can help speed up both induction and emergence from anesthesia. When using nitrous oxide, care should be taken by the end of the case to ensure adequate ventilation with oxygen-enriched breathing gas after turning off the nitrous oxide. Because much of the nitrous oxide is released into the lungs during the first 3–5 min after cessation of administration, a combination of hypoventilation and administration of just air may result in hypoxia during emergence.

Sevoflurane is generally the agent of choice for induction of inhalational anesthesia, and may be used for maintenance of anesthesia. However, sevoflurane is associated with a high incidence (up to 10–20%) of severe, short-lasting agitation during emergence.[49] The incidence will be lower when the child emerges with parents standing close by and having received adequate analgesia. The incidence of emergence agitation may be lower with desflurane, and even lower with propofol.[50] Whereas desflurane is unsuited for inhalational induction, it may be an alternative for maintenance after sevoflurane induction, both due to less postoperative agitation and slightly faster emergence and less respiratory depression.[51] An alternative technique is to turn off the inhalational agent earlier and administer a small bolus dose or short-lasting infusion of propofol towards the end of the case to avoid emergence agitation. The use of propofol can also add a short-lasting anti-emetic effect from propofol.

As in all patients, the surgeon should be encouraged to use local anesthesia as much as possible to decrease postoperative pain, and the anesthesiologist may also consider administering a sacral block with bupivacaine for patients having certain procedures (i.e., hernia, perineal surgery, surgery of external genitalia or lower extremities). Furthermore, non-opioids including NSAIDs may be used, and dexamethasone can help not only with emesis prophylaxis but also with pain reduction. The new COX-2 inhibitors have not yet been approved for use in children, but their use will increase as an alternative to traditional NSAIDs when the latter are contraindicated.

The elderly patient

According to the US Census Bureau, individuals over 65 years of age numbered 39.6 million in 2009, or 12.9% of the population. By 2030, they will represent 19% of the US population.[52]

Ambulatory surgery provides unique advantages to this patient population, including the ability to recover in the familiar home environment, cost savings, reduced postoperative cognitive dysfunction (POCD), reduced respiratory events, and a relative reduction in postoperative pain, PONV, and nosocomial infections.[53]

Most commonly performed ambulatory procedures in the elderly include cataract surgery, and to a lesser extent urological procedures, procedures on joints, muscles or tendons, knee arthroscopies, hernia repairs, and nerve decompression (carpal tunnel release).

Preoperative preparation by systems

Respiratory

Physiological changes of aging result in gas transfer defect, ventilation perfusion mismatch, and impaired respiratory responses to hypoxia and hypercarbia. These changes make the elderly more sensitive to respiratory depressants including opioids and benzodiazepines and more prone to postoperative pulmonary complications.

It is generally desirable to either avoid or minimize benzodiazepines and opioids in these patients.

Elderly patients with severe chronic obstructive pulmonary disease should undergo preoperative pulmonary function testing with and without bronchodilators to determine whether they have a reversible component to their disease.[54] Patients with a reversible component of obstructive disease and/or airway hyperreactivity should receive a short (48 h) preoperative course of a beta2-adrenergic agonist and systemic corticosteroid therapy. The short-term use of steroids has not been found to have an adverse effect on wound healing or infection control.[55]

Smoking cessation has been shown to decrease the risk of perioperative complications,[56] and should be strongly encouraged at least 4 weeks before surgery.[57]

Cardiovascular

In the elderly, the combined effects of vascular stiffening and left ventricular hypertrophy lead to diastolic dysfunction, predisposing them to fluid overload and pulmonary edema. Increased vagal tone leads to slow heart rate, so evaluate for sinus node dysfunction. The incidence of coronary artery disease increases with age. Age alone should not be an indicator for preoperative ECG or cardiac work up. The patient's functional capacity should be assessed by careful history, and the presence and severity of comorbidities evaluated before ordering any preoperative cardiac testing.

The aging autonomous nervous system results in increased blood pressure lability, reduced responsiveness to inotropic and chronotropic drugs, and an increased dependence on preload to maintain cardiac output. Preoperative fasting guidelines should be followed to allow these patients to drink clear liquids up until 2 hours before surgery.

These patients can be instructed to continue all of their cardiovascular medications (except ACE inhibitors). Preoperative management of anti-coagulants should be discussed with the patient's prescribing physician and the surgeon.

Renal

Creatinine clearance progressively declines with age. Their ability to handle a sodium load is impaired and decreased concentrating and diluting ability of the kidneys makes them prone to hypernatremia, dehydration, and fluid overload.

Hepatic

Aging is associated with decreased liver mass, which affects the metabolism of many drugs.

CNS

Cerebral atrophy after 60 years of age makes these patients more prone to POCD and more sensitive to anesthetic drugs. They also require lower doses of local anesthetic drugs.

Frailty

The preoperative assessment should include the following.

1. Information about whether the patient uses glasses, hearing aids, and dentures, or ambulatory assist devices such as a walker or cane.
2. Whether the patient needs assistance transferring to a stretcher or bed.
3. Detailed information about transportation needs.
4. Information about the caregiver who will take the patient home and receive discharge instructions.

Intraoperative

No one technique of anesthesia has been shown to be superior in patients in this age group. The choice of anesthetic depends on the type of surgery.

Keep the following in mind when administering a general anesthetic to these patients.

1. These patients are prone to hypothermia due to a decrease in basal metabolic rate and skeletal muscle mass. Keep the patients warm and as completely covered as possible in the preoperative area and in the OR. Use forced air-warming devices during longer procedures.
2. Avoid benzodiazepines, which can contribute to POCD and cause respiratory depression.
3. MAC for volatile anesthetics is reduced by 40% by the age of 80 years.
4. The use of desflurane is associated with earlier recovery than sevoflurane[58] and has been shown to cause less fatigue in the first week after anesthesia in comparison to propofol infusion for maintenance of anesthesia.[59]
5. Nitrous oxide is a useful adjunct in this population due to its rapid elimination and anesthetic and analgesic-sparing effects.[60]
6. The doses of opioids such as fentanyl, alfentanil, and remifentanil should be reduced by 50% for both boluses and infusion dosing by the age of 80 years.
7. The initial dose of propofol should be reduced by 20–40% in the elderly, and the onset of the desired effect may be delayed. The maintenance dose should be reduced by 10–20%. Due to longer circulation times, drugs take longer for peak effect. Wait 2–3 minutes for peak effect before redosing.
8. Blood pressure lability is expected in this age group both after induction and during the maintenance of GA. A small dose of ephedrine (5–10 mg) administered prior to induction could mitigate the hypotension.[61]
9. Use multimodal analgesia techniques as described earlier.
10. The goal is a short-acting anesthetic with no residual depressant effects.
11. The use of small doses of IV sedative–analgesic drugs for MAC techniques minimizes the adverse physiologic effects on major organ systems, resulting in shorter recovery times than general or spinal anesthesia.[62,63] For elderly outpatients undergoing superficial procedures, MAC techniques are an excellent alternative to GA.

Postoperative

These are the important postoperative considerations unique to elderly patients.

Post-operative delirium (POD)

POD is an acute change in cognition and orientation, presenting a few hours, to days after surgery, lasting days to weeks. It occurs in 5–15% of all elderly patients undergoing non-cardiac surgery.[64] Risk factors include age greater than 70 years, alcohol abuse, poor preoperative cognitive and functional status, abnormalities of serum sodium, potassium and glucose, non-cardiac thoracic surgery, or abdominal aneurysm surgery. Pain management using regional anesthesia with multimodal analgesia may help negate these risk factors in the elderly patient and reduce the incidence of postoperative delirium and cognitive dysfunction.[65]

Post-operative cognitive dysfunction (POCD)

POCD is a more subtle impairment in cognitive function, presenting days to weeks after surgery and occasionally lasting up to one year after surgery. It is present in 10–13% of elderly patients at 3 months after non-cardiac surgery.[66] Risk factors include age greater than 60 years, lower educational level, history of previous cerebrovascular accident with no residual impairment and cognitive impairment at discharge. [67]

Studies suggest that minor surgery performed in an outpatient setting has minimal impact on cognition in the elderly population.[68]

Measures to minimize cognitive impairment include the following.

1. Preoperative optimization of treatment of comorbidities.
2. Use of anesthetic agents and techniques which are short-acting and less likely to cause major physiologic derangements.
3. Have a familiar caregiver available at the patient's bedside in the recovery room, preferably before the patient is awake.
4. Replace sensory aids as soon as possible when the patient awakens (hearing aids, glasses, dentures).
5. Discharge planning should be done in the preoperative period and should include assessment of transportation needs, the presence of a familiar, responsible caregiver, and assessment of where the patient will go after discharge (home/nursing home/skilled nursing facility).

The perioperative care of the older patient undergoing ambulatory surgery has been addressed and will need to be reviewed once analysis based on larger data sets becomes available.[69]

The ASA class 3 patient undergoing surgery at an ASC

Definition

Patients of ASA class 1 and 2 are most suitable for surgery as outpatients and for office-based surgery. ASA class 3 patients may be suitable for elective surgery as outpatients depending on the type of the procedure and type of anesthesia. ASA class 4 patients may be suitable to have some minimally invasive elective procedures performed on an outpatient basis in either an ASC or hospital. CMS (Centers for Medicare and Medicaid Services) requires that ASCs have a transfer agreement with a nearby hospital and that the ASC medical staff have admitting privileges at this hospital (CMS Regulations 416.41(b)).[67]

In addition to patients with disease states such as systemic arterial hypertension, or bronchial asthma, patients with complicated diseases that impact multiple organ systems, such as diabetes mellitus, heart disease (CAD, valvular dysfunction, or arrhythmia, congestive heart failure), or poorly controlled hypertension are being considered for surgery as outpatients in an ambulatory setting.

The appropriate location to perform outpatient surgery, either at a free-standing ASC or out-patient surgery in a hospital setting, depends on the complexity of the surgery, the duration and invasiveness of the surgery, the patient's medical condition, and the anticipated recovery profile. For example, during the postoperative phase, some patients may require laboratory tests or subspecialty consultations, which while readily available in a hospital, are not available in a free-standing ASC. These patients may be better served at a hospital.

Preoperative preparation by system

Unlike a normal healthy patient (ASA physical status 1) or those with mild systemic disease (ASA PS 2) that is well controlled, patients with severe systemic illness are classified as ASA PS 3. Their medical condition is usually being managed by one or more consultants. Patients may need to visit their cardiologist, hematologist, or internist for preoperative evaluation and optimization of their treatment. A patient with severe systemic disease that is a constant threat to life is classified as ASA PS 4. When scheduling the surgery, the surgeon may take into account the complexity of the surgery but not the associated medical comorbidities. Similarly, the primary care physician, while having knowledge of the patient's comorbidities, may not understand the ramifications of anesthesia and surgery as an outpatient. The anesthesiologist, as the perioperative physician, should actively optimize the patient in collaboration with the surgeon and the primary care physician.

A prescreening telephone call from the ASC may prevent scheduling of those patients who are not suitable candidates and helps avoid problems on the day of surgery. In addition, during this call, the functional status of the patient is assessed in terms of each system, and whether the disease state is optimally treated and controlled, to identify the possibility of avoidable complications.

Respiratory

Patients may have severe asthma, history of long-term tobacco abuse, COPD, and on treatment at home on oxygen; they may require non-invasive ventilation via CPAP or BIPAP at night or long-term ventilator support via a tracheostomy at home. As long as their coexisting medical illnesses are under appropriate treatment, and currently stable, these patients could undergo certain specific procedures as outpatients in an ASC.

Cardiovascular

Patients with a history of cardiovascular disease can undergo surgery as outpatients; however, if the disease is moderate to severe, the surgery should be done in a hospital setting should the need for continued post-procedure observation arise. In patients with cardiovascular disease, the risk of bleeding and thromboembolism must be evaluated and medications such as aspirin, warfarin, or clopidogrel must be adjusted.[71]

Renal

Patients with end-stage renal disease on hemodialysis may undergo those surgeries that would not cause major fluid shifts as outpatients, in an ASC.

Endocrine

Patients with stable endocrine disorders such as diabetes mellitus treated with oral hypoglycemics or insulin therapy, hypothyroidism on synthroid, or Addison's disease on steroid therapy may undergo surgery at an ASC.

CNS

Patients with sequelae of a cerebrovascular incident, and with paraparesis, or hemiparesis or even quadriparesis may undergo specific procedures as outpatients in an ASC.

Intraoperative management

No one technique of anesthesia is superior and a combination of IV sedation and judicious infiltration of local anesthetic into the operative site by the surgeon may suffice in many of these cases.

The induction and maintenance of anesthesia of the older patient has been addressed in a separate section. In patients with respiratory and cardiovascular diseases, many of the considerations here are similar in that patients have a lower reserve and the doses of many medications may have to be adjusted to the lower end of the prescribed range. The onset to peak effect of all the drugs may be delayed and therefore waiting for the peak effect to occur before redosing must be considered in these patients.

Monitoring

The level of cardiovascular monitoring depends on the patient's overall health, the presence and severity of cardiovascular disease, and the nature of the surgical procedure. Standard monitoring such as NIBP, heart rate, EKG (simultaneous display of lead II for rhythm and lead V for ST segment changes to detect arrhythmia and myocardial ischemia), pulse oximetry, and respiratory rate is necessary.

Airway management in these patients is as dictated by the procedure. Whenever feasible, patients are maintained in an anesthetic plane that allows spontaneous ventilation with the ventilator set to the pressure support mode, to achieve and maintain adequate minute ventilation. This mode maintains venous return to the right heart and thereby maintains cardiac output and prevents profound hypotension.

Fluid management

Fluid therapy has to be carefully titrated in these patients where even 200 ml of fluid more than necessary may precipitate complications. This is in contrast to young patients undergoing outpatient surgery where the literature supports 20 ml/kg of IV fluid loading to prevent PONV.[72]

Analgesia

Analgesia is best achieved with multimodal non-opioid techniques and short-acting opioids (alfentanil) with the goals of avoiding prolonged sedation and achieving early emergence and prompt discharge to their residence.

Postoperative

With adequate preoperative optimization following a preoperative evaluation, ASA PS 3 patients may undergo surgery safely in an ASC.[73]

References

1. Chung F, Yuan H, Yin L, Vairavanathan S, Wong DT. Elimination of preoperative testing in ambulatory surgery. *Anesth Analg.* 2009; **108**(2):467–75.

2. Joshi GP, Chung F, Vann MA, *et al.* Society for Ambulatory Anesthesia consensus statement on perioperative blood glucose management in diabetic patients undergoing ambulatory surgery. *Anesth Analg.* 2010; **111**(6):1378–87.

3. Gan TJ, Diemunsch P, Habib AS, *et al.* Consensus guidelines for the management of postoperative nausea and vomiting. *Anesth Analg.* 2014 Jan; **118**(1):85–113

4. Michelsen I, Helbo-Hansen HS, Køhler F, Lorenzen AG, Rydlund E, Bentzon MW. Prophylactic ephedrine attenuates the hemodynamic response to propofol in elderly female patients. *Anesth Analg.* 1998 Mar; **86**(3):477–81.

5. Gopalakrishna MD, Krishna HM, Shenoy UK. The effect of ephedrine on intubating conditions and haemodynamics during rapid tracheal intubation using propofol and rocuronium. *Br J Anaesth.* 2007 Aug; **99**(2):191–94.

6. Tramèr M, Moore A, McQuay H. Omitting nitrous oxide in general anaesthesia: Meta-analysis of intraoperative awareness and postoperative emesis in randomized controlled trials. *Br J Anaesth.* 1996; **76**(2):186–93.

7. Brimacombe JR. *Laryngeal Mask Anesthesia: Principles and Practice.* Saunders; 2004.

8. Basic Anesthetic Monitoring, Standards for. http://www.asahq.org/For-Members/~/media/For%20Members/documents/Standards%20Guidelines%20Stmts/Basic%20Anesthetic%20Monitoring%202011.ashx (accessed Jan 10, 2014).

9. Temperature Monitoring during Surgical Procedures. http://www.mhaus.org/healthcare-professionals/mhaus-recommendations/temperature-monitoring (accessed Jan 10, 2014).

10. Ali SZ, Taguchi A, Holtmann B, Kurz A. Effect of supplemental pre-operative fluid on postoperative nausea and vomiting. *Anaesthesia.* 2003 Aug; **58**(8):780–84.

11. Magner JJ, McCaul C, Carton E, Gardiner J, Buggy D. Effect of intraoperative intravenous crystalloid infusion on postoperative nausea and vomiting after gynaecological laparoscopy: Comparison of 30 and 10 ml kg^{-1}. *Br J Anaesth.* 2004 Sep; **93**(3):381–85.

12. Romsing M, Moiniche S, Dahl JB. Rectal and parenteral paracetamol, and paracetamol in combination with NSAIDs for postoperative analgesia. *Br J Anaesth.* 2002; **88**:215–26.

13. Hyllested M, Jones S, Pedersen JL, *et al.* Comparative effects of paracetamol, NSAIDs or their combination in postoperative pain management: A quantitative review. *Br J Anaesth.* 2002; **88**:199–214.

14. Kehlet H, Werner MU. Role of paracetamol in the acute pain management. *Drugs.* 2003; **63**:15–22.

15. Graham GG, Graham RI, Day RO. Comparative analgesia, cardiovascular and renal effects of celecoxib, rofecoxib and acetaminophen (paracetamol). *Curr Pharm Des.* 2002; **8**:1063–75.

16. Kehlet H, Dahl JB. Are perioperative nonsteroidal anti-inflammatory drugs ulcerogenic in the short term? *Drugs.* 1992; **44**(Suppl 5):S38–41.

17. Kenny GNC. Potential renal, haematological and allergic adverse effects associated with nonsteroidal anti-inflammatory drugs. *Drugs.* 1992; **44**(Suppl 5):S31–37.

18. Camu F, Van Lersberghe C, Lauwers MH. Cardiovascular risks and benefits of perioperative nonsteroidal anti-inflammatory drug treatment. *Drugs.* 1992; **44**(Suppl 5):S42–51.

19. Romsing J, Moiniche S. A systemic review of COX-2 inhibitors compared with traditional NSAIDs, or different COX-2 inhibitors for post-operative pain. *Acta Anaesthesiol Scand.* 2004; **48**:525–46.

20. Wickerts L, Warrén Stomberg M, Brattwall M, Jakobsson J. Coxibs: Is there a benefit when compared to traditional non-selective NSAIDs in postoperative pain management? *Minerva Anestesiol.* 2011 Nov; **77**(11):1084–98.

21. Subramaniam K, Subramaniam B, Steinbrook RA. Ketamine as adjuvant analgesic to opioids: A quantitative and qualitative systematic review. *Anesth Analg.* 2004 Aug; **99**(2):482–95.

22. Eisenach JC, De Kock M, Klimscha W. Alpha(2)-adrenergic agonists for regional anesthesia. A clinical review of clonidine (1984–1995). *Anesthesiology.* 1996 Sep; **85**(3):655–74.

23. Blaudszun G, Lysakowski C, Elia N, Tramèr MR. Effect of perioperative systemic α2 agonists on postoperative morphine consumption and pain intensity: Systematic review and meta-analysis of randomized controlled trials. *Anesthesiology.* 2012 Jun; **116**(6):1312–22.

24. Clarke H, Bonin RP, Orser BA, Englesakis M, Wijeysundera DN, Katz J. The prevention of chronic postsurgical pain using gabapentin and pregabalin: A combined systematic review and meta-analysis. *Anesth Analg.* 2012 Aug; **115**(2):428–42.

25. Waldron NH, Jones CA, Gan TJ, Allen TK, Habib AS. Impact of perioperative dexamethasone on postoperative analgesia and side effects: Systematic review and meta-analysis. *Br J Anaesth.* 2013 Feb; **110**(2):191–200.

26. Apfel CC, Philip BK, Cakmakkaya OS, *et al.* Who is at risk for postdischarge nausea and vomiting after ambulatory surgery? *Anesthesiology.* 2012; **117**:475–86.

27. Apfel CC, Läärä E, Koivuranta M, Greim CA, Roewer N. A simplified risk score for predicting postoperative nausea and vomiting: Conclusions

from cross-validations between two centers. *Anesthesiology.* 1999 Sep; **91**(3):693–700.

28. Koivuranta M, Läärä E, Snåre L, Alahuhta S. A survey of postoperative nausea and vomiting. *Anaesthesia.* 1997 May; **52**(5):443–49.

29. Cheng CR, Sessler DI, Apfel CC. Does neostigmine administration produce a clinically important increase in postoperative nausea and vomiting? *Anesth Analg.* 2005 Nov; **101**(5):1349–55.

30. Gupta A, Wu CL, Elkassabany N, Krug CE, Parker SD, Fleisher LA. Does the routine prophylactic use of antiemetics affect the incidence of postdischarge nausea and vomiting following ambulatory surgery? A systematic review of randomized controlled trials. *Anesthesiology.* 2003 Aug; **99**(2):488–95.

31. Apfel CC, Zhang K, George E, *et al.* Transdermal scopolamine for the prevention of postoperative nausea and vomiting: A systematic review and meta-analysis. *Clin Ther.* 2010 Nov; **32**(12):1987–2002.

32. Aldrete JA, Kroulik D. A postanesthetic recovery score. *Anesth Analg.* 1970 Nov–Dec; **49**(6):924–34.

33. Chung F. Recovery pattern and home-readiness after ambulatory surgery. *Anesth Analg.* 1995 May; **80**(5):896–902.

34. White PF, Song D. New criteria for fast-tracking after outpatient anesthesia: A comparison with the modified Aldrete's scoring system. *Anesth Analg.* 1999 May; **88**(5):1069–72.

35. Leykin Y, Pellis T, Del Mestro E, Marzano B, Fanti G, Brodsky JB. Anesthetic management of morbidly obese and super-morbidly obese patients undergoing bariatric operations: Hospital course and outcomes. *Obes Surg.* 2006 Dec; **16**(12):1563–69.

36. Flegal KM, Carroll MD, Kit BK, Ogden CL. Prevalence of obesity and trends in the distribution of body mass index among US adults, 1999–2010. *JAMA.* 2012 Feb 1; **307**(5):491–97.

37. Joshi GP, Ankichetty SP, Gan TJ, Chung F. Society for Ambulatory Anesthesia consensus statement on preoperative selection of adult patients with obstructive sleep apnea scheduled for ambulatory surgery. *Anesth Analg.* 2012 Nov; **115**(5):1060–68.

38. Brodsky JB, Lemmens HJ, Brock-Utne JG, Vierra M, Saidman LJ. Morbid obesity and tracheal intubation. *Anesth Analg.* 2002 Mar; **94**(3):732–36.

39. Law JA, Broemling N, Cooper RM, *et al.* The difficult airway with recommendations for management – part 2 – The anticipated difficult airway. *Can J Anaesth.* 2013 Nov; **60**(11):1119–38.

40. Magee CJ, Barry J, Javed S, Macadam R, Kerrigan D. Extended thromboprophylaxis reduces incidence of postoperative venous thromboembolism in laparoscopic bariatric surgery. *Surg Obes Relat Dis.* 2010 May–Jun; **6**(3):322–25.

41. American Society of Anesthesiologists Committee. Practice guidelines for preoperative fasting and the use of pharmacologic agents to reduce the risk of pulmonary aspiration: Application to healthy patients undergoing elective procedures: an updated report by the American Society of Anesthesiologists Committee on Standards and Practice Parameters. *Anesthesiology.* 2011 Mar; **114**(3): 495–511.

42. Rao SL, Kunselman AR, Schuler HG, DesHarnais S. Laryngoscopy and tracheal intubation in the head-elevated position in obese patients: A randomized, controlled, equivalence trial. *Anesth Analg.* 2008 Dec; **107**(6):1912–18.

43. El-Orbany M, Woehlck H, Salem MR. Head and neck position for direct laryngoscopy. *Anesth Analg.* 2011 Jul; **113**(1):103–09.

44. Sacan O, White PF, Tufanogullari B, Klein K. Sugammadex reversal of rocuronium-induced neuromuscular blockade: A comparison with neostigmine–glycopyrrolate and edrophonium–atropine. *Anesth Analg.* 2007 Mar; **104**(3):569–74.

45. Sprung J, Whalley DG, Falcone T, Wilks W, Navratil JE, Bourke DL. The effects of tidal volume and respiratory rate on oxygenation and respiratory mechanics during laparoscopy in morbidly obese patients. *Anesth Analg.* 2003 Jul; **97**(1):268–74.

46. Pelosi P, Gregoretti C. Perioperative management of obese patients. *Best Pract Res Clin Anaesthesiol.* 2010 Jun; **24**(2):211–25.

47. Reinius H, Jonsson L, Gustafsson S, *et al.* Prevention of atelectasis in morbidly obese patients during general anesthesia and paralysis: A computerized tomography study. *Anesthesiology.* 2009 Nov; **111**(5):979–87.

48. Joshi GP, Ahmad S, Riad W, Eckert S, Chung F. Selection of obese patients undergoing ambulatory surgery: A systematic review of the literature. *Anesth Analg.* 2013 Nov; **117**(5):1082–91.

49. Kuratani N, Oi Y. Greater incidence of emergence agitation in children after sevoflurane anesthesia as compared with halothane: A meta-analysis of randomized controlled trials. *Anesthesiology.* 2008 Aug; **109**(2):225–32.

50. Mayer J, Boldt J, Röhm KD, Scheuermann K, Suttner SW. Desflurane anesthesia after sevoflurane inhaled induction reduces severity of emergence agitation in children undergoing minor ear–nose–throat surgery compared with sevoflurane induction and maintenance. *Anesth Analg.* 2006 Feb; **102** (2):400–04.

51. Einarsson SG, Cerne A, Bengtsson A, Stenqvist O, Bengtson JP. Respiration during emergence from anaesthesia with desflurane/N_2O vs. desflurane/air for gynaecological laparoscopy. *Acta Anaesthesiol Scand.* 1998 Nov; **42**(10):1192–98.

52. Lubitz J, Greenberg LG, Gorina Y, Wartzman L, Gibson D. Three decades of health care use by the elderly, 1965–1998. *Health Aff (Millwood)*. 2001 Mar–Apr; **20**(2):19–32.

53. Canet J, Raeder J, Rasmussen LS, *et al.* Cognitive dysfunction after minor surgery in the elderly. *Acta Anaesthesiol Scand*. 2003 Nov; **47**(10):1204–10.

54. Groeben H. Strategies in the patient with compromised respiratory function. *Best Pract Res Clin Anaesthesiol*. 2004 Dec; **18**(4):579–94.

55. Silvanus MT, Groeben H, Peters J. Corticosteroids and inhaled salbutamol in patients with reversible airway obstruction markedly decrease the incidence of bronchospasm after tracheal intubation. *Anesthesiology*. 2004 May; **100**(5):1052–57.

56. Thomsen T, Tønnesen H, Møller AM. Effect of preoperative smoking cessation interventions on postoperative complications and smoking cessation. *Br J Surg*. 2009 May; **96**(5):451–61.

57. Lindström D, Sadr Azodi O, Wladis A, *et al.* Effects of a perioperative smoking cessation intervention on postoperative complications: A randomized trial. *Ann Surg*. 2008 Nov; **248**(5):739–45.

58. Gupta A, Stierer T, Zuckerman R, Sakima N, Parker SD, Fleisher LA. Comparison of recovery profile after ambulatory anesthesia with propofol, isoflurane, sevoflurane and desflurane: A systematic review. *Anesth Analg*. 2004 Mar; **98**(3):632–41.

59. Vaughan J, Nagendran M, Cooper J, Davidson BR, Gurusamy KS. Anaesthetic regimens for day-procedure laparoscopic cholecystectomy. *Cochrane Database Syst Rev*. 2014 Jan 24; **1**:CD009784.

60. Tang J, Chen L, White PF, *et al.* Use of propofol for office-based anesthesia: Effect of nitrous oxide on recovery profile. *J Clin Anesth*. 1999 May; **11**(3):226–30.

61. Michelsen I, Helbo-Hansen HS, Køhler F, Lorenzen AG, Rydlund E, Bentzon MW. Prophylactic ephedrine attenuates the hemodynamic response to propofol in elderly female patients. *Anesth Analg*. 1998 Mar; **86**(3):477–81.

62. Song D, Greilich NB, White PF, Watcha MF, Tongier WK. Recovery profiles and costs of anesthesia for outpatient unilateral inguinal herniorrhaphy. *Anesth Analg*. 2000 Oct; **91**(4):876–81.

63. Li S, Coloma M, White PF, *et al.* Comparison of the costs and recovery profiles of three anesthetic techniques for ambulatory anorectal surgery. *Anesthesiology*. 2000 Nov; **93**(5):1225–30.

64. Silverstein JH, Timberger M, Reich DL, Uysal S. Central nervous system dysfunction after noncardiac surgery and anesthesia in the elderly. *Anesthesiology*. 2007 Mar; **106**(3):622–28.

65. Halaszynski TM. Pain management in the elderly and cognitively impaired patient: The role of regional anesthesia and analgesia. *Curr Opin Anaesthesiol*. 2009 Oct; **22**(5):594–99.

66. Newman S, Stygall J, Hirani S, Shaefi S, Maze M. Postoperative cognitive dysfunction after noncardiac surgery: A systematic review. *Anesthesiology*. 2007 Mar; **106**(3):572–90.

67. Monk TG, Weldon BC, Garvan CW, *et al.* Predictors of cognitive dysfunction after major noncardiac surgery. *Anesthesiology*. 2008 Jan; **108**(1):18–30.

68. Deiner S, Silverstein JH. Postoperative delirium and cognitive dysfunction. *Br J Anaesth*. 2009 Dec; **103**(Suppl 1):i41–46.

69. White PF, White LM, Monk T, *et al.* Perioperative care for the older outpatient undergoing ambulatory surgery. *Anesth Analg*. 2012 Jun; **114**(6):1190–215.

70. http://www.cms.gov/Regulations-and-Guidance/ Guidance/Manuals/downloads/som107ap_l_ ambulatory.pdf

71. Haeck PC, Swanson JA, Iverson RE, *et al.* Evidence-based patient safety advisory: Patient selection and procedures in ambulatory surgery. *Plast Reconstr Surg*. 2009 Oct; **124**(4 Suppl):6S–27S.

72. Yogendran S, Asokumar B, Cheng DC, Chung F. A prospective randomized double-blinded study of the effect of intravenous fluid therapy on adverse outcomes on outpatient surgery. *Anesth Analg*. 1995 Apr; **80**(4):682–86.

73. Ansell GL, Montgomery JE. Outcome of ASA III patients undergoing day case surgery. *Br J Anaesth*. 2004 Jan; **92**(1):71–74.

Postoperative care

Sekar S. Bhavani, MD

Introduction

Patient recovery from surgery and anesthesia is a continual process and is divided into three phases:

1. Early recovery (phase 1) lasts from the discontinuation of anesthesia until patients have recovered their protective reflexes and motor function usually in a monitored setup, the post-anesthesia care unit (PACU).
2. Intermediate recovery (phase 2) begins following transfer out of the PACU and represents the period during which coordination and physiological function normalize such that the patient can be in a state of "street readiness"[1] or "home readiness"-[2] and be able to be transferred to the day surgical unit (DSU) or hospital ward or home in the company of a responsible adult.
3. Late recovery (phase 3) lasts days to weeks depending on the invasiveness of the procedure until the patient has fully recovered and returned to their baseline state.

Phase 1 recovery

Patients undergoing a surgical procedure under anesthetic care should be carefully monitored and routinely assessed in the postoperative period in order to prevent an adverse outcome. The adverse outcome could be due to the underlying disease process, surgical trauma, or perioperative anesthetic management. This can be prevented to a large extent by appropriate selection of patients, careful monitoring in the recovery unit, and early recognition and management. This strategy allows us to identify patients at risk, intervene and correct any life-threatening conditions in a timely fashion, to identify patients who need further monitoring during overnight stay, and prevent unscheduled readmissions following discharge. This periodic assessment should ideally include:

1. temperature,
2. cardiovascular assessment,
3. respiratory assessment,
4. neurological assessment, including consciousness and cognitive skills,
5. neuromuscular blockade and regional blockade assessment,
6. pain,
7. postoperative nausea and vomiting (PONV),
8. hydration status and hematological status.

Temperature

Hypothermia and hyperthermia are both associated with an adverse outcome. Hypothermia has been associated with increased incidence of shivering, delayed emergence from anesthesia, prolongation of neuromuscular blockade,[3] cardiac events including arrhythmias and myocardial ischemia,[3–5] delayed wound healing,[6,7] immunosuppression,[3,4] surgical wound infections,[3,6,7] coagulation defects, increased need for transfusion,[3,4,7,8] and patient dissatisfaction.

Hypothermia is caused by a combination of peripheral vasodilatation and redistribution of body heat, suppression of the normal thermogenic mechanisms by anesthetics and muscle relaxants, and loss of heat due to exposure to a colder environment. This results in a colder core temperature and peripheral vasoconstriction as the patient recovers from the effects of anesthesia. It should be realized that neuraxial anesthesia can also produce significant losses that are comparable to those observed during general anesthesia.[9]

Practical Ambulatory Anesthesia, ed. Johan Raeder and Richard D. Urman. Published by Cambridge University Press. © Cambridge University Press 2015.

Shivering

Postoperative shivering is an involuntary clonic movement of different muscles, often seen in the post-anesthesia care unit (PACU). The incidence has been described to be anywhere between 6% and 66%.[10] It is a frequent problem after general anesthesia and is less commonly seen after regional anesthesia and propofol-based techniques as opposed to inhalational techniques.

The etiology of postoperative shivering could be part of a thermoregulatory mechanism and thus associated with peripheral vasoconstriction, or non-thermogenic in nature as seen in normothermic patients with peripheral vasodilatation. The shivering in hypothermic patients could be explained as an attempt of the body to maintain normothermia due to a decrease in the core body temperature. The pathogenesis in normothermic patients has been hypothesized to be due to postoperative pain,[11,12] the effects of anesthetics,[13] hypercapnia or respiratory alkalosis, as part of a systemic inflammatory reaction to the stress of surgery,[14] or earlier recovery of spinal reflex activity as compared to the brain and sympathetic over-activity.[10,13] Three independent risk factors that were identified by multivariate analysis included younger age, endoprosthetic surgery, and lower core body temperature.[12]

Effects of shivering

Shivering is not only distressing to patients but also increases the oxygen requirements, increases CO_2 production, and is associated with an increased sympathetic response. This results in tachycardia, tachypnea, and increased heart rate, blood pressure, and cardiac output. Although never demonstrated, it could theoretically increase the risk of an adverse cardiac event in patients with a compromised coronary circulation. It can also induce pain due to stretching and disruption of the surgical wounds. Shivering in addition interferes with monitoring of the vital signs and pulse oximetry in the PACU.

Prevention and management

Prevention of perioperative hypothermia will reduce the incidence of post-anesthetic shivering.

1. As patients mainly lose heat through radiation and convection on the skin surface,[9] a simple maneuver of covering the exposed surfaces of the body and wrapping the extremities in children would significantly decrease such a loss.
2. As the initial loss due to redistribution usually occurs in the first hour, preoperative skin surface warming for an hour prior to surgery has been shown to be helpful during short procedures.[15]
3. Raising the operating room temperature would also address radiation and convection losses.

Medical treatment

1. Evaluate the patient and confirm the core temperature.
2. If the patient is hypothermic, initiate rewarming. Perioperative warming using a forced air-warming unit has been shown to be the most efficient.[10]
3. When transfusion of a large volume of crystalloid or colloid or of cold blood products is needed, intravenous solution rewarming can prevent the patient from cooling down.[9]
4. In addition, radiant heat systems efficiently prevent post-anesthetic shivering by increasing the skin temperature of the exposed parts.
5. There are many effective drugs for preventing or stopping post-anesthetic shivering and they act at different sites. These include the commonly used opiates: μ-receptor agonists (morphine, fentanyl, sufentanil, meperidine), tramadol, α2-agonists (clonidine and dexmedetomidine), anticholinergics (chlorpromazine), NMDA antagonists (ketamine), $5HT_3$ antagonist (ondasetron, granisetron), cholinesterase inhibitors (physostigmine), doxapram, nefopam, magnesium, steroids, etc.
6. Of the opioids, meperidine has the best effect at low doses, i.e., 10–20 mg IV in an adult.
7. Clonidine (as a bolus) and dexmedetomidine infusion lower the threshold for cutaneous vasoconstriction and shivering.[10] The α2-agonists work centrally to prevent shivering. Tramadol, ketanserin, nefopam, and ondasetron act by inhibiting the serotonin uptake centrally. Physostigmine, nefopam, and doxapram act by facilitating the inhibitory pathways. The mechanism of action of magnesium is not known.

Hyperthermia

Hyperthermia can be thought of as a failure of the normal thermoregulation and associated elevation of core body temperature above the normal diurnal range of 36–37.5°C.

Effects of hyperthermia

An increase in the body temperature results in an increase in the basal metabolic rate, increased oxygen consumption, tachycardia, tachypnea, hypercarbia, and a reduced mixed venous oxygen saturation. The increased oxygen demand can aggravate pre-existing cardiac or pulmonary insufficiency. For every degree increase above 37°C the basic metabolic rate increases by 13%. Very high temperatures above 42°C may lead to multiple organ failure.

Malignant hyperthermia (MH) is a rare genetic disorder that can be triggered by exposure to the depolarizing NMB (succinylcholine) or exposure to volatile inhaled anesthetic agents. The term "malignant hyperthermia" is misleading and hyperthermia may be a late finding. It is important to recognize the symptoms and signs of MH (resistant hypercarbia in intubated patients, tachycardia, metabolic and respiratory acidosis, hyperkalemia, and evidence of rhabdomyolysis). It can rapidly prove fatal unless it is recognized early and dantrolene therapy is initiated.

Prevention of hyperthermia

1. Preoperative evaluation with emphasis on:
   a. family history of MH,
   b. allergies,
   c. drug interactions,
   d. management of infections with appropriate antibiotics.
2. Intraoperative monitoring for early detection.
3. Meticulous aseptic technique when invasive access is considered.
4. Prophylactic antibiotics when indicated.

Management

1. Reconfirm and monitor core temperature if possible.
2. Continue to monitor the patient in the PACU.
3. Acetaminophen IV or PO can be given for control of fever.
4. Cold sponging can help but may interfere with monitoring and access.
5. Ice packs can be placed in the axilla, groin, and neck.
6. Cold gastric lavage and cooling blankets can also be used as appropriate. Shivering may occur when active cooling methods are used and it can be suppressed with meperidine, clonidine, or benzodiazepines.
7. Appropriate management for the conditions that have similar presenting signs (MH, neuroleptic malignant syndrome, thyroid crisis) should be initiated if they are the suspected cause of fever. This can help to prevent morbidity/mortality.

Cardiovascular assessment

The cardiac monitoring for an ambulatory setup is no different from that for a routine surgery. The ECG, noninvasive blood pressure, and a pulse oximeter should be routinely monitored during emergence and recovery every 5 minutes.[16] Most recovery units do not need to have the provision for continuous diagnostic ECG and ST segment monitoring, but they should have the facility to monitor the ECG for rate, rhythm, and changes that might alert us to the need for advanced monitoring. Facility for a standard 12-lead ECG should, however, be immediately available.[16]

The heart rate should be carefully monitored in the perioperative period. Any cause for bradycardia (less than 50 BPM) or tachycardia (greater than 120 BPM) should be sought and treated as appropriate.

Bradycardia should be considered clinically significant and warrants treatment if there is evidence of compromised cardiac output causing symptomatic hypotension. Always compare the monitored to historical data if available.

1. Look for a differential diagnosis and correct possible causes of symptomatic bradycardia.
2. Sinus bradycardia can occur as a result of increased vagal tome or due to sympathetic paralysis, as quite frequently seen when opioids (e.g., remifentanil) are given in higher doses than needed for surgery.
3. Look at the rhythm and determine the presence of a block. Rule out complete heart block, as it may be an ominous sign.
4. Atropine (0.5–1.0 mg IV) may be administered initially, but if the patient is unstable, initiate a cardiac consultation.

In the initial evaluation of tachycardia, rule out hemodynamic instability (hypotension, shortness of breath, signs of heart failure, MI, shock, altered mental status). It would be wise to initiate rescue and management in the presence of instability.

Hypertension

The usual causes should be considered, which include patients who did not receive their antihypertensive medications preoperatively; anxiety, pain, hypoxemia, and hypercarbia should also be considered. An iatrogenic cause, such as administration of medications that can raise blood pressure, should also be considered. It is important to remember the epinephrine effect from local anesthetics given, and the sympathomimetic effect of desflurane given too fast and high.

Hypotension

Common causes of hypotension include residual anesthetic agents, other medications that can lower the blood pressure, hypovolemia, hemorrhage, loss of sympathetic tone as sometimes seen with spinal or epidural anesthesia, impaired venous return seen in tension pneumothorax, myocardial dysfunction, and cardiac arrhythmias. Remember that anaphylaxis may start with hypotension as the only clinical sign.

Management

1. Monitor vital signs every 5 minutes for 15 minutes and every 15 minutes until time of discharge.
2. Look at past records and medications. Review the medications used intraoperatively and rule out an allergic reaction.
3. Routine care should be included in addition to cardiac monitoring and oxygen supplementation. Consider blood gas analysis and a metabolic profile (looking for hypoxia, hypercarbia, metabolic acidosis, hypokalemia, hypomagnesemia, or drug toxicities). Rule out pain and anxiety.
4. Administer pain medications, oxygen supplementation (as appropriate).
5. Consider a 12-lead ECG and obtain a cardiac consultation.
6. Initiate preoperative cardiac medications if appropriate.
7. Evaluate the rhythm and see if the arrhythmia is shockable.
8. Consider cardioversion if the patient becomes unstable.
9. Consider transfer to a facility for further evaluation for cardiac ischemia. 12-Lead ECG and 3 sets of cardiac enzymes at 8-hour intervals and initiate cardiovascular support and admission to the facility if you suspect an adverse event.

Hemodynamic stability is a requisite prior to discharge from the PACU. The patients should be hemodynamically stable, on no inotropic support, and within ±20 of baseline vital signs prior to discharge from the PACU. Sometimes the preoperative BP may be increased due to stress, requiring modification of the ±20 rule. In those situations, if other causes of elevated blood pressure have been ruled out the patient may be discharged if other criteria are met.

Respiratory assessment

The majority of healthy patients undergoing ambulatory surgery can be safely transported from the operating room to the PACU while breathing room air. Older patients (> 60 years), obese patients (> 100 kg), and patients who have received nitrous oxide until the end of anesthesia may be at increased risk for oxygen desaturation when breathing room air on transport to the PACU and may require oxygen supplementation. In addition, patients with underlying lung disease or severe systemic disease may need oxygen supplementation. Once the patient arrives in the PACU, a repeat assessment should be performed and a plan for recovery and discharge should be formulated. Respiratory assessment should not only include assessment of the respiratory rate but also the mechanics of breathing (including the rhythm, chest wall and abdominal wall motion, depth of breathing), assessment for obstruction in the upper or lower airway, and oxygen saturation. If there is a significant concern for postoperative respiratory failure, an arterial blood gas analysis may be appropriate. Patients with inadequate ventilation may present with anxiety, confusion, dyspnea, tachypnea, and increased sympathetic nervous system activity – resulting in perspiration, tachycardia, and hypertension. They may also present with mental status changes.

The use of a pulse oximeter is mandatory in this setting. It can provide a late warning of hypoxemia, which is usually preceded by a period of hypoventilation or compromised airway. When patients are supplied with oxygen (mask or nasal cannula), the pulse oximeter may provide adequate values until there is a sudden drop of oxygen concentration in the blood. If supplemental oxygen is not used or is used at lower concentration, there may be a more gradual drop in oxygenation that can be detected earlier when hypoventilation occurs. Therefore, one option for an earlier detection of hypoventilation in a postoperative patient is to use respiratory rate monitoring by either a capnograph or other available device.

Pathogenesis

The respiratory depression seen in the early recovery period may be due to the residual effect of the anesthetic, depression of the ventilator centers due to the effects of hypoxemia and hypercarbia, incomplete reversal of the neuromuscular drugs, excessive use of sedatives and opioids, or a neurological event. Hypoxemia and hypercapnia may develop during transfer to the PACU when supplemental oxygen has been discontinued. Another important aspect to consider is decreased stimulation following surgery and extubation, and the effects of opioids used in the intraoperative period that may lead to hypoventilation. The use of NSAIDs, acetaminophen, local anesthetics, nerve blocks, and regional anesthesia can play a very significant role in preventing this effect and having an opioid-sparing effect.

Obstructive sleep apnea (OSA), obesity, and increased intra-abdominal pressure may interfere with the mechanics of breathing and produce respiratory insufficiency. Upper airway obstruction due to pre-existing neurological deficit, incomplete neuromuscular reversal, inability to clear secretions, and laryngospasm may all also contribute to the postoperative respiratory difficulty, due to chest wall splinting.

Airway obstruction

Airway obstruction in the perioperative period may be caused by multiple factors. This may involve the upper or lower airway and can quickly overwhelm the respiratory reserve of patients who are recovering from anesthesia.

In most cases the cause of upper respiratory obstruction is due to the tongue falling back and obstructing the oropharynx. Less common causes include laryngospasm, secretions, blood or vomitus in airway, or external pressure (i.e., neck hematoma). When this obstruction is partial, the patient may develop stridor. When the obstruction becomes severe, there may be mental status changes with gasping breaths. In addition, there may be a paradoxical movement of the chest and abdomen with inspiratory efforts. Auscultation of the chest would confirm the absence of breath sounds.

Management

1. Assess the patient to confirm the diagnosis and determine the cause. Talk to the patient, check chest/stomach movement, check warm air out of mouth/nose during expiration, and count the respiratory rate.
2. Rule out any upper airway obstruction due to secretions, laryngospasm.
3. Auscultate the chest and confirm bilateral equal air entry and rule out bronchospasm.
4. Assess for neuromuscular weakness in case NBs were used and reversal was administered.
5. Continue to monitor the patient's oxygen saturation and if indicated also monitor exhaled CO_2 and obtain an arterial blood gas analysis, if indicated.
6. Rescue the patient with oxygen supplementation.
7. Have the patient sit upright so that the work of breathing is decreased should the hemodynamics and nature of surgery permit.

8. Treat the reversible causes as appropriate (anemia, hypovolemia).
9. If you suspect upper respiratory obstruction due to the tongue falling back, do a jaw thrust and head tilt.
   a. Use an oral or nasal airway.
   b. Consider laryngospasm if obstruction persists. Clear the secretions and blood if present from the oropharynx.
   c. Try jaw thrust and use positive pressure mask ventilation.
   d. If this fails to break the laryngospasm, consider using a small dose of succinylcholine (10–20 mg) and positive pressure ventilation with 100% oxygen to prevent hypoxemia or negative pressure pulmonary edema. If succinylcholine is contraindicated, propofol may be administered.
   e. Consider endotracheal intubation to protect the airway.
10. If the patient has a history of OSA, consider CPAP.
11. Control pain by minimizing opioid medications and using alternate techniques as appropriate.
12. If aspiration is suspected or the patient does not respond to the above management, consider admission for observation, evaluation, and support.

The patient should be arousable, able to maintain the airway, cough and clear secretions, breathe without tachypnea, and maintain an oxygen saturation of > 92% on room air prior to discharge from the recovery unit, except in cases with known pulmonary disease and everyday baseline oxygenation.

Assessment of neuromuscular function

The assessment of neuromuscular blockade is particularly important in patients who have received intermediate-acting non-depolarizing neuromuscular blocking agents and patients who have a pre-existing underlying neuromuscular dysfunction. When there is marked weakness following the use of a succinylcholine or mivacurium, the possibility of cholinesterase deficiency should be investigated and the airway supported, if required.

Postoperative muscle weakness can lead to inability to maintain and protect the airway, inability to cough and clear secretions, hypoventilation, and postoperative respiratory insufficiency (hypoxia and hypercapnia). This can manifest as delayed wakening, drowsiness, mental status changes, confusion and agitation, aspiration, and hemodynamic instability.

Vigilance and recognition of the weakness can prevent adverse outcome.

Evaluation

Simple bedside evaluation should include sustained head elevation test (for >5 seconds), elevation of the leg in patients who cannot elevate the head, return of hand grip strength to the baseline, ability to bite down on a tongue depressor, or a train-of-four ratio of more than 70–90% on a peripheral nerve stimulator. If a patient can achieve an inspiratory force of negative 40 cm of water, a tidal volume of 10–12 ml/kg, they are much less likely to need ventilator support.

Management

1. Management of the incomplete reversal may involve a watchful wait for the effect of the neuromuscular blockade to regress, administration of reversal, if indicated, or control of the airway should respiratory failure be imminent.
2. The lowest efficacious dose of neostigmine should be used to prevent some of the side effects and decrease the incidence of PONV (0.015–0.025 mg/kg).[17]
3. Sugammadex is a selective reversal agent capable of reversing deeper neuromuscular block induced by rocuronium or vecuronium. However, it is not yet approved for use in the United States.

Neurological assessment

Neurological assessment should include a careful search for new mental status changes.[16] These may present as delayed wakening, postoperative agitation, and psychological changes such as anxiety or panic attacks, weakness, or coma. Consciousness involves awareness to time, space, and person. One of the main requirements for discharge from an ambulatory facility is the return to the baseline conscious level.

Somnolence

Postoperative delayed awakening is an uncommon outcome after routine anesthesia for ambulatory anesthesia. However, a number of factors including patient-related, anesthetic-related, and systemic diseases can all affect the length of emergence and recovery from anesthesia.

Management

1. Check the vital signs and confirm diagnosis.
   a. Assess the airway, breathing, and cardiovascular status.
   b. Check the temperature.
   c. Check the SaO_2.
2. Assess the neurological status.
3. Rescue the patient and protect the airway. Administer oxygen, if indicated.

Table 9.1 Risk factors for delayed emergence.

Patient-related	Extremes of age
	Genetic factors that delay metabolism of commonly used anesthetics or muscle relaxants
	Severe hepatic or renal disease that interferes with the metabolism and excretion of the medications
	Very rare, but reported: prolonged emergence (hours) from propofol without any other symptoms
Intraoperative-related	Prolonged operation time
	Use of muscle relaxants
	Pharmacodynamic and pharmacokinetic properties, context-sensitive half-lives, drug potentiation, interactions and metabolism of muscle relaxants, opioids, anesthetics, and benzodiazepines and anticholinergics
Cardiovascular	Hypotension, hypertension
	Severe cardiovascular instability, shock, cardiac arrest
Respiratory	Hypoxia, hypercapnia
Neurological	Stroke, post-seizure
	Intracranial event
Metabolic	Hypoglycemia, hyperglycemia
	Hyponatremia, hypernatremia
	Hypothermia
Systemic	Severe hepatic or renal dysfunction
	Hypothyroidism

4. Carefully review the historical data for systemic diseases, medications, and intraoperative anesthetic records.

5. Assess for neuromuscular blockade reversal. Support the airway and consider reversal, if indicated.

6. Assess the pupils to rule out a neurological event or opioid overdose. If you suspect opioid overdose, consider naloxone (increments of 0.1 mg IV, repeated after 3–4 min if no response). May repeat every 2–3 min as needed. Higher doses may be needed in case of buprenorphine overdosing. Monitor to prevent relapse of symptoms. May cause nausea and vomiting, reversal of analgesia, delirium, agitation, tachycardia, hypotension or hypertension, tremors, tachypnea, and acute opioid withdrawal symptoms). If you suspect benzodiazepine overdose, consider flumazenil (0.2 mg repeated every minute to a maximum dose of 1 mg or until the desired effect is seen. Flumazenil may cause seizures in susceptible patients, blurred vision, and headache).

7. If possible, obtain an arterial blood gas analysis and a basic metabolic profile. Correct any metabolic derangements.

8. Check blood glucose.

9. If you suspect a neurological event, consider a CT scan/MRI.

10. If you suspect anticholinergic crisis, consider physostigmine administration.

Postoperative delirium

Postoperative delirium may occur in any patient after general anesthesia, but occurs more frequently in the elderly or in patients with an alcohol, drug, or opioid abuse problem. The incidence reported has varied between 4% and 53%.[18] It is also commonly seen in children. It may be seen in as many as half of elderly patients after general anesthesia,[18] and is more common after emergency procedures and extensive surgery. As most of these changes occur after 24–48 hours, they may not be evident in the PACU, but are likely to become an issue after discharge from the hospital. It may be very subtle and present with inability to concentrate and may present as memory fluctuations and silent delirium. This may also be associated with decline in cognitive function. In some patients, it may present as agitation, hyperactivity, and mania, while in others it may be associated with catatonia and withdrawal.

Risk factors for delirium:[19,20]

- Increased age
- Male gender
- ASA class III
- Rapidity of development of the physical insult
- Preoperative alcohol abuse
- Preoperative cognitive impairment
- Preoperative depression
- Presence of multiple comorbidities – hepatic or renal impairment
- Visual or hearing impairment
- Electrolyte imbalance
- Hypoalbuminemia
- Vascular surgery and orthopedic surgery
- Emergency surgery[18]

Management

1. Preventive measures[21]

   a. Appropriate environmental stimuli
   b. Preoperative counseling
   c. Maintenance of oxygen delivery by supplemental oxygen, preventing anemia, and maintaining volume status
   d. Decreasing the dose of opioids and anticholinergics and avoiding benzodiazepines in geriatric patients
   e. Multimodal pain management with less dependence on opioids
   f. Maintaining bowel and bladder function
   g. Early mobilization

2. Several drugs that target receptors thought to play a role in delirium have been tried and they include drugs effective against the cholinergic (donepexil and rivastigmine), dopaminergic (haloperidol), serotonergic (quetiapine, risperidone, olanzapine), and noradrenergic system (dexmedetomidine) and GABA$_A$ receptors (benzodiazepines for alcohol withdrawal-related delirium).[21]

In general, haloperidol may be tried initially. If alcohol withdrawal is suspected, then benzodiazepine treatment is recommended.

Pain assessment and management

Pain is a subjective and unpleasant experience resulting from tissue damage or potential tissue damage and is mediated through pain receptors and pain nerve fibers. Postoperative management of pain in an ambulatory setting is more challenging as we need to balance the need for analgesics to assure patient comfort and the need for discharge to, and recovery at home. The concept of multimodal analgesia involves finding a balance with a combination of opioid and non-opioid analgesics (local analgesics, non-steroidal anti-inflammatory drugs [NSAIDs], and/or acetaminophen) and combining them with non-pharmacological techniques that act at both the central and peripheral sites (regional blocks with or without indwelling catheters). The goal is to improve pain control while eliminating the opioid-related side effects that lead to delay in discharge and readmission into the hospital.[22–27] Pain control not only allows for better patient satisfaction but also prevents the development of chronic pain syndromes.

The Joint Commission mandates pain control as an important component of routine patient care in 2000, and in 2002 a numerical scale of 1–10 was introduced and mandated to be used in the PACU.[28] Frasco et al. showed that this initiative led to an increased use of opioids to control the pain but failed to demonstrate an increased incidence of adverse events or delayed discharge from the PACU.[28] A study by Vila and colleagues, however, showed that this was associated with more than a twofold increase in the incidence of opioid-induced sedation.[29] A more detailed discussion on pathogenesis and management can be found in Chapters 4 and 14.

Postoperative and post-discharge nausea and vomiting

Postoperative nausea and vomiting is one of the most frequent distressing side effects following an ambulatory surgical procedure.[30] Although it is non-fatal in healthy adults, it is associated with considerable patient distress, delayed PACU discharge, and higher costs. Patients rated vomiting and gagging on the endotracheal tube to be more distressing than incisional pain.[31]

Definition

Nausea is defined as a sensation of unease and discomfort in the upper abdomen with an urge to retch or vomit. It often, but not always, precedes vomiting. The pathogenesis is not completely understood. Nausea being a subjective symptom may be difficult to sort out in children and in patients with communication difficulties. Nausea may be reinforced by unpleasant sensations such as smell, taste, pain, and anxiety.

Vomiting is defined as a forceful expulsion of the contents of the stomach through the mouth or the nose. Retching is similar to vomiting but occurs when there are no stomach contents expelled. Vomiting and retching are objective signs.

Consequences

Protracted vomiting can lead to delayed oral intake due to the physiological response to nausea and vomiting leading to increased salivation, sweating, dehydration, electrolyte imbalances, tachycardia, hypotension, cardiac arrhythmias and, in susceptible patients, coronary insufficiency. The interruption of nutrition and oral drugs might lead to unforeseen consequences or the need for admission and institution of intravenous drug therapy. The mechanical stress of retching and vomiting can lead to Mallory Weiss tear, esophageal rupture, muscular strain, bleeding and hematoma formation, disruption of surgical repair and skin grafts,[32] and increased intraocular and intracranial pressures. The onset of vomiting in a patient emerging from anesthesia also increases the risk of aspiration due to failure to protect the airway. The extra workload will lead to higher hospital and insurance costs, delayed discharge from the PACU, and unplanned admissions. All of these lead to poor patient satisfaction scores that can affect reimbursements.

Management of PONV and prevention of PDNV

The management is divided into three stages.
1. Identify patients at high risk.
2. Reduce the baseline risk factors.
3. Intervene with medications and alternate techniques, when appropriate.

Identification of patients at risk

Given the morbidity and financial implications, there is a very strong incentive to proactively prevent PONV in susceptible patients in an ambulatory setting. However, not all patients have the same risk profile for PONV, and hence it is important to identify the high-risk patients in whom it is likely to do the most good and avoid the untoward side effects of the anti-emetic medications and associated costs of care. In a meta-analysis to establish independent and potentially causal predictors for PONV, Patel and colleagues concluded that the most reliable independent predictors of PONV were female gender, history of PONV or motion sickness, non-smoker, younger age, duration of anesthesia with volatile anesthetics, and postoperative opioids.[33]

The contributing factors for PONV can be broadly classified under: patient-related factors,

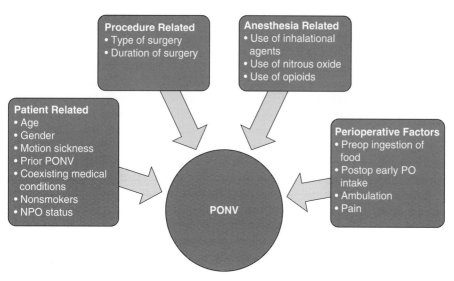

Figure 9.1 Contributing factors for PONV.

surgery-related, anesthesia-related, and perioperative management issues (Figure 9.1).

Reducing the baseline risk

The management of PONV should start with prevention. After identifying patients at a higher risk for PONV, it is important that we first reduce the baseline risk that can lead to PONV. This reduction of risk in mild cases and in patients with a low risk may be sufficient to avoid PONV. These include the following.[34]

1. The use of regional anesthesia when feasible.
2. The use of propofol and TIVA in place of inhalational agents.
3. Avoidance of nitrous oxide.
4. Limiting the use of opioids in the perioperative period and the use of alternate modalities for pain control.
5. Using prophylactic anti-emetics.
6. Adequate perioperative hydration.

Medications and interventions

A clinical decision to initiate anti-emetic measures is dependent on the characteristics of the patient and the clinical scenario. The use of routine anti-emetic prophylaxis is not recommended but should be used only when the patient's risk is sufficiently high and the benefits of therapy are clear.[34,35] The benefits may be obvious in some situations where vomiting might pose a high medical risk due to the surgical procedure

(gastric or esophageal surgery, intraocular procedures), underlying medical condition (increased ICP, IOP) or when the risk of aspiration is high (wired jaws, altered mental status). We need to be aware of the benefits and side effects of the medications as the latter may outweigh their perceived benefits due to associated medical conditions (e.g., prolonged QTc). The patient's preferences also weigh into the decision process.

Algorithm for PONV management

1. Prophylaxis in low-risk patients (1 risk factor, risk score < 10%): prophylaxis is rarely justified. The risks of treatment (sedation, headache, low BP, QT prolongations, Torsade's de pointes, etc.) should be weighed against the patient's preference and medical concerns due to vomiting (e.g., a middle--aged male smoker having a microlaryngoscopy).
2. Moderate-risk patients (2–3 risk factors, risk score 20–40%): consider 1 or 2 anti-emetic drugs or measures (e.g., total intravenous anesthesia [TIVA] with opioid and no other anti-emetic drugs, or 4 mg of dexamethasone and block to minimize opioid consumption). An example is a middle-aged, non-smoking female with no other known risk factors undergoing a laparoscopic gynecologic surgery.
3. High-risk patients (> 3 risk factors, risk score > 60%): consider combination treatment (e.g., regional anesthesia instead of GA, or TIVA with additional anti-emetic).

Treatment guidelines suggest that outpatients should receive longer-acting anti-emetic measures.

Different mechanisms of anti-emetic strategies have additive effects. For a more detailed discussion, readers are referred to Chapters 4 and 14.

Postoperative fluid management and hydration

Postoperative hydration status should be optimized prior to discharge from the PACU. This might involve administering IV fluids or blood and blood components. An indirect way to assess the fluid status is to assess urine output. The amount and type of fluids administered will depend on the patient characteristics (age, preoperative blood count, coagulation parameters), intraoperative course (massive fluid shifts, blood loss) and postoperative hemodynamics. Normally the IV crystalloids are continued into the perioperative period until the oral intake is established and no significant nausea and vomiting exists.

Postoperative renal function and urine output

The current recommendations do not support the need to monitor urine output and voiding in the PACU routinely in all patients, but it may be useful in selected patients.[16] However, monitoring of voiding, although not considered a discharge criterion, would still be useful particularly in patients who have had instrumentation of the urogenital tract or pelvic surgery.

Drainage and bleeding

Monitoring of bleeding and discharge is recommended in the perioperative period for early detection of complications that might need admission, transfusion, or return to the operating room.

Discharge criteria

The last few decades have seen an exponential increase in the number and complexity of surgical procedures done in an ambulatory environment driven by innovations in surgical technique, better anesthetic drugs, improvement in perioperative monitoring techniques, and economic and societal pressures.[36,37] The presence of a well-designed discharge criterion would help the nursing staff assess and manage the patients better, allow to quantitate the progress of recovery, avoid delay to discharge, and allow for comparison between centers. These criteria have been endorsed by and mandated by both the Joint Commission and other accrediting and regulatory bodies. However, there are some limitations to standard criteria as they are not applicable to all patients, surgical procedures, anesthetic techniques, and patient-related specific factors. It is also important to have historical data available

regarding baseline vital signs as they might be inaccurate on the day of surgery due to anxiety.[38]

Aldrete scoring system

Aldrete and Kroulik in 1970 proposed the Post-Anesthetic Recovery Score (PARS), a method analogous to the universally adopted APGAR score which included activity, respiration, circulation, state of consciousness, and color for evaluating patients after anesthesia for their fitness to be discharged from PACU. Numerical scores of 2, 1, or 0 were given depending on their absence or presence. The numbers given to each sign were then added. A score of 10 indicated a patient in the best possible condition. Totals of 8 or 9 were noted to be acceptable for discharge from the recovery room to a step-down unit or ASU, where phase II recovery continued. Total scores of 7 or less in most cases indicated a need for continued close observation.

After the introduction of pulse oximetry, it quickly became obvious that it provided an easy and accurate method of evaluation of the oxygenation of the patients.[1,39,40] This led to the introduction of the modified Aldrete scale, where the color index was replaced by pulse oximeter values. A cut-off of 92% was arrived at by the work of Downs et al., who showed that when the SaO_2 was 92% or higher on room air, there was no need for routine supplemental oxygen.[41]

The PARS system only allowed us to transition the patient from phase I to phase II care. In order to meet the requirements for discharge to home (phase III), Aldrete proposed another modification and included five additional components, namely: appearance of the dressing, severity of pain, ability to stand and ambulate, tolerance of oral fluids, and ability to urinate to reflect "street fitness".[1] Patients were considered fit to be discharged home when their total score is 18 or higher.[1]

However, the limitations of the above scoring system became apparent, because in cases of subarachnoid or epidural (lumbar or caudal) anesthesia, patients may be unable to void for some time, even after obtaining full recovery of sensory and motor functions.

Post-anesthetic discharge scoring system

Chung et al.[2] proposed the Post-Anesthetic Discharge Scoring System (PADSS). This discharge criterion was proposed to assess patients' "home-readiness" prior to discharge into the care of a responsible adult. It mainly incorporated five parameters: vital signs; activity and mental status; control of pain, nausea, and vomiting; surgical bleeding; and

Table 9.2 Modified* Aldrete score.

Criteria	2	1	0
Activity	Moves all four extremities voluntarily or on command	Moves two extremities voluntarily or on command	None
Respiration	Breathes normally, coughs easily	Dyspnea, shallow or limited breathing	Apneic
Circulation	BP ± 20 mm of baseline	BP ± 20–50 mm of baseline	BP ± 50 mm of baseline
Consciousness	Fully awake	Arousable	Not responding
Oxygen saturation*	Maintains $SaO_2 > 92\%$ on room air	Maintains $SaO_2 > 90\%$ on supplemental oxygen	Unable to maintain $SaO_2 > 90\%$ even on supplemental oxygen
Color	Pink	Pale, "dusky," or "blotchy" discoloration, as well as jaundice	Cyanotic

Modified from Aldrete, J. A. and Kroulik, D.; A post anesthesia recovery score: *Anesthesia and Analgesia* 1970; 49(6): 924–34.

Table 9.3 Additions made to the PAR scoring system for "street fitness".

Criteria	2	1	0
Dressing	Dry and clean	Wet but stationary	Growing area of wetness
Pain	Pain free	Mild pain controlled with oral medications	Severe pain requiring parenteral medications
Ambulation	Able to standup and walk	Vertigo when erect	Dizziness on supine
Feeding	Able to drink fluids	Nauseated or still fasting	Nausea and vomiting
Urine output	Voided	Unable to void but comfortable	Unable to void but uncomfortable

Modified from Aldrete, J. A. The post-anesthesia recovery score revisited (letters to editor). *J Clin Anesth* 1995; 7: 89–91.

Table 9.4 Post-Anesthetic Discharge Scoring System.

Criteria	2	1	0
Vital signs	Within ± 20% of baseline	Within ± 20–40% of baseline	Greater than 40% of baseline value
Activity and mental status	Oriented × 3 and has a steady gait	Oriented × 3 OR has a steady gait	Neither
Pain, nausea and vomiting	Minimal	Moderate having required treatment	Severe requiring treatment
Surgical bleeding	Minimal	Moderate	Severe
Intake and output	Has had PO fluids AND voided	Has had PO fluids OR voided	Neither

Modified from Frances Chung, Vincent W.S. Chan, Dennis Ong, A Post-Anesthetic Discharge Scoring System for Home Readiness after Ambulatory Surgery. *J Clin Anesth* 1995; 7:500–06.

intake and output.[2] Numerical scores of 2, 1, or 0 were given depending on set criteria and the numbers given to each sign were then added. A score of 9 or above indicated a patient to be "home-ready".

Discharge criteria have continued to evolve and have been amended by various authors with a greater understanding of the outcome following ambulatory anesthesia and the reasons for readmission following discharge. In addition, waiting for complete resolution of blocks or neuraxial anesthesia resulted in delay. Some of the current modifications are discussed below.

Separation of pain and nausea and vomiting

Pain and nausea and vomiting were the two most common reasons for readmission following discharge from the ambulatory center. In order to give the required weightage when considering discharge, it was realized that they had to be considered separately on their own merits.

Removal of the criteria for need to urinate before discharge

The risk factors for postoperative retention of urine include a history of prior postoperative urinary retention, neuraxial anesthesia (spinal and epidural), surgery on the urogenital tract, pelvis and the anal canal, anticholinergics, and underlying medical conditions.[42–46] Urinary retention may lead to bladder over-distension, resulting in atony and inability to void following discharge from the ambulatory center.

1. Thus, patients in low-risk categories should not be required to void before discharge.

2. In patients who did not have a urinary catheter placed during surgery, the IV fluids should be used judiciously in order to prevent bladder over-distension.[43]

3. It has been suggested that ultrasound monitoring can be used to facilitate the timing of catheterization in patients at high risk of retention.[42] In case scanning facilities are not available, the bladder should be evacuated if the patient has not voided by the time he has reached the other criteria for discharge.

4. Patients who have been catheterized or who have not voided by the time of discharge should be encouraged to return to the facility or the emergency room should they fail to void in 8 hours.

Removal of the criteria for need to tolerate oral feeds

The requirement of drinking clear fluids should not be part of a discharge protocol and may only be necessary for selected patients.[16] Elimination of this criterion can shorten the stay without adversely affecting outcome following ambulatory anesthesia.[47] In a large study of almost 1000 patients, Schreiner et al.[48] showed that in pediatric patients it was unnecessary to make drinking a requisite for discharge from the day surgery center. The goal for perioperative fluid management should be to administer sufficient intravenous fluids to cover the calculated preoperative deficit, the intraoperative maintenance, and the intraoperative losses, thus preventing dehydration.[48]

The current modification that is used as a discharge criterion is the modified PADSS which

Table 9.5 Modified PADSS.

Criteria	2	1	0
Vital signs	Within ± 20% of baseline	Within ± 20–40% of baseline	Greater than 40% of baseline value
Activity	Steady gait, no dizziness	Able to ambulate with assistance	Unable to ambulate
Nausea and vomiting	None or minimal and controlled with PO medications	Moderate and treated with IV medications	Severe and poorly controlled
Pain	Minimal (0–3)	Moderate (4–6) required treatment	Severe (7–10) requiring treatment
Surgical bleeding	None or minimal	Moderate	Severe

Modified from Frances Chung, Vincent W.S. Chan, Dennis Ong, A Post-Anesthetic Discharge Scoring System for Home Readiness after Ambulatory Surgery. *J Clin Anesth* 1995; 7:500–06; P. Palumbo *et al.*, Modified PADSS (Post Anaesthetic Discharge Scoring System) for monitoring outpatients discharge. *Ann Ital Chir* (epub before publication); Lucio Trevisani *et al.*, Post-Anaesthetic Discharge Scoring System to assess patient recovery and discharge after colonoscopy. *World J Gastrointest Endosc* 2013; 5(10):502–07.

includes: vital signs, ambulation, nausea and vomiting, pain, and surgical bleeding.

Patients scoring ≥ 9 for two consecutive measurements are considered fit for discharge home.

Before the discharge can be fulfilled, the patient should be free of their IV cannula and dressed in their own clothes. The patient should have an adult escort with them on the way home and at home until the next day. The patient and chaperone should have been counseled and given written information about the following:

1. Information about the surgical procedure.
2. Not driving until the next day, not operating any heavy equipment, not taking important decisions or signing documents, not drinking alcohol.
3. Advice on appropriate daily activities, rehabilitation, training, and precautions.
4. Information about wound care, change of dressings, care of the limb that is still numb and when showers can be taken, etc.
5. Information about common side effects and concerns: some stained blood in the dressing, type of expected pain (e.g., in the shoulder after a laparoscopy), minor fever during the first 24–48 h, and some neurological symptoms if a local anesthetic block has been given.
6. Information about unexpected symptoms that should prompt the patient to contact health personnel: fresh bleeding from a wound, fainting, increasing fever after day 2, increasing size of, or pain at the site of surgery, problems with pain, nausea, vomiting, and voiding.
7. Instructions on how to deal with pain prophylaxis and extra medication for pain or PONV. The instructions should be accompanied by any medications the patient may need until at least the next day, when someone can go to the pharmacy (also provide prescriptions for extra analgesics needed after day 2). Alternatively, it can be arranged for the patient to buy these drugs before surgery.
8. Clear instructions on where to call (the surgeon, the unit, the hospital, other health personnel) for 24-h service in case of problems and questions.
9. Declaration of necessary sick leave for authorities and employer.
10. Appointment for an outpatient follow-up consultation when appropriate.

Discharge criteria after regional anesthesia

Regional anesthesia has gained popularity for some cases as they not only provide good intraoperative analgesia but also good postoperative pain control, thus having an opioid-sparing effect. In addition, there are no cognitive side effects that may be seen after a general anesthetic. However, regional anesthesia poses some problems. There may be no sensation along the dermatome supplied by the nerve blocked. The patients may thus be needlessly kept in the PACU as the block may take hours to completely resolve if the standard discharge criteria are used. There is always the risk for postdural puncture headache after an epidural or evidence of transient radicular symptoms following an intrathecal block. Occasionally patients who have had their procedure under an epidural or spinal may experience bladder distension and urinary retention. This is more common when long-acting intrathecal anesthetic agents are used. Clinical studies show that the use of shorter-acting local anesthetics for spinal or epidural anesthesia is associated with a lower frequency of bladder catheterization and has not been associated with urinary retention in outpatient surgery.[44]

WAKE is modeled after the 10-point modified Aldrete score, with additional "Zero Tolerance Criteria."[49] Readers are directed to refer to the detailed description in the original article. The WAKE criteria can also be used in patients who have undergone their procedure under a general anesthetic or monitored anesthesia care.

Post-discharge care

Postoperative care ranges from no measures beyond appropriate on-call availability 24 h a day, to outpatient consultation.

Post-discharge nausea and vomiting

The presence of PDNV can delay return to work following discharge from the hospital. During the stay in the PACU, most patients receive IV drugs for control of their PONV. Most of these drugs, however, have a short duration of action. The true incidence is not known as patients may not report the event or may not seek medical attention as in most cases it is self-limiting. In a systematic study of the literature, Wu et al. found that the incidence of nausea and vomiting was 17% (range 0–55%) and 8%(0–16%), respectively.[50,51] One of the difficulties in knowing the exact incidence is that almost 36% of the patients who develop PDNV do not have any symptoms while in the hospital. The presence of these symptoms may delay return to work, but the exact economic impact is not known.[50]

Table 9.6 WAKE criteria compared to Aldrete scoring system.

Criteria	Aldrete criteria	WAKE criteria	Score
Activity	Moves all four extremities voluntarily or on command	Purposeful movement of one upper extremity and one lower extremity	2
	Moves two extremities voluntarily or on command	Purposeful movement of NO upper extremity and one lower extremity	1
	None	No purposeful movement	0
Respiration	Breathes normally, coughs easily	Coughs and deep-breathes freely, and/or on command	2
	Dyspnea, shallow or limited breathing	Involuntarily cough only; unsupported airway	1
	Apneic	Tachypnea, dyspnea or apnea, and/or requiring airway support	0
Circulation	BP ± 20 mm of baseline	Within 20% of preoperative baseline, not orthostatic	2
	BP ± 20–50 mm of baseline	Within 20–40% of preoperative baseline, not orthostatic	1
	BP ± 50 mm of baseline	Less than 40% of preoperative baseline, and/or orthostatic	0
Consciousness	Fully awake	Awake, follows commands; easily aroused when called	2
	Arousable	Arouse to persistent stimuli, protective reflexes are present, follows commands	1
	Not responding	Obtunded or persistently somnolent No protective reflexes	0
Oxygen saturation	Maintains SaO_2 > 92% on room air	95% or (preoperative reading − 2) without supplemental O_2	2
	Maintains SaO_2 > 90% on supplemental oxygen	95% or (preoperative reading − 2) with supplemental O_2	1
	Unable to maintain SaO_2 > 90% even on supplemental oxygen	<95% or (preoperative reading − 2) ± supplemental O_2	0

Modified from Jeffrey G. Moorea, Scott M. Rossa, and Brian A. Williams, Regional anesthesia and ambulatory surgery. *Curr Opin Anesthesiol* 2013; 26:652–60.

Table 9.7 Zero tolerance criteria.

Criteria	Yes	No
Pain as appropriately adjusted to patient's baseline pain scores (with movement) at the surgical site	Yes	No
PONV	Yes	No
Shivering	Yes	No
Pruritus	Yes	No
Orthostatic hypotension	Yes	No

Modified from Jeffrey G. Moorea, Scott M. Rossa, and Brian A. Williams, Regional anesthesia and ambulatory surgery. *Curr Opin Anesthesiol* 2013; 26:652–60.

Risk factors for PDNV

In a meta-analysis to establish independent and potentially causal predictors for PONV, Apfel and colleagues concluded that the most reliable independent predictors of PONV were female gender, history of PONV or motion sickness, non-smoker, younger age, duration of anesthesia with volatile anesthetics, and postoperative opioids.[33] White *et al.* in 2009 showed that a higher Apfel risk score was associated with a higher incidence of vomiting in the first 24 h, but the incidence of late (24–72 h) emetic symptoms was unrelated to the patient's Apfel risk score.[52]

Management

Multimodal pharmacologic therapy with long-acting anti-emetics is essential in PDNV management following ambulatory anesthesia. The addition of non-pharmacologic therapy such as acu-stimulation should be considered in PDNV management.

In addition, the use of multimodal analgesia that includes non-opioid analgesics and ambulatory continuous peripheral nerve blocks may allow for a postoperative analgesia and reduce the opioid-induced PDNV.

A more detailed discussion can be found in Chapters 4 and 12.

On-call availability

It is absolutely essential for the safety and success of ambulatory practice to have a well-defined and clear setup for where the patient or relatives can call in case of questions or problems 24 h a day. As the ambulatory unit by definition is closed for part of the day, an alternative location must provide a readily accessible, friendly, and up-to-date telephone service. For office-based practice, small units and special cases, this may be the surgeon's cell phone, but this may be demanding for the surgeon and sometimes also unreliable as cell phones and signal coverage may fail. A better system is for the service to be provided at a nearby emergency unit with full access to patient data and surgical reports.

Phone call from the unit or the hospital the day after surgery

Many units make routine calls to all ambulatory patients the day after surgery, whereas others only do so for selected cases. The idea is to ensure that all questions and instructions are followed, to hear about any problems or questions, and also to obtain data for quality assurance. If a call is planned, it may be wise to tell the patient about the calling routine, not only to allow them the chance to prepare their own questions but also to avoid any anxiety prompted by an unexpected call from the hospital. A nurse, surgeon, or an anesthesiologist may make the call. It may be sensible to have a structured setup for questions and also to have the option for the patient to come forward with spontaneous input. With a "next-day" call most immediate problems will be dealt with adequately, but such a call will not be informative about the occurrence of infection or thrombosis, which usually happen on day 3 or later; therefore, their usefulness is limited when evaluating some important outcomes. If the patient does not answer, it may be reasonable to leave a message on an answer phone, try to reach the patient later on, or speak with someone else at home who is aware of the patient's condition.

Some useful questions for the patient or caregiver might include the following:

a. Any problems (pain, nausea?) while traveling home?
b. Extent of pain, use of analgesics, and satisfaction with the medication regimen?
c. Any nausea or vomiting?
d. Any problems with the wound and dressings?
e. Problems with eating, drinking, urination or bowel function?
f. Degree of mobilization?
g. Quality and amount of night sleep, daytime sleep, or sedation?
h. Need for contact with healthcare professionals?

Written questionnaire for the patient

This is more a tool for quality assurance for the unit, as the patient will not get rapid feedback on worrisome answers for many days. Nevertheless, a questionnaire may be very useful for this purpose as it is more standardized than an interview and will be less time-consuming for the personnel at the ambulatory unit. The questionnaire may be sent with the patient or sent to them afterwards. It may be for next-day completion, or for completion after 1–2 weeks or even after 1–3 months, in order to obtain more outcome data. To be successful, the questionnaire should not be too cumbersome (yes/no answers, short answers) and a prestamped envelope addressed to the unit should accompany it. Alternatively, an electronic link can be emailed to the patient. Lack of patient response can cause problems and may be handled by sending a gentle reminder, and motivating the patient to answer before leaving the unit.

Postoperative outpatient consultation

As this is potentially time-consuming for both the doctor and the patient, there should be a health indication for such a consultation, although it may also be part of a more dedicated quality assurance or a research project. The benefit with a visit is that much more information can be obtained, because some types of information are difficult to gather by mail or phone, such as wound healing, absence of infection, standardized degree of rehabilitation, etc.

References

1. Aldrete, J.A., The post-anesthesia recovery score revisited. *J Clin Anesth*, 1995. **7**(1): 89–91.

2. Chung, F., V.W. Chan, and D. Ong, A post-anesthetic discharge scoring system for home readiness after ambulatory surgery. *J Clin Anesth*, 1995. **7**(6): 500–06.

3. Reynolds, L., J. Beckmann, and A. Kurz, Perioperative complications of hypothermia. *Best Pract Res Clin Anaesthiol*, 2008. **22**(4): 645–57.

4. Sanchez de Toledo, J. and M.J. Bell, Complications of hypothermia: interpreting 'serious,' 'adverse,' and 'events' in clinical trials. *Pediatr Crit Care Med*, 2010. **11**(3): 439–41.

5. Frank, S.M., *et al.*, Perioperative maintenance of normothermia reduces the incidence of morbid cardiac events. A randomized clinical trial. *JAMA*, 1997. **277**(14): 1127–34.

6. Kurz, A., D.I. Sessler, and R. Lenhardt, Perioperative normothermia to reduce the incidence of surgical-wound infection and shorten hospitalization. Study of Wound Infection and Temperature Group. *N Engl J Med*, 1996. **334**(19): 1209–15.

7. Sessler, D.I., Complications and Treatment of Mild Hypothermia. *Anesthesiology*, 2001. **95**(2): 531–43.

8. Schmied, H., *et al.*, Mild hypothermia increases blood loss and transfusion requirements during total hip arthroplasty. *Lancet*, 1996. **347**(8997): 289–92.

9. Sessler, D.I. and M.M. Todd, Perioperative Heat Balance. *Anesthesiology*, 2000. **92**(2): 578.

10. Alfonsi, P., Postanaesthetic shivering: epidemiology, pathophysiology, and approaches to prevention and management. *Drugs*, 2001. **61**(15): 2193–205.

11. Horn, E.P., *et al.*, Postoperative pain facilitates nonthermoregulatory tremor. *Anesthesiology*, 1999. **91**(4): 979–84.

12. Eberhart, L.H., *et al.*, Independent risk factors for postoperative shivering. *Anesth Analg*, 2005. **101**(6): 1849–57.

13. Sessler, D.I., *et al.*, Spontaneous Post-anesthetic Tremor Does Not Resemble Thermoregulatory Shivering. *Anesthesiology*, 1988. **68**(6): 843–50.

14. Yared, J.P., *et al.*, Dexamethasone decreases the incidence of shivering after cardiac surgery: a randomized, double-blind, placebo-controlled study. *Anesth Analg*, 1998. **87**(4): 795–99.

15. Camus, Y., *et al.*, Pre-induction skin-surface warming minimizes intraoperative core hypothermia. *J Clin Anesth*, 1995. **7**(5): 384–88.

16. Apfelbaum, J.L., *et al.*, Practice guidelines for postanesthetic care: an updated report by the American Society of Anesthesiologists Task Force on Postanesthetic Care. *Anesthesiology*, 2013. **118**(2): 291–307.

17. Alfille, P.H., *et al.*, Control of perioperative muscle strength during ambulatory surgery. *Curr Opin Anaesthesiol*, 2009. **22**(6): 730–37.

18. Shim, J.J. and J.M. Leung, An update on delirium in the postoperative setting: prevention, diagnosis and management. *Best Pract Res Clin Anaesthesiol*, 2012. **26**(3): 327–43.

19. Chaput, A.J. and G.L. Bryson, Postoperative delirium: risk factors and management: continuing professional development. *Can J Anaesth*, 2012. **59**(3): 304–20.

20. Steiner, L.A., Postoperative delirium. Part 1: pathophysiology and risk factors. *Eur J Anaesthesiol*, 2011. **28**(9): 628–36.

21. Steiner, L.A., Postoperative delirium. part 2: detection, prevention and treatment. *Eur J Anaesthesiol*, 2011. **28**(10): 723–32.

22. Hebl, J.R., *et al.*, A pre-emptive multimodal pathway featuring peripheral nerve block improves perioperative outcomes after major orthopedic surgery. *Reg Anesth Pain Med*, 2008. **33**(6): 510–17.

23. Schug, S.A. and C. Chong, Pain management after ambulatory surgery. *Curr Opin Anaesthesiol*, 2009. **22**(6): 738–43.

24. Elvir-Lazo, O.L. and P.F. White, The role of multimodal analgesia in pain management after ambulatory surgery. *Curr Opin Anaesthesiol*, 2010. **23**(6): 697–703.

25. Elvir-Lazo, O.L. and P.F. White, Postoperative pain management after ambulatory surgery: role of multimodal analgesia. *Anesthesiol Clin*, 2010. **28**(2): 217–24.

26. White, P.F., Pain management after ambulatory surgery – where is the disconnect? *Can J Anaesth*, 2008. **55**(4): 201–07.

27. Chung, F., E. Ritchie, and J. Su, Postoperative pain in ambulatory surgery. *Anesth Analg*, 1997. **85**(4): 808–16.

28. Frasco, P.E., J. Sprung, and T.L. Trentman, The impact of the Joint Commission for Accreditation of Healthcare Organizations pain initiative on perioperative opiate consumption and recovery room length of stay. *Anesth Analg*, 2005. **100**(1): 162–68.

29. Vila, H., Jr., *et al.*, The efficacy and safety of pain management before and after implementation of hospital-wide pain management standards: is patient safety compromised by treatment based solely on numerical pain ratings? *Anesth Analg*, 2005. **101**(2): 474–80, table of contents.

30. Imasogie, N. and F. Chung, Risk factors for prolonged stay after ambulatory surgery: economic considerations. *Curr Opin Anaesthesiol*, 2002. **15**(2): 245–49.

31. Macario, A., *et al.*, Which clinical anesthesia outcomes are important to avoid? The perspective of patients. *Anesth Analg*, 1999. **89**(3): 652–58.

32. Steely, R.L., *et al.*, Postoperative nausea and vomiting in the plastic surgery patient. *Aesthetic Plast Surg*, 2004. **28**(1): 29–32.

33. Apfel, C.C., *et al.*, Evidence-based analysis of risk factors for postoperative nausea and vomiting. *Br J Anaesth*, 2012. **109**(5): 742–53.

34. Gan, T.J., *et al.*, Consensus guidelines for the management of postoperative nausea and vomiting. *Anesth Analg*, 2014. **118**(1): 85–113.

35. Gan, T.J., *et al.*, Society for Ambulatory Anesthesia guidelines for the management of postoperative nausea and vomiting. *Anesth Analg*, 2007. **105**(6): 1615–28, table of contents.

36. Urman, R.D. and S.P. Desai, History of anesthesia for ambulatory surgery. *Curr Opin Anaesthesiol*, 2012. **25**(6): 641–47.

37. Brown, I., *et al.*, Use of postanesthesia discharge criteria to reduce discharge delays for inpatients in the postanesthesia care unit. *Journal of Clinical Anesthesia*, 2008. **20**(3): 175–79.

38. Ead, H., From Aldrete to PADSS: Reviewing discharge criteria after ambulatory surgery. *J Perianesth Nurs*, 2006. **21**(4): 259–67.

39. Chung, F., Are discharge criteria changing? *J Clin Anesth*, 1993. **5**(6 Suppl 1): 64S–68S.

40. Soliman, I.E., *et al.*, Recovery scores do not correlate with postoperative hypoxemia in children. *Anesth Analg*, 1988. **67**(1): 53–56.

41. Downs, J.B., Prevention of hypoxemia: the simple, logical, but incorrect solution. *J Clin Anesth*, 1994. **6**(3): 180–81.

42. Pavlin, D.J., *et al.*, Voiding in patients managed with or without ultrasound monitoring of bladder volume after outpatient surgery. *Anesth Analg*, 1999. **89**(1): 90–97.

43. Pavlin, D.J., *et al.*, Management of bladder function after outpatient surgery. *Anesthesiology*, 1999. **91**(1): 42–50.

44. Mulroy, M.F., *et al.*, Ambulatory surgery patients may be discharged before voiding after short-acting spinal and epidural anesthesia. *Anesthesiology*, 2002. **97**(2): 315–19.

45. Ng, K.O., *et al.*, Urinary catheterization may not be necessary in minor surgery under spinal anesthesia with long-acting local anesthetics. *Acta Anaesthesiol Taiwan*, 2006. **44**(4): 199–204.

46. Ruhl, M., Postoperative voiding criteria for ambulatory surgery patients. *AORN J*, 2009. **89**(5): 871–74.

47. Beatty, A.M., *et al.*, Relevance of oral intake and necessity to void as ambulatory surgical discharge criteria. *J Perianesth Nurs*, 1997. **12**(6): 413–21.

48. Schreiner, M.S., *et al.*, Should children drink before discharge from day surgery? *Anesthesiology*, 1992. **76**(4): 528–33.

49. Williams, B.A. and M.L. Kentor, The WAKE(c) score: patient-centered ambulatory anesthesia and fast-tracking outcomes criteria. *Int Anesthesiol Clin*, 2011. **49**(3): 33–43.

50. Wu, C.L., *et al.*, Systematic review and analysis of postdischarge symptoms after outpatient surgery. *Anesthesiology*, 2002. **96**(4): 994–1003.

51. Melton, M.S., S.M. Klein, and T.J. Gan, Management of postdischarge nausea and vomiting after ambulatory surgery. *Curr Opin Anaesthesiol*, 2011. **24**(6): 612–19.

52. White, P.F., *et al.*, The relationship between patient risk factors and early versus late postoperative emetic symptoms. *Anesth Analg*, 2008. **107**(2): 459–63.

Chapter 10

Anesthetic techniques for subspecialty surgery

Niraja Rajan, MBBS, Srikantha Rao, MD, MS, and Johan Raeder, MD, PhD

Common themes

This chapter deals with anesthesia for patients undergoing a few specific procedures. Unique surgical and anesthetic considerations associated with each type of procedure are discussed. A simple anesthetic plan for each category of procedure is provided. A few general principles are listed below.

- Preoperative evaluation

  - Pay attention to common coexisting medical illnesses such as arterial hypertension and diabetes mellitus and ensure that these patients have taken their scheduled medication.

- Premedication

  - While patients remain NPO for solid foods 6–8 hours prior to surgery, clear liquids up until 2 hours prior to surgery are acceptable.[1]

  - Patients anxious about the procedure may benefit from oral benzodiazepines such as 1–2 mg of lorazepam, either the night before or morning of surgery. The oral regimen can be supplemented with IV benzodiazepines, such as 1–2 mg of midazolam, prior to surgery when necessary, and especially in those with an anxiety trait.

  - Treat any preoperative pain using the patient's established medication regimen.

  - Regional anesthesia and analgesia

    - The site for the block is marked and a "Patient Safety Time-out" is performed and documented before performing any blocks with due consideration to the patient's anticoagulation status.

- Induction

  - An IV catheter is placed in the appropriate limb, closest to the anesthesiologist in case the OR table is turned 90 or 180 degrees. The non-invasive blood pressure cuff, placed on the same or opposite limb has to be sized appropriately for large patients. Blood pressure should be measured in the sitting position and marked as "baseline" in patients undergoing shoulder surgery.

- Maintenance

  - Anesthesia is maintained using oxygen with air or oxygen with nitrous oxide, along with an inhaled anesthetic agent or using a Total Intravenous Anesthetic (TIVA) technique or a combination of the two.

  - Analgesia is achieved using non-opioid drugs (i.e. acetaminophen, NSAIDs), local anesthetic infiltration (when feasible) and IV opioids, the latter carefully titrated.

  - Regional analgesia techniques are used if the block has not already been performed prior to surgery in the patient holding area.

- Emergence

  - During emergence the patient needs to meet standard extubation criteria.

  - The removal of the laryngeal mask airway (LMA) or endotracheal tube can occur while the patient is still anesthetized (i.e., so-called "deep extubation") or more awake, depending on the procedure and the desire to minimize coughing and bucking during emergence.

- Discharge instructions

  - The patients are discharged to a familiar responsible caregiver with specific instruction to continue oral analgesics at regular intervals for at least 48 hours after discharge, given the slow onset to peak effect of oral analgesics.

Practical Ambulatory Anesthesia, ed. Johan Raeder and Richard D. Urman. Published by Cambridge University Press.
© Cambridge University Press 2015.

· They are instructed to be cognizant of postural hypotension and its consequences.

ENT procedures

Procedures on the ear, nose, or throat typically performed at ASCs include myringotomy and grommet tube insertion, tympanomastoidectomy, stapedectomy, sinus surgery, septoplasty, tonsillectomy, adenoidectomy, vocal cord injections, and polypectomy.

Preoperative

Patients should be screened for their suitability to be operated on at an ASC. Pediatric patients less than 3 years of age presenting for a tonsillectomy may have associated OSA (obstructive sleep apnea) and are not good candidates for outpatient surgery.[2,3] With adenoidectomy, the lower age limit for ambulatory care is usually 2 years.[4] Patients with severe asthma similarly may benefit from having their procedure done at an ambulatory unit or hospital with longer postoperative observation.

A clear method of communication, such as lip-reading or a sign language interpreter, may be necessary in hearing-impaired patients undergoing middle or inner ear procedures.

The patients who present for nasal surgery tend to suffer from chronic allergies and/or repeated upper respiratory tract infections. They may have associated gastroesophageal reflux and asthma. During the preoperative interview, it is important to remind these patients to breathe through their mouth upon emergence.

Premedication

Anxiolytics should be used with caution in patients with OSA. Tonsillectomy patients are cautioned about the use of NSAIDs in the preoperative period due to risk of bleeding, whereas COX-2 inhibitors are safe in this respect. Postoperatively, when hemostasis is established, there are no studies showing increased bleeding risk with traditional NSAIDs.[5] A review from the Cochrane Collaboration found that NSAIDs, excluding ketorolac, did not significantly alter postoperative bleeding compared with placebo.[4]

Intraoperative

The usual technique for most ENT procedures is general anesthesia (GA). Airway management is via (flexible) LMA or an endotracheal tube (i.e., oral RAE tube or other specialized tube) and is based on surgeon and anesthesiologist preference. Dexamethasone is given in higher doses in ENT surgery (10 mg) for both PONV and pain prophylaxis, and to reduce edema and perhaps pain. In middle ear surgery, nitrous oxide use should be avoided. Total intravenous anesthesia may help decrease PONV, because many ENT procedures are associated with increased PONV risk.

The operating table may be turned away from the anesthesiologist, by either 90 or 180 degrees, during surgery. IV lines, breathing circuits and monitoring cables must be routed appropriately.

To reduce bleeding after nasal surgery, arterial pressure is lowered using a deeper plane of anesthetic during surgery or administering labetalol 20 minutes before or small doses of esmolol just prior to extubation. The venous pressure is lowered by placing the head in the elevated position during surgery and extubating the patient in this position, and capillary bleeding is reduced by using topical vasoconstrictors. These may have side effects and the surgeon should be cognizant of the cardiovascular side effects of the vasoconstrictors used in the operative field.

During emergence and extubation, throat packs that may have been used by the surgeon in some of these procedures should be removed and their removal documented before extubation. Extubating the patient while still in a deep plane of anesthesia, to avoid the coughing and straining that often accompany ENT procedures, must be weighed against the potential risk of laryngospasm or pulmonary aspiration, and is based on the expertise and preference of the anesthesiologist. Using short-acting drugs such as esmolol, deliberate hypotension may be induced during emergence prior to extubation to minimize bleeding.

Postoperative

PONV is very common after these procedures and all ENT patients should receive at least two prophylactic anti-emetics, such as dexamethasone and ondansetron, in addition to risk reduction strategies. Post-tonsillectomy bleeding is a surgical complication. Patients are observed in the recovery room for two or more hours and are given instructions to seek immediate attention in case of bleeding after discharge. This may necessitate return to the OR, and patients are advised to remain within a 1–2 hour range of an appropriate hospital. Surgery to treat bleeding following a tonsillectomy is an emergency; patients are treated with full stomach considerations during induction of GA.

Laparoscopic surgery

Laparoscopic abdominal and pelvic surgery, while anatomically minimally invasive, is potentially physiologically disruptive. The carbon dioxide insufflated into the abdominal cavity must eventually be excreted, and poses problems once the body buffer capacity is exceeded (about 200 liters), especially in patients with poor lung function. The peak CO_2 levels may occur up to 2 hours after surgery with the patient in the recovery room who may appear somnolent. Anesthesiologists need to work with the surgeons to reduce the hemodynamic effect of insufflated CO_2, elevated intra-abdominal pressure, and reduced chest wall compliance, especially in obese patients[6,7] in lithotomy position (fluid overload) with steep head-down position (respiratory embarrassment, high airway pressures). It is also important to devise ventilation strategies to avoid barotrauma and volutrauma.

Preoperative

The patient should be warned about the occurrence of shoulder pain (referred pain) from diaphragmatic irritation by insufflated CO_2. Many of the patients presenting for pelvic surgery have depression, anxiety, and chronic pain and may be on multiple anxiolytics and antidepressants, including serotonin-specific reuptake inhibitors. The anesthesiologist must be aware of the potential for drug interactions leading to serotonin syndrome when certain other medications such as meperidine, fentanyl, and promethazine are administered to these patients.[8]

Intraoperative

Attention must be paid to position the patient appropriately in order to avoid positional injuries. Pad all pressure points, especially when tucking the arms. In surgeries performed in the lithotomy position, be aware of positioning injuries in patients with back pain. Foot drop may occur from the lithotomy pole impinging upon the common peroneal nerve. The fingers on the hands tucked next to the hips are at risk of crush injury when the leg portion of the table is lowered or raised during surgery.

In general, during surgery on the external genitalia, GA is preferable to local or spinal anesthesia.

Postoperative

Visceral pain associated with pelvic endometriosis is compounded by pain caused by the surgical removal of these lesions from the peritoneal surfaces. In such patients, NSAIDs given IV soon after induction of anesthesia may be useful in reducing postoperative pain. There also may be a component of chronic pelvic pain that needs to be addressed in a few patients using multimodal analgesia with adjunct analgesics, such as gabapentin, magnesium, and ketamine.

These patients are at high risk for PONV and are managed with risk reduction strategies and two or more prophylactic agents such as dexamethasone and ondansetron. The use of NSAIDs may lower the requirement for IV opioids, reducing the likelihood of PONV.

Eye

A large number of ophthalmological procedures are performed on outpatients. Common procedures include cataract extraction, glaucoma procedures, procedures involving the cornea and conjunctiva such as corneal transplants, and strabismus correction. Patients range in age from the very young to the elderly. Patients for cataract and glaucoma surgery tend to be older and have multiple comorbidities. Patients for strabismus surgery tend to be pediatric and may have associated neurologic syndromes.

Ophthalmological procedures are minimally invasive, do not cause hemodynamic instability, and are therefore considered low-risk procedures.

Preoperative

Preoperative testing is not required in patients undergoing cataract surgeries.[9] Children undergoing strabismus surgery may have underlying neurologic conditions and may be susceptible to MH. This should be determined during the preoperative screening process.

Premedication

An anxiolytic is given when indicated either orally or IV. Mannitol IV is given to reduce intraocular pressure in patients undergoing certain glaucoma and corneal procedures, at the discretion of the surgeon.

Intraoperative

Most superficial ophthalmological procedures can be successfully performed under mild sedation with topical local anesthetic. Procedures requiring retrobulbar blocks can be performed under moderate to deep sedation (alfentanil and/or propofol) for the establishment of the block, followed by anxiolysis as required for the rest of the procedure. Older patients with prolonged circulation times benefit from pretreatment with 5–10 mg ephedrine, flushing the IV line with 20 ml of flush and waiting a full 90 seconds before redosing propofol. General anesthesia is indicated for strabismus surgery, deeper ophthalmic procedures, uncooperative or claustrophobic patients, and when patients prefer to remain unconscious. If neuromuscular blocking drugs are needed, be aware of potential problems of raised intraocular pressure with succinylcholine. For the same reason, nitrous oxide should not be used during procedures in which intraocular gases have been used, such as surgery to correct retinal detachment.

Emergence

Attention must be paid to ensure a smooth emergence using techniques similar to those described in the ENT section. Short-acting opioids (alfentanil) before extubation prevent coughing (with its attendant increased intraocular pressure) and the benefits of deep extubation must be weighed against its risks.

Unique considerations

PONV

All patients undergoing eye surgery are at high risk of PONV and should receive multi-therapy with two or more agents for prophylaxis, accompanied by other risk reduction strategies.

Oculocardiac reflex

This reflex is elicited by pressure on the globe or manipulation of extraocular muscles. It manifests as bradycardia or may be accompanied by dysrhythmias ranging from junctional rhythm, ectopic atrial rhythm, AV block, or ventricular bigeminy or asystole. It may also be elicited by a retrobulbar block, ocular trauma, or by pressure on the ocular tissue in an empty orbit. The afferent limb is trigeminal and the efferent limb is vagal. Hypercarbia and hypoxemia and inadequate depth of anesthesia augment or exaggerate this reflex. Management strategies include maintenance of adequate anesthetic depth and ventilation. Close monitoring and asking the surgeon to cease stimulation usually suffice and the heart rate and rhythm return to baseline within 20 seconds. The reflex usually fatigues after repeated stimulation. Atropine is administered IV for persistent severe bradycardia or serious arrhythmias. The surgeon should cease ocular manipulation prior to the administration of atropine. Prophylactic atropine is not recommended because it may itself cause a variety of arrhythmias.

Complications of retrobulbar and peribulbar block

Retrobulbar and peribulbar blocks are well suited for most ophthalmologic procedures involving the anterior chamber. They provide both akinesia and anesthesia of the eyeball. They are usually performed by the surgeon. Common complications are retrobulbar hemorrhage and hematoma, systemic local anesthetic toxicity (when there is inadvertent intravascular injection), oculocardiac reflex, and possible spinal anesthesia. The anesthesiologist must be watchful to diagnose and treat any of these potential complications during the performance of the block.

Complications

Please see Table 10.1.

Orthopedics

This encompasses a wide range of procedures on both upper and lower extremities. They vary from very superficial low-risk procedures (trigger finger release, carpal tunnel release) to intermediate-risk, longer-duration procedures (shoulder arthroscopy with rotator cuff repair or hip arthroscopy).

The patient population can range from young and healthy patients undergoing sports injury-related procedures to older patients with significant comorbidities. Most outpatient orthopedic procedures tend to have minimal blood loss and do not cause major hemodynamic derangements. A tourniquet is used in many procedures and its use may cause pain ("tourniquet pain") that is more likely to be severe if the tourniquet is applied for more than one hour. There is a potential for limb ischemia during tourniquet application and bleeding and hypotension following tourniquet deflation.

Position

Upper extremity hand and wrist procedures are performed with the patient supine and the operative hand on a hand table abducted 90 degrees; the table may be turned 45–90 degrees. Elbow procedures are performed with the patient either in supine or lateral decubitus position. Shoulder procedures are performed mostly with the patient sitting. Most lower extremity procedures are performed with the patient supine or prone.

Preoperative

Preadmission testing usually depends on the patient's comorbidities. The procedures themselves seldom warrant additional testing.

Table 10.1 Complications of retrobulbar block.

Symptoms and signs	Onset time	Mechanism	Treatment
Hypotension Bradycardia Nausea	2–30 minutes	Oculocardiac reflex	Stop the stimulus Increase fiO$_2$ IV fluids Atropine IV if persistent
Seizures Apprehension Perioral numbness Tinnitus	Immediate	Intravascular local anesthetic	Airway ventilatory support Benzodiazepines IV, Propofol IV Supportive as needed
Proptosis	Immediate	Retrobulbar hemorrhage	Gentle pressure to the eye for 20–30 minutes Reschedule surgery
Shivering	Few minutes	Absorption of local anesthetic along optic nerve sheath into CNS	Supportive
Apnea, bradycardia Amaurosis Loss of consciousness Cardiac arrest	2–40 minutes	Injection of local anesthetic into the brainstem	Airway and circulatory support Usually resolves in 1–3 hours

Premedication

Elective orthopedic surgery is often undertaken only after the patient is committed to a smoking cessation program. As many of these patients might have recently started tobacco cessation, they may be more anxious and hence require oral or IV anxiolytics.

Antibiotics

Many of these patients receive hardware implants. Hence, it is vital that prophylactic antibiotics be administered prior to tourniquet inflation to reduce the occurrence of postoperative surgical site infections.

Regional or local anesthesia

Many of these procedures are amenable to local or regional anesthesia, which could be performed in the preoperative holding area or block room, allowing the block to be well established prior to transporting the patient to the OR. Ankle blocks need not be done awake but could be done after induction of general anesthesia, as they are painful and involve multiple injections. With ultrasound guidance, other blocks may also be safely performed in the anesthetized patient.[10,11]

Intraoperative

Anesthetic technique

Depending on the surgical procedure, options include regional anesthesia, local anesthesia, infiltration or IVRA supplemented with mild to moderate sedation, or GA using standard ASA monitoring and maintenance IV fluids. PONV prophylaxis is recommended. Axillary nerve blocks are used for surgery below the elbow, while infraclavicular blocks are used for surgery on the arm and interscalene block for shoulder surgery.

In patients undergoing hand surgery such as carpal tunnel release or distal hand surgery, a brief duration of GA that allows the surgeon to perform a field block followed by deep sedation may be adequate in most patients, while a few may require GA for the entire surgery.

In patients undergoing shoulder surgery in the sitting position, meticulous attention must be paid to BP measurement and management to avoid cerebral hypoperfusion.

In patients undergoing knee arthroscopy, intra-articular injection of local anesthetic, supplemented with intravenous sedation may be sufficient for most patients, while GA using an LMA may be necessary in a few patients.

Postoperative

Pain management remains a challenge in these patients and the use of multimodal agents is strongly recommended to facilitate discharge. See Chapter 7 for additional details. Patients who receive upper extremity nerve blocks are discharged with a sling supporting the arm until return of motor function. Patients who receive a femoral and sciatic nerve block are discharged with crutches until return of motor function.

Urology

A large number of urological procedures are performed on an outpatient basis. These include cystoscopies, bladder biopsies, TURBTs, TURPs, prostate biopsies, procedures imaging the urinary tract, lithotripsies, ureteral stent placement or removal, vasectomy or its reversal, a wide variety of procedures on the external genitalia, hydrocelectomy, orchiopexy, and procedures for SUI, to name just a few.

As all of these procedures are minimally invasive, they constitute a low cardiac risk. The procedures tend to be of short duration, usually under 2 hours, with minimal hemodynamic derangement.

Patients range in age from the pediatric to geriatric and could be healthy or have multiple comorbidities. Many patients with spinal cord injuries or spina bifida need repeated urologic procedures.

Intraoperative patient position varies depending on the procedure. Many of these procedures are performed with the patient in the lithotomy position. Transrectal ultrasound-guided prostate biopsies are performed in the left lateral decubitus position.

Preoperative

Pre-admission testing (PAT)

PAT depends on patient comorbidities and should follow established guidelines listed elsewhere in this book. These procedures are low-risk, minimally invasive and do not require routine PAT unless significant comorbidities are present.

Premedications

1. Benzodiazepines may be administered orally or IV for anxiolysis.
2. Antibiotics as indicated, based on the procedure.
3. Oxybutynin, a muscarinic receptor antagonist, may be administered orally in patients at risk for bladder or ureteral spasms.

Intraoperative

Anesthetic technique is either GA or moderate to deep IV sedation depending on the procedure. GA using short-acting agents is preferred with attention to PONV and analgesia (see Chapter 5). LMA is the preferred method of securing the airway unless contraindicated. Often in older patients who are edentulous, mask ventilation may be difficult and seating the LMA may be challenging. Infiltration of local anesthetics by the surgeon as a nerve block, field block, or at the site of surgery is encouraged whenever possible. Short-acting spinal anesthesia may also be an option, with either lidocaine, mepivacaine, or low-dose bupivacaine with fentanyl.

As bipolar cautery is now used by surgeons during TURP, saline is acceptable for bladder irrigation, hence hyponatremia is not a concern. Hypothermia may occur if a large volume of cold fluid is used to irrigate the bladder. Monitor the patient's core temperature and use warm irrigation fluid and a forced air warming blanket to prevent hypothermia.

Postoperative

The complications that occur frequently following urological surgery are bleeding and urinary retention.

Bleeding

Bleeding is a complication after some procedures such as TURBT or TURP. Some of these patients may have been on chronic anticoagulants prior to surgery. Bleeding is usually detected in the recovery room by observation of the color of urine draining from the urinary catheter. A small amount of bleeding is expected after these procedures. Unusually, amounts of bleeding characterized by bright red blood in the urinary catheter may necessitate bladder irrigation or a return to the operating room. Patients who do not have a urinary catheter and who notice an excessive amount of bleeding when they void should be catheterized before being discharged.

Urinary retention

Postoperative urinary retention (POUR) is a common complication in older men especially after urological procedures. Other high-risk procedures include anorectal surgery and hernia repair. Predisposing medical conditions include benign prostatic hyperplasia and concurrent neurologic conditions such as cerebral palsy, multiple sclerosis, diabetic neuropathy, and spinal cord lesions. Anticholinergics, sympathomimetics, and neuraxial blockade may predispose to POUR by causing detrusor muscle relaxation. Inadequate pain control may contribute to POUR. Excessive IV fluid administration can cause POUR by bladder overdistension. POUR can cause pain, hypertension, hypotension, bradycardia, and PONV and prolong the time to discharge.

POUR is diagnosed by a combination of clinical evaluation, ultrasound examination for bladder volume, and bladder catheterization.

High-risk patients are managed by bladder catheterization if their urinary bladder volume exceeds 600 ml in the PACU. They may then be discharged home with instructions to contact their surgeon if they are unable to void after several hours at home or experiencing severe suprapubic pain.

Low-risk patients do not need to void prior to discharge.[12]

ECT

Electroconvulsive therapy is indicated for the treatment of medication-resistant depression and is also beneficial in mania and catatonia. The mechanism of action is not exactly known. An electrical current is applied to the brain via electrodes either unilaterally or bilaterally with the aim of inducing generalized epileptiform activity monitored by both EEG and observed tonic–clonic seizures, either general or in a limb isolated by a tourniquet. Optimal seizure duration is unclear, but is targeted to be at least 30 seconds. ECT produces physiological effects on the central nervous system and cardiovascular system.

Cardiovascular effects start with initial parasympathetic stimulation, causing bradycardia and hypotension lasting 10–15 seconds. This is followed by sympathetic stimulation characterized by hypertension, tachycardia, and sometimes arrhythmias. The resulting increase in myocardial oxygen consumption coupled with decreased myocardial oxygen supply can cause myocardial ischemia and infarction.

Central nervous system effects include increase in intracranial pressure, cerebral blood flow, and cerebral metabolic oxygen requirement. Cognitive effects include disorientation, short-term memory impairment, and impaired attention. Intelligence and judgment are unaffected.

Other effects include clinically insignificant increase in intraocular pressure and intragastric pressure; long bone fractures, myalgias, increased salivation, dental damage, nausea, and amnesia can also occur.

ECT has a low mortality rate despite being performed in a high-risk population.

Preoperative

ECT is usually performed under GA at a non-OR location, usually in a hospital setting near the PACU. Appropriate resuscitation equipment and drugs should be immediately available and ASA standards for monitoring and recovery should be met. Contingency plans for transfer to a critical care facility must be made for patients with ASA physical status 3 or higher.

Patients with severe depression tend to be poor historians and also have a variety of comorbidities that may not be well controlled due to self-neglect.

Relative contraindications to ECT should be identified on preoperative interview. These include the following:

- Myocardial infarction or cerebrovascular accident within the past three months.
- Elevated intracranial pressure.
- Poorly stabilized congestive heart failure.
- New-onset DVT (until anticoagulated).
- Cerebral aneurysm.
- Major fractures.
- Pheochromocytoma.
- Retinal detachment.
- Cochlear implants (consider unilateral ECT).
- Severe hypertension: blood pressure should be checked before start of the procedure. If baseline pressure is already high (above 180/110), a blood pressure lowering medication should be considered prior to the start of the procedure.

The patient's coexisting medical illnesses should be treated appropriately and the patient optimized prior to commencing ECT.

Sedative, anxiolytic premedications usually interfere with seizure generation and should be avoided.

Intraoperative

The goals of the anesthetic are to provide unconsciousness and muscle relaxation for the duration of the induced seizure, minimizing the adverse physiological effects of this seizure without interfering with seizure efficacy and rapid emergence.[13]

Most available intravenous induction agents except ketamine are suitable for ECT.[14] Barbiturates, such as methohexital or thiopenthal (currently not available in the US), are preferred by some because they do not mask the convulsions to the same degree as propofol. Etomidate can also be used as an induction agent. Neuromuscular blocking drugs are used to reduce injuries from seizures. Succinylcholine is commonly used by some practitioners, usually after precurarization with a non-depolarizing agent. In patients in whom succinylcholine is contraindicated, there is no good alternative which has a rapid onset of action and very short duration. Once sugammadex gets an FDA approval in the US, it can be used to reverse rocuronium or vecuronium even minutes after the administration of these paralytics. Adjuncts may be used to either reduce the dose of induction agent (remifentanil/alfentanil), prolong the duration of the seizure (caffeine IV), control adverse parasympathetic effects (glycopyrrolate) or treat sympathetic effects (esmolol). Prophylactic administration of non-cardioselective beta antagonists (esmolol and propranolol) is not recommended.

After preoxygenation and IV induction, a tourniquet applied on an upper or lower extremity is inflated above arterial pressure, and then a short-acting neuromuscular blocking drug is administered. Ventilation is assisted via bag-mask system (moderate hyperventilation may be useful in lowering the convulsion threshold) and a bite block is inserted. After the electrical stimulus and during the seizure, the airway is maintained and breathing is gently assisted until resumption of adequate spontaneous ventilation.

Postoperative

Emergence agitation is common and can be avoided by using a secluded recovery area with a familiar caregiver present during emergence. Small doses of midazolam can be administered for severe anxiety during emergence. Mild headache and/or myalgia may also occur, but usually responds well to a minor analgesic, such as acetaminophen.

Patients are discharged to the care of a familiar caregiver.

Dental surgery

Most dental procedures are performed in an office setting with local anesthesia without any sedation. Patients requiring sedation or GA usually have underlying medical conditions that preclude them from being performed under local anesthesia alone. These include mentally challenged, uncooperative, severely anxious or psychiatric patients. Other patients are cardiac surgery patients getting dental clearance. These patients may have severe comorbidities and are high-risk for cardiac complications. It may be beyond the capabilities of the dental office to care for these patients and they are usually taken care of in a hospital setting but as outpatients.

Preoperative

If the patient is cooperative but very anxious, an anxiolytic by mouth may be useful. Otherwise, the anxiolytics are better controlled by intravenous titration in the office before the beginning of the procedures. Antibiotics, including those for infective endocarditis prophylaxis, are administered when indicated.

Intraoperative

The type of anesthesia depends on the extent of dental surgery and the patient. The very uncooperative mentally challenged patient may require intramuscular ketamine 5–10 mg/kg which induces hypnosis in approximately 5–10 minutes after which IV access is established. In needle-phobic patients who cooperate with an inhalational induction using a mask, after an oral premedication, IV access is established after they are rendered unconscious. Anesthesia could be maintained by continuous IV infusion of propofol or an inhalational agent via an LMA or a nasotracheal tube or a combined technique. Throat packs are usually inserted to protect the airway from blood and secretions and must be removed at the end of the procedure and their removal diligently documented. During emergence observe closely for laryngospasm and airway obstruction and bleeding.

During sedation with spontaneous ventilation a nasal cannula with two ports, one for oxygen delivery and one for capnography and respiratory rate monitoring, is very useful, in addition to pulse oximetry, ECG monitoring, and BP measurements.

Postoperative

Infiltration of local anesthetic by the surgeon is encouraged during surgery, to facilitate pre- and postoperative analgesia. PONV prophylaxis is provided with one or more drugs as these patients are at a high risk for PONV.

The high-risk patient (heart failure for cardiac transplant, or valvular disease for valve replacement surgery) for dental clearance prior to cardiac surgery typically requires dental extractions. This is usually performed with minimal sedation and local anesthesia.

Endoscopy

Many gastrointestinal (GI) procedures are performed in the endoscopy or GI suite, which may be connected to a hospital, or is a free-standing center.

The American Gastroenterologists Association reports that 98% of endoscopists administer sedation for upper and lower endoscopies.[15] They use a wide variety of sedation techniques including IV propofol.[16] The AGA calls for anesthesiologist involvement with patients in ASA categories IV and V or if they have had prior adverse or inadequate response to sedation.

Common GI procedures include upper endoscopy, sigmoidoscopy, colonoscopy, endoscopic retrograde cholangiopancreatography, esophageal dilation, stenting, and percutaneous endoscopic gastrostomy tube placement. Patients may have a large number of comorbidities including gastroesophageal reflux, hepato-renal disease with porto-pulmonary hypertension, and esophageal varices. Patients requiring the involvement of an anesthesiologist usually have limited end-organ reserve and require deep sedation or general anesthesia.

Intraoperative

Patients who are likely to be at increased risk for aspiration must be identified preoperatively and may require endotracheal intubation to protect the airway. A topical local anesthetic spray to the faucial pillars and posterior pharyngeal wall facilitates the passage of the endoscope when upper GI procedures are performed under sedation and reduces the MAC when they are performed under GA.

Anesthesia could be maintained by continuous IV infusion of propofol or an inhalational agent via an endotracheal tube or a combined technique.

Also, the use of ketamine after a small dose of benzodiazepine, eventually combined with low-dose propofol infusion, may be a useful technique in order to ensure adequate spontaneous ventilation.

Postoperative

These procedures are usually brief and cause minimal to no post-procedure discomfort. PONV prophylaxis with at least one drug is recommended.

Non-operating room anesthesia

A large number of procedures requiring sedation and anesthesia are being performed outside the OR. These include the diagnostic and interventional radiology suites, cardiac catheterization and electrophysiology labs, and gastroenterology suites. Anesthesiologists must be cognizant of the potential hazards or unique features of these locations in order to maintain the same high standard of care as the OR. Anesthetic considerations and patient characteristics remain the same, but due to the location there may be constraints relating to space and available equipment and personnel.

Closed claims review for anesthesia claims relating to locations outside the OR showed more substandard care and greater severity of injury.[17] The guidelines provided by the ASA in their statement on non-OR locations should be followed.[13]

ASA standards of monitoring should apply to all these cases.[18,19] Many locations have an awkward layout from an anesthesiologist's perspective and were designed for their primary role rather than as an anesthetizing location. The equipment may be outdated or obsolete.

Personnel at these non-OR locations are not trained to assist with anesthetic aspects of patient care. Open communication between team members before and throughout the procedure is essential for providing high quality of patient care. The anesthesiologist must also ensure that an adequate number of anesthesia personnel are available at the remote location.

Preoperative

The patient must be evaluated, comorbidities optimized, NPO status confirmed, and informed consent obtained by the anesthesia team.

The anesthetizing location must comply with building and safety codes. It is required to have a written valid plan for evacuating a patient in case of a disaster. Sufficient space must be available to accommodate equipment and personnel and allow access to the patient. Ensure that sufficient electrical outlets are available for the anesthesia machine, monitoring, and resuscitative equipment. Check for a battery-powered illumination source and adequate illumination of the patient and anesthesia machine.

The following equipment must be available and in working condition: oxygen source and back up supply, suction apparatus, scavenging system for waste anesthetic gases, anesthetic drugs, standard monitoring equipment, self-inflating hand resuscitation bag, emergency cart with defibrillator and emergency drugs, equipment for infusion and airway control, and transport equipment including portable monitors, oxygen source, and stretchers to transport the patient to the PACU.

Adequate number of trained staff to support the anesthesiologist, reliable means of two-way communication to request assistance, and at least one person trained in ACLS in addition to the anesthesiologist should be available.

Intraoperative

The anesthetic techniques vary from minimal sedation to general anesthesia. Mild to moderate sedation is often provided by non-anesthesiologists in these situations. This is a great opportunity for Anesthesiology Departments to take the lead and not only provide anesthesia in selected patients in the non-OR setting, but help the hospital administration to develop policies and quality assurance review mechanisms for non-anesthesiologists to safely provide sedation. Anesthesiologists could oversee the training of these personnel to ensure that they receive adequate training and possess the necessary skills to provide mild to moderate sedation safely.[20]

Anesthesiologists care for patients requiring monitored anesthesia care. Standard monitoring should be used.

Postoperative

Patients may require transportation over long distances to the recovery room in these situations. Prior to transport, the patient must be stable and accompanied by the anesthesia provider to the recovery area. Monitoring and supplemental oxygen may be required for transportation. Patients may be discharged from the recovery area once criteria are met.

References

1. American Society of Anesthesiologists Committee. Practice guidelines for preoperative fasting and the use of pharmacologic agents to reduce the risk of pulmonary aspiration: application to healthy patients undergoing elective procedures: an updated report by the American Society of Anesthesiologists Committee on Standards and Practice Parameters. *Anesthesiology*. 2011 Mar; **114**(3):495–511.

2. Coté CJ, Posner KL, Domino KB. Death or neurologic injury after tonsillectomy in children with a focus on obstructive sleep apnea: Houston, we have a problem! *Anesth Analg*. 2013 Jul 10.

3. Schwengel DA, Sterni LM, Tunkel DE, Heitmiller ES. Perioperative management of children with obstructive sleep apnea. *Anesth Analg*. 2009 Jul; **109**(1):60–75.

4. Baugh RF, Archer SM, Mitchell RB, *et al*. Clinical practice guideline: tonsillectomy in children. *Otolaryngol Head Neck Surg*. 2011 Jan; **144**(1 Suppl):S1–30.

5. Ravi, R, Howell, T. Anaesthesia for paediatric ear, nose, and throat surgery. *Contin Educ Anaesth Crit Care Pain*. 2007 Vol 7 (2).

6. Nguyen NT, Wolfe BM. The physiologic effects of pneumoperitoneum in the morbidly obese. *Ann Surg*. 2005 Feb; **241**(2):219–26.

7. Joshi GP, Ahmad S, Riad W, Eckert S, Chung F. Selection of obese patients undergoing ambulatory surgery: a systematic review of the literature. *Anesth Analg*. 2013 Nov;**117**(5):1082–91.

8. Rastogi R, Swarm RA, Patel TA. Case scenario: opioid association with serotonin syndrome: implications to the practitioners. *Anesthesiology*. 2011 Dec; **115**(6):1291–98.

9. Balk EM, Earley A, Hadar N, Shah N, Trikalinos TA. *Benefits and Harms of Routine Preoperative Testing: Comparative Effectiveness*. Rockville, MD: Agency for Healthcare Research and Quality (US); 2014 Jan.

10. Marhofer P, Harrop-Griffiths W, Kettner SC, Kirchmair L. Fifteen years of ultrasound guidance in regional anaesthesia: part 1. *Br J Anaesth*. 2010 May; **104**(5):538–46.

11. Marhofer P, Harrop-Griffiths W, Willschke H, Kirchmair L. Fifteen years of ultrasound guidance in regional anaesthesia: Part 2 – Recent developments in block techniques. *Br J Anaesth*. 2010 Jun; **104**(6):673–83.

12. Baldini G, Bagry H, Aprikian A, Carli F. Postoperative urinary retention: anesthetic and perioperative considerations. *Anesthesiology*. 2009 May; **110**(5):1139–57.

13. Vishal Uppal, Jonathan Dourish, Alan Macfarlane. Anaesthesia for electroconvulsive therapy. *Contin Educ Anaesth Crit Care Pain*. 2010 Vol **10** (6): 192–96.

14. Hooten WM, Rasmussen KG Jr. Effects of general anesthetic agents in adults receiving electroconvulsive therapy: a systematic review. *J ECT*. 2008 Sep; **24**(3):208–23.

15. Cohen LB, Delegge MH, Aisenberg J, *et al*. AGA Institute review of endoscopic sedation. *Gastroenterology*. 2007 Aug; **133**(2):675–701.

16. Byrne MF, Baillie J. Nurse-assisted propofol sedation: the jury is in! *Gastroenterology*. 2005 Nov; **129**(5):1781–82.

17. The risk and safety of anesthesia at remote locations: the US closed claims analysis. *Curr Opin Anaesthesiol*. 2009 Aug; **22**(4):502–08.

18. https://www.asahq.org/For-Members/~/media/For %20Members/Standards%20and%20Guidelines/2014/ STATEMENT%20ON%20NONOPERATING%20 ROOM%20ANESTHETIZING%20LOCATIONS.pdf

19. https://www.asahq.org/For-Members/~/media/For% 20Members/documents/Standards%20Guidelines% 20Stmts/Basic%20Anesthetic%20Monitoring%202011 .ashx

20. American Society of Anesthesiologists Task Force on Sedation and Analgesia by Non-Anesthesiologists. Practice guidelines for sedation and analgesia by non-anesthesiologists. *Anesthesiology*. 2002 Apr; **96**(4):1004–17.

Pediatric anesthesia

Fatima Ahmad, MD

Pediatric ambulatory surgery has a long-standing record of safety, as children generally represent a healthy cohort of the patient population. However, some children have complex syndromes and major morbidity. Additionally, there are many pediatric surgical procedures that do not require postoperative hospitalization and can be done efficiently in an ambulatory set up. The success is highly dependent on a team approach where child life specialists, perioperative nurses, surgeons, and anesthesiologists all work together to achieve the best results by making the experience comfortable, non-threatening, and pleasant for both the parents and the children.

Psychologically also, ambulatory surgery is more suitable for children as they recover from surgery in the comfort and security of their home environments as compared to more stressful inpatient hospital surroundings.[1] The downside of efficiency and cost-effectiveness of pediatric ambulatory surgery is the recruitment of increasing numbers of patients with chronic medical problems. Careful patient selection by the anesthesiologist is crucial to continue this record of safety. Although the incidence of life-threatening complications in this population is low, some perioperative issues may require overnight hospital admission.

Pediatric anesthesia is considered a distinct subspecialty due to significant anatomic and physiological differences between children of different ages and adults. The most important anatomic characteristics in children that are relevant to anesthesia are related to airway. Their large tongue size relative to oral cavity can easily lead to airway obstruction in the presence of sedation, as natural muscle tone may be reduced. Being obligate nose breathers, any unfavorable upper airway conditions like inflammation or excessive secretions can make the work of breathing difficult. The pliability and smaller diameter of the trachea makes it more prone to occlusion if the neck is overly extended or flexed. Even a small amount of swelling of tracheal mucosa can lead to significant obstruction in airflow. The selection of an appropriately sized endotracheal tube and ensuring an airleak around the tube cuff is important for this reason. Another measure is to consider using the LMA whenever appropriate. This can help avoid tracheal irritation, although increased attention should be given to avoiding abundant pharyngeal secretion or gastric regurgitation.

Physiologically, the pediatric cardiovascular system is prominent by its many characteristics that differ from adults. The pediatric cardiac compliance is low as compared to adults, so cardiac output is highly dependent on the heart rate. Bradycardia in a child usually results from hypoxia, and by lowering cardiac output, it can create a dangerously hypoxic low output state. In addition, with the rib cage being unable to increase the anteroposterior diameter and small, overcrowded abdomen hindering the diaphragm's ability to move downward, the pulmonary reserve becomes very limited.

Children are also easily susceptible to hypothermia due to limited fat reserves and larger surface area to volume ratio. Special efforts are mandatory to keep them normothermic.

Pharmacokinetics of various drugs differ significantly in children as compared to adults. This may be due to immaturity of enzyme systems and clearance mechanisms and altered protein binding during the first 1–2 years of life, leading to increased bioavailability and prolonged half-life of certain drugs. In children above this age, the dose need of hypnotic agents and inhalational agents is increased as compared with adults, whereas the need for opioids is approximately similar per kg of weight.

Practical Ambulatory Anesthesia, ed. Johan Raeder and Richard D. Urman. Published by Cambridge University Press.
© Cambridge University Press 2015.

Due to some of the factors mentioned above, the safe provision of anesthetic care is highly dependent on the clinical skills of the anesthesiologist. Credentialing criteria for personnel providing pediatric anesthesia at free-standing surgery centers may differ from hospital setups as situations differ with respect to immediate availability of skilled help. The American Society of Anesthesiologists *Statement on Practice Recommendations for Pediatric Anesthesia*[2] clearly delineates the criteria required to be privileged to perform pediatric anesthesia. In addition, PACU nurses skilled in taking care of pediatric patients should be available on facility. PALS certification for these nurses is highly recommended. In addition to skilled personnel, the facility should be equipped with state-of-the-art specialized pediatric equipment and drugs. These include items for airway management, positive pressure ventilation systems, and temperature maintenance devices, intravenous fluid administration supplies, monitoring equipment per ASA standards, specialized difficult airway management devices, and pediatric crash carts, among others.

Common pediatric ambulatory surgeries

The commonly performed procedures in ambulatory surgery centers are listed below.

- ENT surgeries, i.e., myringotomy and tube insertion, tonsillectomy, adenoidectomy, frenulectomy.
- Dental surgeries.
- General and urologic surgeries, i.e., inguinal herniorrhaphy, circumcision, orchiopexy, hypospadias repair.
- Gastrointestinal endoscopies.
- Ophthalmologic procedures, strabismus repair.
- Orthopedic surgeries on extremities.
- Plastic cleft lip repair and removal of skin lesions.

Patient selection and commonly faced challenges

Similar to preoperative evaluation of patients getting surgeries in the hospital setup, outpatient pediatric evaluation should be focused on a detailed health assessment, physical examination and necessary lab work.

In many surgery centers, a preliminary telephone screening is done by a nurse as soon as the surgery is booked and the anesthesiologist reviews the data.

Most of the children are ASA physical status 1 or 2 and this initial review is sufficient. For ASA physical status 3 patients, this initial screening helps to determine if further referral to a primary physician is indicated for optimization for their clinical conditions. On the day before surgery they are called again to reinforce fasting guidelines and to determine if there is a change in their conditions. These calls help to reduce cancellations on the day of surgery when the patient is thoroughly evaluated again by the anesthesiologist performing the case. Some of the common controversies and challenges faced in pediatric population are discussed below.

Upper respiratory tract infection (URI)

Children with symptoms of URI have increased risk of respiratory complications including laryngospasm,[3] bronchospasm,[4] and postoperative oxygen desaturation.[5] The URIs can result in airway hyperactivity that lasts for up to 6 weeks after infection.[6] Generally, afebrile patients with uncomplicated URI, clear secretions, and no major comorbid conditions are safe to proceed.[7] The sick febrile child with purulent secretions, persistent cough, lethargic appearance, and lower respiratory symptoms, such as wheezing, should, if possible be postponed for at least 4 weeks,[6] or referred to an inpatient setting if the surgery is needed sooner. In patients with nasal congestion and slight nonproductive cough for procedures requiring intubation, other risk factors such as history of asthma, prematurity, parental smoking, and surgery on the airways should be taken into account. The anesthetic management should focus on minimizing secretions, adequate hydration, and avoidance of airway stimulation under light anesthesia.[6]

Patient age and history of prematurity

Full-term infants can be done as outpatients once they are 2–4 weeks of age.[8] By this time, symptoms of physiologic jaundice have decreased, ductus arteriosus has closed, pulmonary vascular resistance has reached a normal level and risk of postoperative apnea has declined. Preterm infants have increased risk of apneic events in the immediate postoperative period and require at least 12-hour monitoring for up to 60 weeks of post-conceptual age.[9] The risk is increased if there is a history of episodes of apnea at home, anemia, and neurological and chronic lung diseases.[10]

Children with obstructive sleep apnea (OSA)

OSA is mostly seen in children presenting for tonsillectomy and adenoidectomy. It is characterized by complete or partial upper airway obstruction during sleep, resulting in hypoxia and hypercarbia and pulmonary hypertension in severe cases. The severity of hypoxemia, hypocarbia, and apnea/hypopnea events on polysomnographic testing relates to increased risk of postoperative respiratory complications. All children with OSA may not have undergone polysomnography and screening tools can be developed according to ASA guidelines.[11] These should focus on BMI, neck circumference, anatomical nasal obstruction, craniofacial abnormalities, tonsillar hypertrophy, history of loud snoring, breath-holding (apnea) during sleep, interrupted sleep, and daytime sleepiness. The risk of postoperative respiratory complications, including fatal events, is higher in children with severe OSA.[12]

These children have increased sensitivity to anesthetic agents, including opioids. They are usually not good candidates for outpatient surgeries, especially tonsillectomy and adenoidectomy procedures, as prolonged continuous monitoring may be required. Children younger than 3 and 2 years of age presenting for tonsillectomy and adenoidectomy, respectively, are also at higher risk for respiratory complications and should not be done in an ambulatory setting.[13]

Congenital heart disease

Children with congenital heart disease often have other coexisting conditions that require surgical management. Many of these procedures are performed on an outpatient basis. This patient cohort is at increased risk of mortality while undergoing non-cardiac surgical procedures.[14]

It is imperative that not only the anesthesiologist should be experienced in handling these kinds of cases, but also the surgery center should be a suitable location for these cases with easy access to skilled personnel and emergently required monitoring and treatment capabilities. Free-standing surgery centers may not be the ideal location for some of these cases. While selecting the patient for outpatient surgery, the anesthesiologist should be thoroughly familiar with the patient's current pathophysiological state, hemodynamic status, and their medications. Generally, it is safe to provide ambulatory anesthetic care to children who have had complete correction of their congenital heart condition and are regularly followed up by their cardiologists, meet their developmental milestones, and do not have exercise restrictions.[15] If the cardiac condition is partially corrected, they may be at increased risk of hypoxemia, systemic hypotension, and poor tolerance to hypovolemia, necessitating hospital admission.

Premedication vs. parental presence at induction

Children often manifest signs and symptoms of severe anxiety in the perioperative period. Both sedative premedication and parental presence at induction have been advocated as methods to reduce perioperative anxiety and increase patient and parental satisfaction. A decision should be made regarding which patients would benefit from one or both of these modalities. Midazolam has been widely used for this purpose. It is a rapid-onset, short-acting drug and provides adequate sedation and anxiolysis within 20 minutes of oral administration of 0.5 mg/kg. Oral clonidine has also been recommended for this purpose in a dose of 2–4 µg/kg. Although it has a slower onset time of up to 45 minutes, it provides better postoperative pain control and decreased incidence of emergence delirium.[16]

Some children may become aggressive or combative in the preoperative period due to pre-existing psychological and developmental behavioral disorders. Sometimes these children resist any attempt at premedication or other modes of anxiolysis. Intramuscular ketamine 4–5 mg/kg has been shown to provide adequate sedation within 5 minutes of administration.[17] Atropine or glycopyrrolate administration along with ketamine decreases the sialagogue effect of ketamine.

Pain control

Regional anesthesia should be strongly considered in pediatric patients. Not only does it provide postoperative pain relief, but also helps to achieve rapid emergence from anesthesia, quicker recovery time, and greater parent satisfaction. Nerve blocks help to reduce requirements of general anesthetic agents and opioids. Occurrence of postoperative nausea and vomiting is also reduced in these patients. The need and suitability of nerve block should be discussed ahead of time with the surgeon and appropriate consent obtained from the parents. The commonly performed blocks in ambulatory surgery include caudal block for urological, lower abdominal and lower extremity surgeries, upper and lower extremity blocks for orthopedic surgeries, and transverse abdominal plane (TAP) and ilioinguinal block for herniorrhaphies and orchipexies. Usually the nerve blocks are performed after induction of general anesthesia in children. Care should be exercised about local anesthetic dosing. The dose of bupivacaine should be limited to 2.0 mg/kg for single shots as children may not have fully developed hepatic metabolic functions and the ability to handle a large drug load. Infants have low serum protein binding of drugs which allows for a higher fraction of free drug. This can result in local anesthetic toxicity at lower blood levels.[18] Nerve blocks should be performed very carefully, preferably under direct vision by using ultrasonography. Local anesthesia into all wounds and also tonsillar beds is also an excellent adjunct in most cases.

Ketorolac and acetaminophen can be used as analgesic adjuncts in suitable situations. Caution should be exercised when administering acetaminophen via different routes as total dose should stay within the maximum allowable dose of up to 100 mg/kg per day.

Hydrocodone and codeine are also widely used to manage moderate pain in children. The analgesic effect of codeine depends on its metabolism to morphine. Due to genetic polymorphism, some children metabolize codeine ultra-rapidly and some are poor metabolizers. Codeine is ineffective in providing analgesia to poor metabolizers and can cause potentially fatal respiratory depression in ultra-rapid metabolizers. The US Food and Drug Administration (FDA) has issued a boxed warning to the drug label of codeine-containing products. It makes a strong recommendation against the use of codeine in children following tonsillectomy and adenoidectomy.[19] An alternative here may be oral oxycodone, which has reliable absorption and direct opioid agonist effect.

In summary, anesthesia to children can be safely provided in the ambulatory surgery center under skilled personnel at well-equipped facilities.

References

1. Bogetz, M. S. (1988). Anesthesia for pediatric outpatient surgery. *Pediatrician*, 16(1–2), 45–55.

2. American Society of Anesthesiologists. *Statement on Practice Recommendations for Pediatric Anesthesia.* Committee of Origin: Pediatric Anesthesia (Approved by the ASA House of Delegates on October 19, 2011).

3. Olsson, G. L., & Hallen, B. (1984). Laryngospasm during anaesthesia. A computer-aided incidence study in 136 929 patients. *Acta Anaesthesiologica Scandinavica*, 28(5), 567–75.

4. Olsson, G. L., & Hallen, B. (1987). Laryngospasm during anaesthesia. A computer-aided incidence study in 136 929 patients. *Acta Anaesthesiologica Scandinavica*, 31, 244–52.

5. Desoto, H., Patel, R. I., Soliman, I. E., *et al.* (1988). Changes in oxygen saturation following general anesthesia in children with upper respiratory infection signs and symptoms undergoing otolaryngological procedures. *Anesthesiology*, 68(2), 276–78.

6. Tait, A. R., & Malviya, S. (2005). Anesthesia for the child with an upper respiratory tract infection: still a dilemma?. *Anesthesia & Analgesia*, 100(1), 59–65.

7. Rolf, N., & Coté, C. J. (1992). Frequency and severity of desaturation events during general anesthesia in children with and without upper respiratory infections. *Journal of Clinical Anesthesia*, 4(3), 200–03.

8. Bajaj, P. (2009). What is the youngest age appropriate for outpatient surgery? *Indian Journal of Anaesthesia*, 53(1), 5.

9. Kurth, C. D., Spitzer, A. R., Broennle, A. M., & Downes, J. J. (1987). Postoperative apnea in preterm infants. *Anesthesiology*, 66(4), 483–88.

10. Walther-Larsen, S., & Rasmussen, L. S. (2006). The former preterm infant and risk of post-operative apnoea: recommendations for management. *Acta Anaesthesiologica Scandinavica*, 50(7), 888–93.

11. Gross, J. B., Bachenberg, K. L., Benumof, J. L., *et al.* (2006). Practice guidelines for the perioperative management of patients with obstructive sleep apnea: a report by the American Society of Anesthesiologists Task Force on Perioperative Management of patients with obstructive sleep apnea. *Anesthesiology*, 104(5), 1081.

12. Morris, L. G., Lieberman, S. M., Reitzen, S. D., *et al.* (2008). Characteristics and outcomes of malpractice claims after tonsillectomy. *Otolaryngology – Head and Neck Surgery*, 138(3), 315–20.

13. Brigger, M. T., & Brietzke, S. E. (2006). Outpatient tonsillectomy in children: a systematic review. *Otolaryngology – Head and Neck Surgery*, 135(1), 1–7.

14. Baum, V. C., Barton, D. M., & Gutgesell, H. P. (2000). Influence of congenital heart disease on mortality after noncardiac surgery in hospitalized children. *Pediatrics*, 105(2), 332–35.

15. Veyckemans, F., & Momeni, M. (2013). The patient with a history of congenital heart disease who is to

undergo ambulatory surgery. *Current Opinion in Anesthesiology*, **26**(6), 685–91.

16. Rosenbaum, A., Kain, Z. N., Larsson, P., Lönnqvist, P. A., & Wolf, A. R. (2009). The place of premedication in pediatric practice. *Pediatric Anesthesia*, **19**(9), 817–28.

17. Tan, L., & Meakin, G. H. (2010). Anaesthesia for the uncooperative child. *Continuing Education in Anaesthesia, Critical Care & Pain*, **10**(2), 48–52.

18. Stow, P. J., Scott, A., Phillips, A., & White, J. B. (1988). Plasma bupivacaine concentrations during caudal analgesia and ilioinguinal–iliohypogastric nerve block in children. Anaesthesia, **43**(8),650–53.

19. US Food and Drug Administration. (2012). FDA Drug Safety Communication: Codeine use in certain children after tonsillectomy and/or adenoidectomy may lead to rare, but life-threatening adverse events or death.

Chapter 12

Aesthetic surgery

Fatima Ahmad, MD

Cosmetic plastic surgery has become an important part of ambulatory surgical procedures over the last decade. It is a purely elective procedure with the aim of achieving observable aesthetically satisfying results. Patients have a general belief that because of their elective nature, plastic surgical procedures should be free of both surgical and anesthesia-related complications. A complication-free surgical course is perceived as a positive and satisfying experience. According to the American Society for Aesthetic Plastic Surgery,[1] board certified doctors performed more than 10 million cosmetic surgical and non-surgical procedures in the United States in 2012, reflecting an increase of 250% since 1997. Out of these, cosmetic surgeries accounted for approximately 1.7 million procedures. These are being done both in ambulatory surgery centers and office-based locations. Some of the common procedures that require the services of anesthesiologists include breast augmentation, liposuction, abdominoplasty, eyelid surgery, rhinoplasty, breast reduction to treat enlarged male breast, ear shaping, neck lift, and facelift (rhytidectomy). Even though these procedures are purely elective, they are still considered a contributing factor to surgical morbidity and mortality in ambulatory patients, especially in the office-based setting.[2] Hence, it is incumbent on anesthesiologists to be familiar with the unique challenges faced in aesthetic surgery.

In this chapter, a brief description of the techniques, complications and anesthetic management of some common cosmetic surgical procedures will be presented.

Facelift (rhytidectomy)

Intuitively, it would be assumed that a successful facelift with a resultant satisfied patient is solely dependent on surgical skill. On the contrary, it has been emphasized in plastic surgery literature that "A well-performed anesthetic makes a smooth postoperative course more likely, but a poorly handled anesthetic can increase the likelihood of postoperative complications and can strain the relationship between surgeon and patient."[3] This indicates not only the importance of intraoperative management but also the impact of anesthetic technique on postoperative complications. A successful result can be obtained by having awareness about the basic techniques and common complications of rhytidectomy.

A rhytidectomy can be performed alone or in combination with other cosmetic procedures on the face such as blepharoplasty, rhinoplasty, and forehead lift. It has evolved over the last century from a cutaneous procedure where redundant facial skin was pulled and excised. Now subcutaneous facelift is typically combined with surgeries on the superficial musculoaponeurotic system (SMAS) and deeper planes including the subperiosteal technique.[4–6] Before the surgery, the face and neck is infiltrated with a solution of local anesthetic and epinephrine in normal saline, prepared in various strengths depending on the surgeons' techniques and preferences.

Complications

Common complications of facelift surgery consist of expanding hematoma, skin sloughing, nerve injury, hypertrophic scarring, and infection. Out of these, postoperative expanding hematoma has the highest frequency with a reported incidence of 0–15%.[7] A delay in its diagnosis and management can lead to facial edema, skin sloughing, scarring, and neuropraxia. A rapidly expanding hematoma, especially from an arterial bleed, can lead to airway compromise and respiratory distress. The usual presenting signs and symptoms

Practical Ambulatory Anesthesia, ed. Johan Raeder and Richard D. Urman. Published by Cambridge University Press.
© Cambridge University Press 2015.

are sudden onset of pain, swelling and bruising. Prompt evacuation of the hematoma is essential for good results. There is no definite consensus of opinion in the plastic surgery literature on factors contributing to post-rhytidectomy hematoma. Besides factors related to surgical techniques leading to hematoma formation, other issues implicated are pre-existing hypertension,[8] sudden perioperative spikes in blood pressure,[7] retching, coughing and vomiting,[9] the patient's level of anxiety and activity after the surgery, platelet and coagulation disorders, and perioperative use of medications that interfere with clotting. Some studies show higher incidence of hematoma in patients receiving general anesthesia[10] while others show none.[11]

The incidence of surgical site infection after face-lift surgery has been reported as 0.6%. In a chart review of 780 post-rhytidectomy patients between 2001 and 2007, five were found to have developed infections. Four of them were MRSA-positive.[12] Albeit the small incidence, morbidity can be significant as it may require wound exploration with irrigation and drainage and hospital admission for intravenous antibiotic administration.

Patient selection and preoperative evaluation

Although ambulatory anesthesia for aesthetic surgery is considered relatively risk-free as compared to other surgical procedures, its safety is intricately linked with coordination among all team members, focused preoperative evaluation, patient selection, and preparation. In addition to the general factors that are considered for suitability of a patient for any ambulatory surgical procedure, there are some additional considerations specific to facelift that help in both patient selection and crafting the anesthetic plan. It goes without saying that careful preoperative evaluation and selection goes a long way towards reducing morbidity.

Preoperative evaluation starts with a detailed medical history and physical examination with emphasis on cardiopulmonary history. History of hypertension should be carefully elicited and surgery should be scheduled in hypertensive patients only if there is well-documented evidence of controlled hypertension. Patients may have been prescribed anti-hypertensive medications but may not be compliant. Blood pressure should be checked and if there is any suspicion of unmanaged hypertension, they should be referred for treatment. Although facelift is considered a low-risk

ambulatory procedure, patients should be optimized from a cardiac standpoint. Intraoperative injection of epinephrine-containing solutions can cause significant tachycardia and hypertension that may be detrimental for a patient with cardiac issues. Epinephrine absorption can continue postoperatively, too, when the patient may not be monitored.

Family and personal history of bleeding tendencies and coagulopathies is very important. Patients should be carefully asked about these issues. A high index of suspicion should be maintained if there is any suggestion of menorrhagia, recurrent nosebleeds, easy bruising, and prolonged bleeding from minor cuts and wounds, and suitable laboratory tests should be ordered. Names of all the prescription and non-prescription medications and herbal supplements should be asked as some of them interfere with normal clotting.

Recent use of diet pills, herbal supplements and weight loss medications may not be voluntarily disclosed by patients due to the attached stigmata. They should be directly asked about these medications because of their various ill effects in combination with anesthetics,[13] such as prolonged hypotension at induction, and arrhythmias, hypoglycemia, and hypotension during maintenance of anesthesia. Hypotension can be due to the catecholamine depletion or direct cardiac depression. Arrhythmogenic effect in the face of epinephrine used for infiltration can have dangerous consequences. Some of these drugs may slow gastric emptying, which can be unsafe in a patient receiving deep sedation with unprotected airway.

Illicit drugs, alcohol abuse, and smoking can also add to morbidity and make intravenous sedation difficult by altering the dosing requirements of anesthetic medications. Use of nicotine in patients undergoing facelift is associated with skin necrosis and hematoma formation.[14] Smoking is also associated with increased sputum production and associated coughing. Not only does this lead to increased blood pressure, but it can also cause laryngospasm in a sedated patient. Preoperative smoking cessation for at least 4–6 weeks is recommended to reduce the risk of an increased intraoperative sputum volume.[15]

A special note should be made about the history of obstructive sleep apnea and obesity as this may impact the anesthetic plan. Similar to anesthetic evaluation for any other procedure, airway exam is mandatory. Overdose, and in some instances normal levels, of intravenous anesthetic agents in unintubated patients can cause airway obstruction that can be disastrous in patients with difficult airways. Because facelift is a totally elective surgery, if there is any concern, surgery should not be scheduled until appropriate consultations have been obtained and all issues resolved.

Anesthetic management

Patient safety is the first and main goal of the anesthesiologist while performing any surgery. It is demonstrated by published data[16] that the risks associated with rhytidectomy and liposuctions are similar to other surgical procedures. Despite the relative safety of elective ambulatory cosmetic surgeries, a 10-year audit of prospectively collected in-office adverse event data[17] from Florida indicates that there were 46 deaths over this period; 56.5% (26/46) of these deaths were associated with cosmetic procedures. The majority of these deaths were in patients who had received general anesthesia, although most of them occurred in non-accredited facilities with substandard care and limited staffing.

In addition to patient safety concerns, the successful performance of facial cosmetic surgery is dependent on a well-formulated anesthetic plan that ensures a motionless patient in a calm and controlled surgical field, a smooth anesthetic emergence without coughing and bucking, avoidance of postoperative nausea and vomiting, and timely readiness for discharge home.

Preoperative sedation for anxiolysis should be used judiciously in these patients and not before the surgeon has completed marking the face. Facial topography is marked in the sitting position immediately before surgery. Benzodiazepines have a relaxant effect on the muscles and can add to drooping, which may interfere with marking. Even the shorter-acting benzodiazepine midazolam has a half-life of 1–4 hours that may be prolonged in the elderly. Once the surgeon has completed marking the face, sedation can be started with midazolam. In some instances, such as blepharoplasties, surgeons may request to avoid benzodiazepines completely. Many plastic surgeons routinely prescribe clonidine 0.1–0.2 mg preoperatively as it helps both to allay anxiety and control blood pressure.[18]

The technique and depth of anesthesia is contingent on the extent and invasiveness of the procedure. It can range in depth from minimal sedation where the patient follows commands to a level compatible with general anesthesia and anything in between. The most important aspect of these surgeries that distinguish them from other procedures is airway avoidance. Not only is the operation table usually turned 90 degrees away from the anesthesia providers, but also the face and neck are in the sterile field and cannot be touched for jaw thrust or lifting the chin up in case of airway obstruction in unintubated patients. This is a vital factor that determines the technique used for airway management. Surgeons should be consulted about the extent of the procedure and their expectation of depth of anesthesia. Do they want a completely motionless patient throughout the case? Some surgeons prefer patients to be in a sedation plane compatible with general anesthesia while they inject and infiltrate tissues with local anesthetic solutions, and awake during other parts of the case when they ask the patients to smile or do other movements to check the integrity of the facial nerve. Oral endotracheal intubation is considered bothersome by some surgeons as the endotracheal tube is in their way and causes distortion of the mouth. Another option may be to use a nasotracheal tube, although this may introduce the risk of nasal bleeding, which may be reduced by careful insertion and lubrication of the tube and mucous membranes of the nose. Surgeons are also concerned about coughing and bucking at emergence with consequent sudden increases in blood pressure. Their expectations should be considered in light of patient characteristics, the final decision being dependent on the anesthesiologist. If the patient has history and features of obstructive sleep apnea and difficult airway, especially potentially challenging mask ventilation, the best option is to electively intubate the airway rather than do it emergently in the middle of the case in a suboptimal and stressful situation. Of course, a valid alternative may be the laryngeal mask airway (LMA), which can help reduce the need for profound general anesthesia and paralysis. However, in peri-oral procedures, distortion of the shape of the lips by the bulky LMA tubing may be undesirable. The risk of aspiration should be assessed, especially in procedures of longer durations. Patients with histories of depression and anxiety can be challenging to sedate, too, as they may have either tolerance to sedatives or altered drug metabolism. Due to these factors, sedatives and hypnotics cannot be titrated effectively as depth of sedation in these patients tends to dwindle between the extremes of fidgeting and apnea but no happy medium; and that too without the luxury of being able to quickly mask ventilate.

Basic American Society of Anesthesiologists standards of monitoring are applicable to all cases to ensure safe provision of anesthesia. Capnography

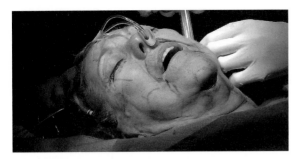

Figure 12.1 Oxygen tubing via nasopharyngeal airway technique.

detection of CO_2 and monitoring of respiration frequency can be achieved in unintubated patients by various methods. Nasal oxygen cannulae with the capability of carbon dioxide sampling and monitoring can be used if agreed with surgeons. Care should be taken during oxygen administration in close proximity to the surgical site when electrocautery is being used. American Society of Anesthesiologists Practice Advisory for the Prevention and Management of Operating Room Fires[19] includes surgeries on face and neck in high-risk procedures as far as operating room fires are concerned. There should be close communication among all team members and an agreed upon emergency plan with specific role and task assignment for everyone in case of a fire. In unintubated patients in our practice, we use a combination of nasopharynegeal airway and nasal oxygen cannula to provide oxygen if needed. The cut ends of a nasal cannula tubing and capnography sample line are inserted into an appropriate size rubber nasopharyngeal airway up to its tip (Figure 12.1). This whole unit is then externally lubricated and advanced into the nostril of a sedated patient. Supplemental oxygen up to 3 liters per minute can be safely used by this technique. Oxygen concentration is determined to be close to ambient air in various areas around the face while using this technique.[20]

Blood pressure is closely monitored and although lower pressure is desirable to decrease the risk of hematoma formation, caution should be exercised in the older patient population with long-standing hypertension as they are prone to cerebral ischemia. Infrared brain oxygen monitor with pads on the forehead may be an expensive but useful option in high-risk patients. Cases of carotid stenosis should be identified and carefully managed. This concern should be discussed with the surgeon and the lowest blood pressure safe for a particular patient should be agreed upon by both

anesthesiologist and surgeon. A sudden increase in blood pressure due to epinephrine absorption can occur. Care should be taken not to manage this with beta-blockers alone as this can give rise to unopposed alpha stimulation, which can lead to severe vasoconstriction in the face of cardiac beta-blockade, resulting in pulmonary edema. If intravascular injection is suspected, the surgeon should be informed immediately. Although surgeons prefer blood pressure to be on the lower side, some of them may request normotensive pressures before flap closure to ensure sufficient hemostasis. Temperature monitoring and maintenance of normothermia, especially in longer cases, not only ensures patient comfort but helps to decrease negative patient consequences. These include bleeding, which can lead to hematoma formation, surgical site infection, morbid cardiac events, and prolongation of postanesthesia discharge time to home.

The maintenance of general anesthetic can be achieved with either inhalational or intravenous agents in intubated patients. Emergence is usually smoother in intubated patients receiving total intravenous anesthesia. In our practice, propofol is nearly always used in conjunction with another medication in subhypnotic doses for this purpose. Ketamine is one of the adjuncts and can be added to propofol in concentrations ranging from 0.25 to 1.5 mg/ml, titrated to patient requirements of sedation or general anesthesia.[21] However, it should be remembered that ketamine causes increased salivation that can lead to coughing and laryngospasm in an unintubated patient. The lower dose range is not associated with postoperative nausea and vomiting or delayed discharge. Another drug combination that has been used successfully is alfentanil and propofol, both for general anesthesia and mild to moderate sedation. Alfentanil is infused over a dose range of 0.2–0.4 µg/kg/min and propofol 25–75 µg/kg/min.[22] It has a faster onset than fentanyl but a shorter duration of action. During deep sedation, it has been shown to cause oxygen desaturation. Remifentanil infusion can also be safely titrated in spontaneously breathing unintubated patients and in intubated patients. It has been shown that the risk of postoperative hypertension is increased after remifentanil-based anesthesia. The underlying mechanism, although not completely understood, has been attributed to abrupt cessation of analgesia or acute opioid tolerance.[23,24] This may be a concern after facelift where there is a risk of hematoma formation, especially in the setting of ongoing absorption of previously infiltrated epinephrine. Blood pressure should be closely monitored and managed accordingly. Anti-emetic prophylaxis is extremely important is plastic surgical procedures as straining during retching and vomiting can also increase blood pressure.

Post-anesthesia recovery room (PACU)

The key points of anesthetic care, including but not limited to blood pressure management, normothermia, and anti-emetic management, should be continued in PACU, too. PACU staff should be directed to watch for any sign of hematoma formation and respiratory distress. In the rare situation of airway obstruction, the wound may have to be opened immediately. Timely diagnosis and evacuation of hematoma not only averts respiratory emergency but also leads to normal healing. An emergency plan should be in place for surgical evacuation of hematoma.[7] Anesthesiologist and operating room nursing personnel should be available until the decision is made to discharge the patient. Equipment to emergently secure the airway should be at hand, operating room set up before staff leaves, and a sterile set of instruments available. Evacuation of hematoma may require intravenous sedation or general anesthesia depending upon the situation and anxiety level of the patient.

Tumescent anesthesia for liposuction

Liposuction is one of the most common ambulatory cosmetic procedures performed in the United States, and tumescent anesthesia is widely used for this purpose. Surprisingly, there is a dearth of articles or any comprehensive guidelines on this topic in anesthesia literature in spite of many of us being involved in the perioperative management of these cases.

Tumescent anesthesia is regional local anesthesia of the skin and subcutaneous tissue. This technique was first described by a dermatologist, Dr. Jeffry Klein.[25] It involves the ballooning of subcutaneous fat with large volumes of dilute lidocaine and epinephrine solution in normal saline or Ringer's Lactate. The concentration of lidocaine ranges from 0.025% to 0.1% as compared to the traditional 0.5–2% used for nerve blocks or field blocks. One milligram of epinephrine is added to each liter of solution with resultant final strength of 1:1,000,000 (1 µg/ml). Approximately 3–4 ml of the infiltrate is infused for each planned milliliter of aspirate. Subcutaneous infiltration of large volumes of this solution produces swelling and firmness (tumescence) of tissues. Fat is detached from the subcutaneous skin with the help of liposuction cannulas and up to several liters of emulsified fat are suctioned or aspirated. Aspiration can be either manual or power-assisted.

The major dichotomy that is faced by anesthesiologists is the dose of lidocaine used for tumescent anesthesia. According to Practice Advisory on Liposuction,[26] "it is generally accepted that a lidocaine dose of up to 35 mg/kg is safe when injected into the subcutaneous fat with solutions containing epinephrine, although doses up to 50 mg/kg have been utilized." This goes against our training of a conventional maximum allowable dose of 7 mg/kg. This dose, when used as 1–2% lidocaine for neuraxial blocks, nerve blocks, and skin infiltration, is constrained by the development of central nervous system toxicity. In comparison, tumescent anesthesia doses have been used in tens of thousands of procedures with minimal harm. This duality of lidocaine dosing has been attributed to the fact that a very dilute solution (1 mg/ml) is slowly infiltrated into a poorly vascularized space. Because liodcaine is relatively lipophilic, it binds to the extensive shallow subdermal fat reservoir in the range of 1 mg of lidocaine per gram of tissue, and some of this is removed when the lipid is aspirated out. This large absorption buffer retains lidocaine in comparison to concentrated (10 mg/ml or 1%) lidocaine, where 1/10 mg is absorbed by the buffer and 9/10 mg remains unbound and can be absorbed in systemic circulation, leading to elevated levels in blood.[27] Epinephrine in the solution has a vasoconstrictive effect that also slows and decreases the systemic absorption of lidocaine, resulting in lower peak blood levels and increased duration of analgesia.[28] It has been shown that after 1% lidocaine injection for epidural block and intercostal nerve block, peak blood levels are achieved in approximately 7 and 8 minutes, respectively.[29] In contrast, lidocaine peaks 8–16 hours after infiltration for tumescent anesthesia.[28]

In addition to difference in peak effect, there is a difference in clearance of lidocaine from systemic circulation, too. Two hours after epidural lidocaine injection, lidocaine blood level is negligible. Measurable levels of lidocaine and its metabolite persist for more than 36 hours after tumescent anesthesia.[27]

Although tumescent doses of lidocaine have been used safely, neurologic and cardiac toxicity can occur due to various reasons. Lidocaine is metabolized in the liver by the CYP 450 enzyme family and toxicity depends on the ratio of its absorption and removal from the blood. Any limit on hepatic clearance can prolong lidocaine persistence in the circulation, resulting in serious toxicity. Various drugs can cause competitive inhibition of the CYP 450 system. Some of these drugs that are commonly used are alprazolam, carbamazepine, erythromycin, losartan, and simvastatin. As hepatic lidocaine clearance is flow-dependent (rather than substrate-dependent), enzyme saturation is a bigger concern than competitive inhibition. This means that a massive lidocaine load can overwhelm the CYP 450. Toxicity from tumescent lidocaine can initially present as cardiac toxicity instead of CNS symptoms as slow rise and prolonged elevated levels progressively depress cardiac conduction and contraction, ultimately leading to circulatory failure. Careful calculation of maximum tumescent lidocaine dose is essential to minimize the risk of toxicity. It is also important not to combine tumescent anesthesia with procedures requiring regular-strength lidocaine (nerve blocks or local infiltration for various procedures).

Volume overload is another important risk associated with tumescent anesthesia. As previously mentioned, a substantial volume of anesthetic solution (3–4 ml infiltrate/ml of planned aspirate) is injected to produce tumescence. This can add up to 800–2000 ml for abdomen, 400–1000 ml for each hip, 500–1200 ml for each lateral thigh, and same volume for each medial and anterior thigh, respectively. Fifty to seventy percent of infiltrate is left behind at completion of procedure and gets absorbed.[26] Fluid overload can result in serious complications such as pulmonary edema and electrolyte imbalance. Communication with the surgeon on fluid management is critical and it is imperative to monitor fluid input and output throughout the case and afterwards. At completion of the procedure, calculation of residual volume helps to determine postoperative care. If large volume liposuction (> 5000 cc of aspirate) is planned, it should be performed as inpatient instead of ambulatory procedure. Patients should be monitored overnight for stability of vital signs and urine output. Large-volume procedures should be done as separate serial procedures.[26]

Intraoperative hypothermia can be another consequence of large-volume tumescent anesthesia and appropriate measures should be taken to prevent and manage it, such as using pre-warmed (37°C) fluid.

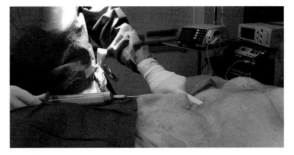

Figure 12.2 Liposuction trocar in close proximity to liver.

Like any other surgical procedure, serious consideration should be given to prophylaxis for deep vein thrombosis which can result in pulmonary embolism. There have been reports of death from fat emboli, too.[26] Fat emboli can occur from both mechanical (absorption of fat globules) and biochemical reasons (inflammation from circulating fatty acids causing damage to pneumocytes).

The choice of anesthesia for tumescent liposuction depends on patient status, site and extent of the procedure, and the patient's level of comfort. Complex procedures are better done under general anesthesia to provide a motionless surgical field and airway control. Liposuction over the abdominal wall is relatively high-risk due to the repetitive motion of the trocar in close proximity to critical viscera such as the liver (Figure 12.2). Any sudden patient movement or coughing can cause hepatic injury so adequate depth of anesthesia is imperative. Epidural and spinal anesthesia in the ambulatory setting might not be suitable for large-area liposuction as sympathectomy from neuraxial anesthesia can lead to vasodilatation and hypotension which is usually managed with intravenous fluid infusion. In this particular situation where the patient is already receiving tumescence fluids, this can increase the risk of fluid overload.

Careful patient selection is critical for this procedure. The history of congestive heart failure and patients on multiple medications should be evaluated in detail and, if possible, medications altering metabolism of hepatic enzyme systems should be stopped ahead of time.

Recovery room nurses should be carefully instructed to monitor signs of fluid overload or local anesthetic toxicity.

Intralipid should be immediately available. There should be a pre-existing emergency patient transfer arrangement with a nearby hospital with the capability to manage local anesthetic toxicity. Active warming of the patient should continue in PACU if needed.

Breast surgery

Breast reduction or breast implant surgery usually requires general anesthesia. Muscle relaxation is not needed in most cases so intubation is not necessary and laryngeal mask airway is sufficient. During the procedure, surgeons may ask the anesthesiologist to put the operating table in a sitting position. The patient's arms should be carefully secured on the arm boards for this reason. The anesthesia circuit should be of adequate length to avoid the risk of extubation while sitting up the patient. Although local anesthetic injection in the field is enough for analgesia in most of the cases, some patients may still feel significant pain, discomfort, or pressure. Thoracic paravertebral block may be helpful in these situations, but is not without inherent risks. This can be discussed ahead of time with the surgeon and if done preoperatively, it helps to decrease intraoperative opioid requirement with its resultant negative consequences. Still, a combination of local anesthetic infiltration and titrated remifentanil or alfentanil infusion may be adequate in the majority of cases. Alfentanil lasts well into the recovery period and contributes to postoperative analgesia.

Factors leading to perioperative morbidity in plastic surgery include some of the following:

- Insufficient preoperative evaluation.
- Failure to monitor respiration.
- Failure to monitor vital signs.
- Poor communication.
- Delay in responding to emergencies.
- Failure to ensure emergency equipment was working properly.
- Local anesthetic overdose.
- Intravascular/intralaryngeal injection of local anesthetic.

References

1. American Society for Aesthetic Plastic Surgery reports over 10 Million Cosmetic Procedures, NEW YORK, NY (March 12, 2013), Statistics, Surveys & Trends, *American Society for Aesthetic Plastic Surgery*, http://www.surgery.org/
2. Vila H Jr., Soto R, Cantor AB, *et al.* Comparative outcomes analysis of procedures performed in physician offices and ambulatory surgery centers. *Arch Surg.* 2003;**138**(9):991–95.
3. Prendiville S, Weiser S. Management of anesthesia and facility in facelift surgery. *Facial Plast Surg Clin North Am.* 2009 Nov;**17**(4):531–38, v.
4. Miller TR, Eisbach KJ. SMAS facelift techniques to minimize stigmata of surgery. *Otolaryngol Clin North Am.* 2007;**40**:391–408.
5. Baker SR. Rhytidectomy. In: Cummings CW, Flint PW, Haughey BH, Robbins KT, Thomas JR. *Otolaryngology: Head & Neck Surgery.* 4th ed. St. Louis, MO: Mosby; 2005: chapter 30.
6. Hamra ST. Composite rhytidectomy. *Plast Reconstr Surg* 1997;**24**(2):1–13.
7. Niamtu J III. *Expanding Hematoma in Face-lift Surgery: Literature Review, Case Presentations, and Caveats 2005* by the American Society for Dermatologic Surgery, Inc. Published by BC Decker Inc. ISSN: 1076–0512 *Dermatol Surg* 2005;**31**:1134–44.
8. Berner RE, Morain WD, Noe JM. Postoperative hypertension as an etiological factor in hematoma after rhytidectomy: prevention with chlorpromazine. *Plast Reconstr Surg* 1976;**57**:314–19.
9. Steely RL, Collins DR Jr, Cohen BE, Bass K. Postoperative nausea and vomiting in the plastic surgery patient. *Aesthetic Plast Surg* 2004;**28**:29–32.
10. Rees TD, Aston SJ. Complications in rhytidectomy. *Clin Plast Surg* 1978;**5**:109–19.
11. Conway H. The surgical face lift – rhytidectomy. *Plast Reconstr Surg* 1970;**45**:124–30.
12. Zoumalan RA, Rosenberg DB. Methicillin-resistant *Staphylococcus aureus*-positive surgical site infections in face-lift surgery. *Arch Facial Plast Surg* 2008;**10**(2):116–23.
13. Jeffers L. Anesthetic considerations for the new anti-obesity medications. *The Internet Journal of Anesthesiology.* 1996 Volume **1** Number 4.
14. Rees TD, Liverett DM, Guy CL. The effect of cigarette smoking on skin-flap survival in the face lift patient. *Plast Reconstr Surg* 1984;**73**(6):911–15.
15. Yamashita S, Yamaguchi H, Sakaguchi M, *et al.* Effect of smoking on intraoperative sputum and postoperative pulmonary complication in minor surgical patients. *Respir Med.* 2004 Aug;**98**(8):760–66.
16. Yoho RA, Romaine JJ, O'Neil D. Review of the liposuction, abdominoplasty, and face-lift mortality and morbidity risk literature. *Dermatol Surg.* 2005 Jul;**31**(7 Pt 1): 733–43; discussion 743.
17. Starling J 3rd, Thosani MK, Coldiron BM. Determining the safety of office-based surgery: what 10 years of Florida data and 6 years of Alabama data reveal. *Dermatol Surg.* 2012 Feb;**38**(2):171–77.

18. Thorne CH, *et al.*, eds. Facelift. In *Grabb and Smith's Plastic Surgery*, Sixth Edition, Chapter 49. Philadelphia, PA: Lippincott Williams and Wilkins, 2006.

19. Practice Advisory for the Prevention and Management of Operating Room Fires. *An Updated Report by the American Society of Anesthesiologists Task Force on Operating Room Fires. Anesthesiology* 2013;**118**(2).

20. Meneghetti SC, Morgan MM, Fritz J, *et al.* Operating room fires: optimizing safety. *Plast Reconstr Surg.* 2007 Nov;**120**(6):1701–08.

21. Badrinath S, Avramov MN, Shadrick M, Witt TR, Ivankovich AD. The use of a ketamine–propofol combination during monitored anesthesia care. *Anesth Analg* 2000 Apr;**90**(4):858–62.

22. Avramov MN, White PF. Use of alfentanil and propofol for outpatient monitored anesthesia care: determining the optimal dosing regimen. *Anesth Analg* 1997 Sep;**85**(3):566–72.

23. Guignard B, Bossard AE, Coste C, *et al.* Acute opioid tolerance: intraoperative remifentanil increases postoperative pain and morphine requirement. *Anesthesiology.* 2000 Aug;**93**(2):409–17.

24. Bilotta F, Lam AM, Doronzio A, *et al.* Esmolol blunts postoperative hemodynamic changes after propofol–remifentanil total intravenous fast-track neuroanesthesia for intracranial surgery. *J Clin Anesth* 2008;**20**(6):426–30.

25. Klein JA. *Tumescent Technique – Tumescent Anesthesia and Microcannular Liposuction.* St. Louis, MO: Mosby, 2000.

26. Iverson RE, Lynch DJ, ASPS Committee on Patient Safety. Practice Advisory on Liposuction. *Plast & Reconstructive Surg* 2004;**113**:1478–90.

27. DeJong RH. Tumescent anesthesia: lidocaine dosing dichotomy. *Intern J Cosmetic Surg Anesth Dermatol* 2002;**4**(1):3–7.

28. Kenkel JM, Lipschitz AH, Shepherd G, *et al.* Pharmacokinetics and safety of lidocaine and monoethylglycinexylidide in liposuction: a microdialysis study. *Plast Reconstr Surg* 2004;**114**(2):516–24.

29. Yokoyama J, Mizobushi S, Nakatsuka H, Hirkawa M. Comparison of plasma lidocaine concentrations after injection of a fixed small volume in the stellate ganglion, the lumbar epidural space, or a single intercostal nerve. *Anesth Analg* 1998;**87**(1):112–15.

Chapter 13

Anesthesia for gastrointestinal endoscopy

John E. Tetzlaff, MD, and Walter G. Maurer, MD

Introduction

With the progressive increase in the volume of ambulatory anesthesia in the United States, more and more of these anesthetics are being provided outside the traditional realm of the operating room with increasing complexity of the surgical procedures and comorbidity in the patients. Minimally invasive procedures are best performed with a minimally invasive anesthetic. These are best performed by an ambulatory anesthetic technique. Of all the arenas where ambulatory anesthetics are being performed outside the operating room (OR), the gastrointestinal endoscopy suite (GES) may be the best example of this rapid expansion of case volume, procedural complexity, and patient comorbidity.[1] Even those anesthesia providers with extensive experience with ambulatory anesthesia may find the environment in the GES to be unusual related to unique elements of this setting, compared to the traditional OR experience. This is related to unique elements of the GES, including design, patient selection, scheduling, advanced endoscopy procedures (AEP), role of the Gastroenterologist as a consultant, variety of cases performed, equipment, anesthetic technique, and recovery from anesthesia.

Design of the gastrointestinal endoscopy suite

Providing anesthesia services for gastrointestinal (GI) procedures began with requests to provide anesthesia in the OR for unusual cases. Routine procedures such as colonoscopy and esophagogastroduodenoscopy (EGD) were scheduled in the OR when difficulty with sedation and/or comorbidity dictated the participation of an anesthesia team.[2] It is also clear that there is considerable variability in the opinions of patients and providers about the level of comfort required for endoscopy.[3,4]

As the volume of GI endoscopy procedures has increased, there has been demand for a setting with the capacity for greater volume. Different gastroenterology groups have approached this in a variety of ways. The simplest (but perhaps least-efficient) approach is for the gastroenterology service to regularly schedule cases in the OR. The advantages including the existence of a scheduling system, the guarantee that each OR is staffed with anesthesia services available, and routine recovery from anesthesia. Disadvantages include the need to move endoscopy equipment to the OR, case turnover time, and distance from the gastroenterology procedural suite where anesthesia services are not required.

An alternative to bringing the GI cases to the OR is bringing the anesthesia services needed to the GES. The gastroenterology endoscopist will favor this option because of the proximity to their offices and to the routine endoscopy cases. It will also be optimal from the equipment standpoint, as transporting scopes, camera pods, and disposables can be avoided. With the increasing complexity of AEP, there is equipment which cannot be transported, including camera towers and customized fluoroscopy devices. This makes bringing anesthesia services directly to the GES reasonable. The issues from the anesthesia service standpoint revolve around efficiency and scheduling. The control of the OR schedule is the focus that influences the structure of anesthesia services. It is widely known that scheduling efficiency decays frequently with cases scheduled outside the OR. Non-operating room anesthesia (NORA) requires dedicated anesthesia personnel, and for team care environments, reduces concurrency. It also requires providing and maintaining anesthesia equipment and availability of anesthesia drugs. This requires considerable effort when the services requested by the gastroenterology endoscopist are

Practical Ambulatory Anesthesia, ed. Johan Raeder and Richard D. Urman. Published by Cambridge University Press.
© Cambridge University Press 2015.

infrequent or irregular. When the need for anesthesia services is regular and the volume predictable, efficiency issues can take care of themselves.

With the increasing volume of routine colonoscopy and EGD patients with difficult sedation issues or severe comorbidity and the number of AEP cases, there is a trend toward creation of optimally designed GES. This presents the anesthesia service with the opportunity to interact with the design and management structure of the new unit. This allows optimal location of anesthetic gas supply, purchase of dedicated anesthesia machines for each location, and some system for dispensing anesthesia drugs. Some of these GES include rooms for AEP and routine cases, and the need for anesthesia service is designed by structure.

Patient selection for the GES

Although the majority of cases in most GES are ambulatory, the creation of a dedicated procedure suite within a hospital will immediately create demand to do these procedures for hospital patients. However, the anesthesia care for the hospital patients often is not substantially different from the ambulatory patient, due to the minimally invasive nature of the procedures.

The highest volume of patients needing anesthesia services are scheduled for routine colonoscopy or EGD with a history of difficult sedation for previous endoscopy.[5] This can involve prior attempts at the procedure that could not be completed or prior procedures that were completed but left the patient with a high level of anxiety leading to the request for deeper sedation. Hospital patients can be scheduled in the GES for screening colonoscopy or EGD prior to listing for heart, lung, or liver transplant. The final group of patients is those scheduled for AEP. The majority are still ambulatory, but with the rapid advancement of endoscopic skills and technology allowing procedures to be performed without surgery, a substantial number of these cases will be done for hospital patients. The common denominator for all is the rapid turnover environment of the GES, where rapid recovery is required, and may be best provided by the anesthesia team.[6]

Advanced endoscopic procedures (AEP)

Most of the AEP have evolved from modifications of routine endoscopy techniques and equipment. The procedures are either diagnostic, therapeutic, or both and listed in Table 13.1. Early therapeutic endoscopic management of GI bleeding was limited by the

Table 13.1 Advanced endoscopic procedures.

Double-balloon enteroscopy (DBE)

Endoscopic ultrasound (EUS)

Endoscopically assisted fine-needle aspiration (FNA)

Endoscopic intestinal dilation

Endoscopic retrograde cholangiopancreatography (ERCP)

Esophageal dilation or stenting

Endoscopic treatment of GI bleeding

Endoscopic drainage of pancreatic pseudocyst

Endoscopic removal of pancreatic or bile duct stones

Endoscopic placement of intestinal feeding tubes

Percutaneous endoscopic gastrostomy (PEG) tube placement

length of the scopes and what they could reach. When GI bleeding sites could not be identified, the only alternative was surgical intervention. This led to the creation of double-balloon endoscopy (DBE). With an outer cannula, and inner and outer balloons, the endoscopist can telescope the gut on itself, greatly increasing the depth that can be reached. With sequential DBE via upper and lower access, it is possible to endoscopically examine the entire length of the GI tract, reaching treatable varices, arteriovenous malformations, or other bleeding lesions. It is possible to dilate any intestinal stricture throughout the entire length of the gut, avoiding surgical procedures in many cases. These can be prolonged procedures and may require deep sedation or general anesthesia.[7]

The diagnostic acuity of endoscopy has been increased by the addition of ultrasound technology. Endoscopic ultrasound (EUS) has been developed to help with the diagnosis of lesions throughout the GI tract, especially for the pancreas and common bile duct.[8] This has been further advanced with the technology for endoscopically aided fine-needle aspiration (FNA). This allows tissue diagnosis of difficult lesions in locations such as the pancreas or biliary tree, where the location of lesions is difficult, the consequences of surgery are serious, and the need for accurate tissue is critical to guide serious therapeutic interventions including chemotherapy and radiation. EUS has been used to evaluate pancreatic lesions and to locate stones within the pancreatic or biliary tracts.

Endoscopy has been combined with balloon dilation techniques to correct strictures within the full length of the gut, from the esophagus to the rectum. The DBE technique to identify the stricture combined with balloon dilation allows treatment of strictures within the distal small bowel, previously only addressed surgically. For recurrent or very tortuous strictures, the balloon dilation is followed by the deployment of a stent. Stent treatment is also used when the stricture is accompanied by fistula. One of the more exciting applications is dilation if needed and stenting of tracheoesophageal fistula, related to esophageal cancer, radiation sequelae, or invasive cancer located in the proximal trachea.

One of the most rapidly expanding roles for AEP involves endoscopic diagnosis and treatment of the biliary tract and pancreas. Endoscopic retrograde cholangiopancreatography (ERCP) allows visualization of the patency of the biliary and pancreatic ducts, identification of stones or masses obstructing either ductal system, as well as identification and treatment of purulent cholangitis with irrigation and stenting. When combined with balloon techniques, strictures of these ductal systems can be dilated and stented. When combined with EUS technology, it is possible to drain giant pancreatic pseudocysts.

Intestinal feeding tubes and percutaneous endoscopic gastrostomy (PEG) tubes are facilitated applications of EGD techniques. Endoscopic placement of feeding and gastric emptying tubes has virtually replaced the surgical approaches in many high-volume gastroenterology centers.

Scheduling within the GES

The scheduling of cases in the GES can present frustration for the anesthesia team because of the significant differences compared to the OR environment. In the operating room (including the ambulatory suite), the scheduling model is closed, which means that for the vast majority of cases, the booking of a case is done by the team of the primary surgeon. In many GES, the scheduling is fully open. This means that the endoscopist is assigned to do cases, most of which are scheduled by other physicians. The scheduling physicians can be other Gastroenterologists, Internists, Colorectal surgeons, and a variety of other physicians within individual centers. This means that the endoscopist is rarely the primary physician for the AEP and often meets the patient minutes before the procedure for consent. This creates a whole spectrum of issues, including the indications for the procedure, the preparation of the patients and

issues with who admits the patient if there is an unplanned complication, such as acute pancreatitis after ERCP. The disconnect between scheduling and deciding if the procedure is indicated often requires interaction between the endoscopist and the scheduling physician and further discussion of risk/benefit considerations with the patient.

Role of the gastroenterology staff physician as a consultant

In the OR, the surgeon is the primary care physician. In the GES, the endoscopist most often is a consultant to another service, gastroenterology or other. The case is scheduled and this creates an obligation for the endoscopist to do the case. There can be friction when there are different opinions about the indications for the procedure or the decision of which procedure to perform. Ultimately, the endoscopist scheduled to do the case decides, but this can leave referring teams disappointed or angry. In addition to scheduling issues, there are management issues that are challenging to resolve, including admission to the hospital and pain control. This creates even more management issues for the anesthesia team, when issues present that are outside the traditional responsibility for gastroenterology such as pain or nausea/vomiting. Arranging admission to the hospital is even more challenging than it is for the endoscopist, whose service has admitting privileges.

Pre-anesthesia preparation

For ambulatory patients scheduled for OR procedures, there is a wide range of approaches to pre-anesthesia testing (PAT). However, there is variability in the approach but no resistance to the idea that the patient must be prepared for surgery. For patients scheduled for AEP with anesthesia participation, this is not a widely recognized element of the process. For those scheduling the cases, there is no prior experience with the routines of preparation for surgery. The endoscopist may be aware, but most of the patients do not meet the endoscopist until the day of the procedure. This creates an obligation for the anesthesia service to create protocols and insist on compliance.[9] Even simple things like NPO guidelines can create conflict. The gastroenterology team will be familiar with conscious sedation and liberal consumption of fluids within 4 hours, or even 2 hours before the procedure. On the other hand, the AEP patient population includes many obese patients, and

Table 13.2 Common comorbidity in GES patients.

Anemia
Cardiomyopathy
Cholangitis
Chronic kidney disease
Coagulopathy
COPD
Coronary artery disease
Gastroparesis
Intestinal obstruction
Liver failure
Neurological disease
Obstructive sleep apnea
Reflux
Valvular heart disease

many with delayed gastric emptying from a variety of causes. The absence of formal PAT makes these instructions even more challenging, given that they must be delivered and explained. Pre-medication and instructions about whether to take chronic medications are routinely handled in the OR environment. This is not handled in a uniform manner in many GES settings, even for medications that either really should or should not be taken on the morning of an ambulatory procedure.

Patients in the GES may have common comorbidities (Table 13.2) related and unrelated to the GI pathology. Many have bleeding and may be anemic. Others have had multiple transfusions and can be difficult to cross-match in preparation for transfusion. If there has been extensive bleeding, or if end-stage liver disease is present[10] coagulopathy is possible. Coagulopathy can also be a consequence of end-stage liver disease, which is also a common cause for various AEP. Risk for aspiration is a continuous issue in AEP patients, related to reflux, gastroparesis, and/or intestinal obstruction. With instrumentation of the pancreatic and biliary ductal system, infection is a possibility, as is spontaneous cholangitis. Sepsis may be the indication for AEP.

Many GES patients are healthy except for their GI pathology. Others have the usual array of comorbidities with anesthetic implications, such as coronary artery disease (CAD), chronic obstructive pulmonary disease (COPD), chronic neurological disease (e.g. Parkinson's disease), chronic kidney disease, and liver disease. The severity of chronic disease and compliance with

treatment must be considered to determine suitability for AEP. With cardiac patients with pacemakers or implanted cardiac defibrillators (ICD), someone should check device function and battery life, and if electro-surgery is planned or anticipated as a part of the endoscopy, the ICD needs to be safely turned off and supplemented by a transcutaneous device until the ICD is turned on again after the procedure. Decisions about chronic cardiac medications should be active and most medications should be taken on the morning of the procedure, except angiotensin-converting enzyme inhibitors, angiotensin receptor blockers, and diuretics. Diabetic patients should have appropriate instructions about insulin and oral hypoglycemic agents, be scheduled early in the day to avoid long NPO intervals, and have glucose measured on arrival to the GES. COPD patients should have a determination of oxygen saturation and observed room air saturation if oxygen-dependent to assist the decision of how to manage the airway. Medications for chronic reflux should be continued including on the day of the procedure.

Given the nature of the GES and how patients are selected for anesthesia, many of the recommendations above may be partially or completely neglected. This will require the anesthesia team to quickly assess the patient and determine if the patient is suited to receive an anesthetic.

Equipment

In contrast with the OR, there is less standardization of what equipment is available to provide anesthesia support for AEP. In the ideal situation, everything available for OR anesthesia would also be available for anesthesia service in the GES. In the reality of many GES, the anesthesia team must bring what it needs to ensure suction, positive pressure oxygen, airway equipment, anesthesia and resuscitation drugs, and the tools to provide American Society of Anesthesiologists standard monitoring. Tools for management of the difficult airway are important, as is the option to place invasive monitoring in the event of a complication. Although not widely acknowledged by the endoscopists, the use of capnography should be considered an essential part of any sedation for AEP.[11,12]

Anesthetic techniques for procedures in the GES

The starting point for decisions about anesthetic technique for AEP is the choice of how to handle the airway.

Simple endoscopy requires very little analgesia and moderate sedation is adequate. Other AEP can be more complex and have different levels of stimulus. For these cases, the choice is between deep sedation and general anesthesia.[13] Compared to conscious sedation, deep sedation/general anesthesia may actually improve the quality of the procedural outcome for EUS/FNA.[14] Although the separation can be almost semantic, the traditional dividing line is whether endotracheal intubation is required. The decision to intubate involves a number of issues. For patients with chronic gastroparesis or esophageal food impaction, the risk of aspiration is relatively high and intubation is frequently chosen. Some anesthesiologists believe that the prone position, which is frequently chosen by the endoscopist for ERCP, is an indication for endotracheal intubation, although others are willing to proceed with deep sedation without intubation. A strong indication to intubate comes with the plan to drain giant pancreatic pseudocyst, purulent cholangitis, or high-volume irrigation to remove multiple small common duct stones. Obesity is an area where some providers will choose endotracheal intubation, although again, other providers will defer intubation until clinically indicated. In fact, the endoscope often acts like an oral airway, relieving obstruction from backward shifting of the tongue. When in doubt about stomach contents, there is the option to create excellent topical anesthesia and minimal sedation and enter the stomach with a small endoscope. If empty, the level of sedation can be deepened and the procedure completed. If liquid is encountered, it can be emptied prior to proceeding. If solids are encountered, the procedure can be aborted and rescheduled after proper prep, of if emergent, the scope is removed and the patient intubated with a rapid sequence technique. When proper screening is deployed, propofol-based deep sedation without intubation for a variety of AEP was performed without airway compromise.[15]

For most AEP cases, analgesic requirements are minimal and the possibility of patient movement is accepted within reason by the endoscopist because of their experience with mild sedation that they administer for routine cases. The starting point is drying of secretions (glycopyrrolate) followed by topical anesthesia with either benzocaine or lidocaine. The 2% viscous lidocaine gel achieves excellent topical anesthesia of the whole oropharynx if gargled and swallowed, and greatly reduces the level of stimulation with insertion of the endoscope. Drying secretions prior to performing topical anesthesia will increase the quality of the topical anesthesia although advanced planning is required in a busy, rapid-turnover GES. The use of ketorolac is another premedication or component of the sedation technique. The analgesia achieved with ketorolac will reduce the need for opioid and provide a foundation for post-procedure analgesia.[16] This is particularly relevant for the patient with chronic pain related to the GI tract. Ketorolac may have a role in the reduction of post-procedure acute pancreatitis after ERCP, although this outcome is still under review.[17] Unfortunately, ketorolac should be avoided with bleeding, coagulopathy, or renal insufficiency, commonly found in AEP patients. In such cases a COX-II inhibitor may be a valid alternative, either celecoxib, etrocoxib (both have to be given orally before the procedure) or iv parecoxib (currently not FDA-approved in the US). The majority of AEP patients will receive premedication with midazolam (1–2 mg) to relieve anxiety about the procedure and to contribute to moderate or deep sedation, if chosen.

When endotracheal intubation is planned, the anesthetic plan is dictated by disposition plans. For a hospital patient, the options are unlimited. For the ambulatory patient, total intravenous anesthesia (TIVA) or rapid-emergence inhaled agents (desflurane or sevoflurane) can be selected. Opioids can be added, although long-acting opioids such as hydromorphone should be reserved for chronic pain patients and for the treatment of acute pain after the procedure when the patient must be admitted for pain control of acute pancreatitis.

When intubation is not chosen, the technique will be either moderate sedation, deep sedation, or general anesthesia without an endotracheal tube. Propofol is most commonly selected, either alone or in combination with opioids or other intravenous agents. The most common additive is fentanyl, previously identified as a common premedicant at the start of sedation. Alfentanil is also a choice in a mixture with propofol. Alfentanil has a more rapid onset (1–2 min) and shorter duration (5–10 min after bolus) than fentanyl and may be beneficial when pain is acute and short-lasting. However, the risk of sudden respiratory problems may be less with the slower-acting profile of fentanyl bolus. A propofol/alfentanil mixture provides rapid onset of sedation (faster than propofol alone) with opioid-induced blocking of the stimulation of endoscopic intubation. Increasingly, ketamine is also being mixed with propofol or used as a bolus adjunct analogous to how fentanyl is used during the procedure, such as immediately prior to insertion of the endoscope or during peak stimulation moments during ERCP. Ketamine may have a distinct role in the management of patients with severe chronic pain of GI origin.[18] Dexmedetomidine can be used as a sole agent, with the advantage of hemodynamic stability and avoidance of respiratory depression. The disadvantage of dexmedetomidine is the 20-minute loading dose prior to achieving sedation, the occasional hyper-/hypotension encountered during the loading dose, and the prolonged emergence. Some users of dexmedetomidine will use a small dose of midazolam to ensure amnesia.

Regardless of whether deep sedation or endotracheal anesthesia is selected, it is important to take active steps to avoid nausea/vomiting after the procedure. One of the technical elements of endoscopy is inflation of the gut with air to improve the endoscopic viewing of structures and identifying lesions. Saline is often injected to clear the field when the GI prep is less optimum or to clear blood when there has been bleeding. The endoscopist will make every effort to remove gases and/or liquid, but remaining distention is emetogenic. Recent endoscopy technique has been modified to include insufflation with carbon dioxide instead of air.[19,20] This is designed to reduce post-procedure nausea, vomiting, and pain related to insufflation without compromise of the airway or hypercarbia in patients with normal pulmonary reserves.[21,22] Using propofol as the primary sedative brings with it mild anti-emetic properties. Most providers use other prophylaxis including the 5HT-3 antagonists and/or dexamethasone. Patients who start with pain or have a very invasive procedure are likely to emerge from sedation or anesthesia with pain. Acetaminophen plus ketorolac or fentanyl may be sufficient, but chronic severe pain may require morphine or hydromorphone prior to emergence.

Recovery from anesthesia after GES procedures

Any patient who receives care by the anesthesia team should have care post-anesthesia. In some settings, this means the post-anesthesia care unit (PACU) that serves the OR. The care is good but the efficiency is poor. This leads to a push to have PACU care within the GES. This may be feasible when the GES is designed from scratch, but less ideal in existing units where anesthesia has been invited to provide services.

Regardless, the setting must provide appropriate Level 1 and Level 2 PACU care, which includes hemodynamic monitoring, observation of the airway, oxygenation and ventilation, recognition and treatment of nausea/vomiting, and pain control. Criteria must be established for ambulation, fluid, and the need to void prior to discharge for selected patients. A protocol for admission to the hospital should be established, as well as clear definitions of whether the gastroenterology or anesthesia team responds to the various issues. There should be clear protocols for investigating post-procedure GI issues such as acute pancreatitis, bleeding, or perforation at some point in the gut.

References

1. Liu H, Waxman DA, Main R, Mattke S. Utilization of anesthesia services during outpatient endoscopies and colonoscopies and associated spending in 2003–2009. *JAMA* 2012;**307**:1178–84.

2. Aisenberg J, Cohen LB. Sedation in endoscopic practice. *Gastrointest Endoscopy Clin N Am* 2006;**16**:695–708.

3. Barriga J, Sachdev MS, Royall L, Brown G, Tombazzi CR. Sedation for upper endoscopy: comparison of midazolam versus fentanyl plus midazolam. *Southern Med J* 2008;**101**:362–66.

4. Basson MD. Choosing sedation for upper endoscopy. *Southern Med J* 2008;**101**:345–46.

5. Alharbi O, Rabeneck L, Paszat L, *et al*. A population-based analysis of outpatient colonoscopy in adults assisted by an anesthesiologist. *Anesthesiology* 2009;**111**:734–40.

6. Shah B, Cohen LB. The changing face of endoscopic sedation. *Expert Rev Gastroenterol Hepatol* 2010;**4**:417–22.

7. deVilliers WJS. Anesthesiology and gastroenterology. *Anesthesiol Clin* 2009;**27**:57–70.

8. Albashir S, Stevens T. Endoscopic ultrasonography to evaluate pancreatitis. *Cleveland Clinic J Med* 2012;**79**:202–06.

9. Hausman LM, Reich DL. Providing safe sedation/analgesia: an anesthesiologist's perspective. *Gastrointest Endoscopy Clin N Am* 2008;**18**:707–16.

10. Bamji N, Cohen LB. Endoscopic sedation of patients with chronic liver disease. *Clin Liver Dis* 2010;**14**:185–94.

11. Kodali BS. Capnography outside the operating rooms. *Anesthesiology* 2013;**118**:192–201.

12. Waugh JB, Epps CA, Khodneva YA. Capnography enhances surveillance of respiratory events during procedural sedation: a meta-analysis. *J Clin Anesth* 2011;**23**:189–96.

13. Goulson DT, Fragneto RY. Anesthesia for gastrointestinal endoscopic procedures. *Anesthesiol Clin* 2009;**27**:71–85.

14. Ootaki C, Stevens T, Vargo J, *et al.* Does general anesthesia increase the diagnostic yield of endoscopic ultrasound-guided fine needle aspiration of pancreatic masses? *Anesthesiology* 2012;**117**:1044–50.

15. Cote GA, Hovis RM, Ansstas MA, *et al.* The incidence of sedation-related complications with propofol use during advanced endoscopic procedures. *Clin Gastroenterol Hepatol* 2010;**8**:137–42.

16. De Oliveria GS, Agarwal D, Benzon HT. Perioperative single dose ketorolac to prevent postoperative pain: a meta-analysis of randomized trials. *Anesth Analg* 2012;**114**:424–33.

17. Elmunzer BJ, Scheiman JM, Lehman GA, *et al.* A randomized trial of rectal indomethacin to prevent post-ERCP pancreatitis. *N Engl J Med* 2012;**366**:1414–22.

18. Gharaei B, Jafari A, Aghamohammadi H, *et al.* Opioid-sparing effect of preemptive bolus low-dose ketamine for moderate sedation in opioid abusers undergoing extracorporeal shock wave lithotripsy: a randomized clinical trial. *Anesth Analg* 2013;**116**:75–80.

19. Suzuki T, Minami H, Komatsu T, *et al.* Prolonged carbon dioxide insufflation under general anesthesia for endoscopic submucosal dissection. *Endoscopy* 2010;**42**:1021–29.

20. Takano A, Kobayashi M, Takeuchi M, *et al.* Capnographic monitoring during endoscopic dissection with patients under deep sedation: a prospective, crossover trial of air and carbon dioxide insufflations. *Digestion* 2011;**84**:193–98.

21. Bretthaurer M, Selp B, Aasen S, *et al.* Carbon dioxide insufflation for more comfortable endoscopic retrograde cholangiopancreatography: a randomized, controlled, double-blind trial. *Endoscopy* 2007;**39**:58–64.

22. Dellon ES, Hawk JS, Grimm IS, Shaheen NJ. The use of carbon dioxide for insufflation during GI endoscopy: a systematic review. *Gastrointest Endosc* 2009;**69**:843–49.

Management of emergencies in ambulatory setting

Fatima Ahmad, MD

The most important thing for managing any emergent situation is its anticipation and preparedness ahead of time. Every surgery center and office should have a pre-existing plan to handle both surgery- and anesthesia-related emergencies such as malignant hyperthermia, local anesthetic toxicity, anaphylaxis, aspiration, airway fire, and cardiac arrest, among others. Management strategies should be reviewed regularly by all staff members and periodic drills should be performed, as these events are not very common.

It has been stated that the incidence of malignant hyperthermia (MH) in the United States is on the rise and in-hospital mortality remains elevated and higher than previously reported.[1] This may be a valid argument for only using TIVA techniques in the office based setting, and avoiding the use of suxamethonium unless called for in an emergency situation. With such practice, MH protocols may be simplified considerably from what is described below.

Denborough first described MH in 1962 when he reported recurrent deaths in the members of a family after exposure to anesthesia.[2] Since then, a lot has been written in the literature about MH. MH is the expression of a pharmacogenetic variation in some individuals, which gives rise to a life-threatening hypermetabolic response to triggering agents such as volatile anesthetic gases and succinylcholine. The resultant fatal syndrome, aptly called MH crisis, is characterized by unexplained increase in end-tidal CO_2 concentration, rigidity of the trunk or total body, spasm of the masseter muscle (trismus), tachycardia, tachypnea, mixed respiratory and metabolic acidosis, increase in body temperature, myoglobinuria, and hyperkalemia with resultant arrhythmias. If not treated in time, and sometimes even when treated properly, this can rapidly progress to death.

Although hyperthermia is one of the main signs of MH, it might not be the first sign. It is extremely important for the anesthesiologist to recognize the early signs of MH, especially an increase in end-tidal CO_2 concentration. It is also vital to monitor the temperature of patients undergoing general anesthesia except for very short procedures. The most common cause of death in this situation is either acute hyperkalemia or disseminated intravascular coagulation from very high body temperature.

Not only should there be an agreed-upon plan between the surgeon and anesthesiologist to anesthetize a known MH-susceptible patient, all the members of the office team should also be well trained and prepared to handle an MH crisis. There should be an existing arrangement for emergent transfer with a nearby hospital that meets state and federal accreditation. Depending upon patient population, this hospital should include pediatric or adult critical care. According to the Malignant Hyperthermia Association of the United States (MHAUS)[3] "Transfer Plan for Suspected MH Patients", this hospital should have the following capabilities:

- continuous temperature and cardiopulmonary monitoring;
- administration of therapeutic options including non-invasive/invasive cooling, continuous sedation and antidote therapy (dantrolene by bolus and maintenance therapy with at least 36 vials available for crisis treatment);
- dysrhythmia treatment;
- hemodialysis; and
- available consultants including anesthesia, critical care, hematology, surgery, nephrology, neurology, and medical toxicology.

Practical Ambulatory Anesthesia, ed. Johan Raeder and Richard D. Urman. Published by Cambridge University Press.
© Cambridge University Press 2015.

A transfer of care guide, jointly developed by MHAUS, the Ambulatory Surgery Foundation, the Society for Ambulatory Anesthesia, the Society for Academic Emergency Medicine, and the National Association of Emergency Medical Technicians, also recommends for the transport team to be adequately equipped. They specifically recommend capabilities of ventilatory support, cardiopulmonary and temperature monitoring, fluid resuscitation, medication administration, and phone communication.[4]

There have been instances when patients developed MH during surgery in ambulatory setup and later died in the hospital. This could have happened due to inability to continue treatment and inadequate monitoring during the process of transferring to the hospital. According to a study done by Rosero *et al.* there are about 500–600 MH cases per year in the US and mortality from MH is about 5% where the patient was admitted for routine elective surgery.[1] In comparison to this, the mortality is 20% for patients who are transferred to the hospital from free-standing facilities.

MHAUS[3] has established definitive protocols for treating MH and these are considered the standard of care. According to MHAUS, "Dantrolene is the only currently accepted specific treatment for MH." Hence, it is imperative to administer dantrolene rapidly in adequate doses. Management of metabolic acidosis, cooling the patient, and treating hyperkalemia and arrhythmias are other vital steps. Dantrolene should be administered as soon as the diagnosis is made.[5] The starting dose is 2.5 mg/kg and it can be repeated up to a cumulative dose of 10 mg/kg. However, if there is no response to higher doses, an alternative diagnosis should be considered. Dantrolene is supplied in 70 ml vials containing 20 mg dantrolene sodium and 3 g mannitol. It is reconstituted with 60 ml sterile water. It is poorly soluble in water and difficulties are experienced in rapidly preparing intravenous solutions in emergency situations. Thirty-six vials of dantrolene should be available wherever MH-triggering agents are used. Dantrolene should be administered by continuous rapid intravenous push, preferably via a big vein (but treatment should not be delayed for this reason).

Goals of MH crisis management in office

Early recognition of the signs and symptoms: educate and update your staff through "in-servicing".

Rapid treatment/MH cart/kit: 36 vials of dantrolene, sterile water, and the other supplies should be present at easily accessible designated locations known by all concerned personnel.

Response plan to implement the MHAUS recommended therapies quickly and efficiently: this plan should be practiced by both the anesthesiologists and nursing staff.

Periodic drills: review the response program. The frequency of drills at your site may be determined by your staff experience and turnover.

Transfer agreement with accepting hospital

A major difference in the management of MH in an office setup as compared to a hospital is the limited availability of personnel and resources. As recommended by MHAUS, multiple tasks need to be performed at the same time, quickly and efficiently. These tasks should be specifically assigned to different members of the staff, outlined on a worksheet using a checklist format. Responding members should pick up the appropriate worksheet(s) that are kept on the MH cart/kit and perform the tasks outlined. A sample of various checklists based on MHAUS recommendations is provided below.

Anesthesiologist's MH crisis checklist

Signs of Malignant Hyperthermia Identified, surgical team informed.

> MH 24 hour Hotline in USA:
> 1-800-MH-HYPER (1-800-644-9737)
> MH 24 hour Hotline outside USA:
> 1-315-464-7079

Initiate treatment

Discontinue volatile anesthetic agents and succinylcholine

Hyperventilate with 100% oxygen, high flows (at least > 10 l/min)

Call for MH cart/kit

Instruct surgeon to close the wound/irrigate wound with cold saline if possible

MH cart/kit in room and worksheets distributed

Mix and administer dantrolene

Continuously monitor ECG, end-tidal CO_2, and core temperature

Draw arterial, central, or venous blood gas sample (if possible)

Check K^+, Ca^{2+}, Na, glucose (if possible)

Treat acidosis

Treat hyperkalemia

Treat dysrhythmias/follow ACLS guidelines (avoid calcium channel blockers)

Cool hyperthermic patient (not lower than 38°C)

Infuse cold saline, turn off warming device

Place nasogastric tube and lavage the stomach with cold saline

Irrigate wound with cold saline

Place Foley catheter, collect urine sample for myoglobin, lavage with cold saline

Invasive lines in place if available/needed

Other labs drawn (if possible)

CPK

Serum myoglobin

Urine myoglobin

PT/PTT, fibrinogen, FSP, D-DIMER, CBC with platelets

Lactic acid

Urine output > 2 cc/kg/h

Talk to family

Transfer arrangements

Give detailed report to receiving hospital /physician

Ambulance with ACLS capabilities

Accompany the patient if possible

Circulator/scrub nurse MH crisis checklist

(1) Bring MH cart/kit, nursing supplies (bag), code/crash cart and defibrillator to the crisis area.

(2) Get materials to help surgeon close wound.

(3) Help mix dantrolene if necessary.

(4) Prepare and place ice bags over groin and axilla.

(5) Place Foley catheter, obtain urine for myoglobin, and then begin cold saline lavage, if necessary.

(6) Take telephone worksheet to the secretary/clerk/recovery nurse.

(7) Await further assignment.

After patient is stable

Restock nursing supplies in refrigerator and on MH cart/kit.

Recovery nurse checklist

(1) Prepare monitors and bed space for the patient in recovery area (if applicable).

(2) Ensure defibrillator, code cart, and ice are available at the bed space.

(3) Offer assistance to circulator/scrub nurse (if possible).

(4) Call the emergency phone numbers, receiving hospital, ACLS ambulance.

(5) Write down contact person's name.

(6) Call available medical and nursing personnel.

(7) Call clinical laboratory (if specimens are being sent).

After patient is stable

Confirm receiving hospital is ready to receive the patient and update the receiving hospital on patient transfer.

Anesthesiologist's post-crisis checklist

(1) Ensure restocking of dantrolene for MH cart/kit and supplies.

(2) Ensure MH cart/kit has been returned to designated location.

(3) Report to MHAUS.

(4) Counsel family and patient:

- Explain implications of MH and further precautions
- Recommend follow-up muscle biopsy
- Provide a letter describing events
- Carefully mark the chart: include volatile anesthetic gases and succinylcholine in the allergies section of the chart
- Inform patient about MHAUS ID-Tag Program.

Refer patient to: MHAUS

P.O. Box 1069
39 East State Street
Sherburne, NY 13460-1069
(607) 674-7901
(800) 98-MHAUS
E-mail: mhaus@norwich.net

MH cart/kit supplies checklist

Dantrolene 36 vials (each is diluted with 60 ml sterile water)

Sterile water vials

8.4% sodium bicarbonate 50 ml × 2

Furosemide 40 mg/amp × 2 ampules

D50 50 ml vials × 2

10% calcium chloride 20 ml vial × 2

2% lidocaine HCl 20 ml vial × 2

60 ml syringes × 3 (to dilute dantrolene)

Mini Spike IV additive pins × 2 and Multi Ad fluid transfer sets × 2 (to reconstitute dantrolene)

Angiocaths (for IV access and arterial line)

NG tubes: sizes appropriate for your patient population

Pressure bag

Irrigating syringes × 2 (for NG irrigation)

Large clear plastic bags for ice

Bucket for ice

Ambu bag for transportation

Esophageal temperature probes

A line/CVP/transducer kits

D5W 250 ml × 1

Microdrip IV set × 1 (infusion pump preferable)

3 ml syringes or ABG kits

Blood specimen tubes/urine specimen tubes

Anesthesia cold supplies

From refrigerator: supplies labeled "**for Malignant Hyperthermia Crisis only**"

– 1000 ml bags cold normal saline × 3
– Regular insulin 100 U/ml × 1 (refrigerated)

Nursing supplies

Large Steri-drape (for rapid draping of wound)

Three-way irrigating Foley catheters: sizes appropriate for your patient population

60 cc Toomy irrigating syringe × 2

Large clear plastic bags for ice × 4

Small plastic bags for ice × 4

Tray for ice

Management of MH-susceptible patient

MH-susceptible patients can be safely anesthetized at ambulatory centers and offices using non-triggering agents, such as propofol, remifentanil, and other opioids, and, in case of neuromuscular block needed, any non-depolarizing drug. The anesthesia machine should be prepared according to the manufacturer's recommendation. $EtCO_2$ and temperature monitoring is imperative. After an uneventful anesthetic, prolonged patient monitoring in the recovery room is not necessary.[6] Discharge instructions should include the recommendation of going to hospital if temperature elevation or dark-colored urine is noted.

Local anesthetic toxicity

Local anesthetic toxicity is a potential complication of nerve blocks, epidural blocks, tumescent anesthesia, and procedures where large volumes of local anesthetics are being administered. If not adequately managed, this can lead to catastrophic results.

Local anesthetic toxicity can result from inadvertent intravascular injection, systemic absorption of large doses of local anesthetics from peripheral nerve block injection, infiltration at surgical sites, or tumescent anesthetic for plastic surgery procedures. Addition of epinephrine to nerve block solution can act as a marker in case of intravascular injection by increasing the heart rate that can alert the clinician.[7] It has been shown in the literature that highly lipid-soluble and extensively protein-bound local anesthetics such as bupivacaine are more cardiotoxic than less lipid-soluble agents such as ropivacaine, levo-bupivacaine, lidocaine, mepivacaine, and prilocaine.[8]

Diagnosis

All patients receiving nerve blocks should have heart rate, pulse oximetry, and blood pressure monitored during the procedure as early detection of symptoms of local anesthetic toxicity leads to prompt interventions and better chances of successful treatment. Monitoring should be continued for at least 30 minutes after the block as signs of toxicity may manifest slowly in some situations. The symptoms range from ringing in the ears, perioral numbness, metallic taste, and dizziness to peripheral motor twitching, altered level of consciousness, and seizures leading to coma and respiratory arrest. Cardiac symptoms initially manifest as tachycardia, hypertension, and arrhythmias, progressively leading to hypotension, ventricular fibrillation, and cardiovascular collapse.[9]

Preventive measures

These include diligent monitoring, carefully calculated doses to stay within the safe limits, and frequent gentle aspiration to check for unintended intravascular needle placement. Local anesthetic should be injected in small increments with the patient being assessed between dosing increments. Direct communication with the patient to evaluate the mental status is important. As mentioned previously, the addition of epinephrine 1:200,000 to local anesthetic can act as a marker of unintentional intravascular injection by increasing the heart rate. Nerve blocks should be performed in locations where all rescue equipment is within reach. In our surgery center, in addition to monitoring capabilities, we have a block cart in the area which is well stocked with emergency medications, induction drugs, and airway supplies. Ambu bag, working suction catheter, crash cart, and defibrillator should be immediately available. The recommended antidote for local anesthetic toxicity, 20% lipid infusion, should be available at all locations where local anesthetics are being used in large doses.[9]

Management

Once the diagnosis of Local Anesthetic Systemic Toxicity (LAST) is made, immediate management, as recommended by the American Society of Regional Anesthesia and Pain Management (ASRA), should be initiated. ASRA emphasizes that the pharmacological management of LAST differs from other cardiac arrest situations.[9] They recommend early treatment with 20% intralipid as it can prevent cardiovascular collapse. As in any other crisis situation, immediate help should be called for. Due to the limited number of people in ambulatory centers, specific tasks should be immediately assigned to everyone. All nurses in the center should be aware of the location where 20% lipid emulsion is stocked. Airway should be secured immediately and patient ventilated with 100% oxygen. Seizures

should be treated with a benzodiazepine, preferably, as propofol can make a hypotensive collapse situation worse. ACLS should be initiated if indicated and prolonged effort may be needed in case of bupivacaine toxicity. The family should be informed of the situation. A pre-existing transfer arrangement with a nearby facility with capabilities for cardiopulmonary bypass should be in place. That facility should be alerted regarding the situation.

American Society of Regional Anesthesia and Pain Medicine

Checklist for Treatment of Local Anesthetic Systemic Toxicity

---

The Pharmacologic Treatment of Local Anesthetic Systemic Toxicity (LAST) is Different from Other Cardiac Arrest Scenarios

---

❑ **Get help**
❑ **Initial focus**
❑ **Airway management:** ventilate with 100% oxygen
❑ **Seizure suppression:** benzodiazepines are preferred; **AVOID propofol** in patients having signs of cardiovascular instability
❑ **Alert** the nearest facility having **cardiopulmonary bypass** capability
❑ **Management of cardiac arrhythmias**
❑ **Basic and Advanced Cardiac Life Support (ACLS)** will require adjustment of medications and perhaps prolonged effort
❑ **AVOID vasopressin, calcium channel blockers, beta-blockers, or local anesthetic**
❑ **REDUCE individual epinephrine doses to < 1 μg/kg**
❑ **Lipid Emulsion (20%) Therapy** (values in parentheses are for 70 kg patient)
❑ **Bolus 1.5 ml/kg** (lean body mass) intravenously over 1 minute (~100 ml)
❑ **Continuous infusion 0.25 ml/kg/min** (~18 ml/min; adjust by roller clamp)
❑ **Repeat bolus** once or twice for persistent cardiovascular collapse
❑ **Double the infusion rate** to 0.5 ml/kg/min if blood pressure remains low
❑ **Continue infusion** for at least 10 minutes after attaining circulatory stability
❑ **Recommended upper limit:** Approximately 10 ml/kg lipid emulsion over the first 30 minutes
❑ **Post LAST events** at www.lipidrescue.org and report use of lipid to www.lipidregistry.org

Anaphylaxis

National Institute of Allergy and Infectious Disease/ Food Allergy and Anaphylaxis Network has defined anaphylaxis as a serious allergic reaction that is rapid in onset and may cause death.[10] It can be caused by exposure to medications or other substances used in the perioperative period. It is an IgE-mediated reaction, leading to the release of histamine and other biochemical mediators. These mediators in turn cause a series of events, ranging from mild symptoms such as itching and skin redness to generalized mucocutaneous swelling, low blood pressure, increased heart rate, constriction of gastrointestinal smooth muscle, and bronchoconstriction. A variety of substances can cause anaphylaxis. The substances commonly implicated during the perioperative period include antibiotics, non-depolarizing muscle relaxants, induction agents, opioids, local anesthetics, chlorhexidine, intravenous contrast agents, and latex.[11]

Prevention

During preoperative evaluation, a careful history of allergies and previous allergic reactions should be elicited. Some facilities use allergy bands wrapped around the patient's wrist that lists the names of substances causing allergies. In our institution, mentioning the allergies as part of the preoperative time-out list is mandatory with all OR personnel present and attentive to the situation. Latex precautions must be observed in latex-sensitive patients.

Diagnosis

Early diagnosis of the symptoms of anaphylaxis is important as the condition can rapidly deteriorate into a life-threatening situation. In an anesthetized patient, a drop in blood pressure can lead to impalpable pulses. Oxygen saturation may drop due to bronchospasm with subsequent difficulty in ventilation and increased peak airway pressures. Ultimately, full cardiovascular collapse can ensue.

Management

The main goal of treatment is hemodynamic support and improved oxygenation. Depending on the severity of the situation, extra help may have to be called. The surgeon should be informed and advised to shorten the procedure if possible.

The following steps are recommended in the management of perioperative anaphylaxis:

The agent suspected of causing the reaction should be immediately removed from the vicinity.

- Epinephrine: for mild to moderate reactions, epinephrine, titrated in small doses, 10–200 µg, may be administered as needed. For more severe reactions, full ACLS doses of 1 mg should be given and repeated as necessary.
- Airway/oxygen: the airway should be secured if not previously done and 100% oxygen should be administered.
- Bronchospasm: inhaled albuterol or salbutamol helps to treat the bronchospasm. In the case of severe bronchospasm, epinephrine should be titrated in. Corticosteroids may be given; although their effect is delayed.
- Fluid resuscitation: because histamine causes severe vasodilatation, fluid resuscitation is critical, especially in severe anaphylactic reactions. Crystalloid or colloid boluses should be rapidly administered titrated to the patient's response.
- Venous return can be improved by tilting the operating table or patient bed in a head-down position.
- H-1 receptor antagonists are also recommended in the management of anaphylaxis.
- Refractory anaphylaxis: in situations unresponsive to epinephrine, phenylephrine, norepinephrine, and vasopressin should be considered.[11]
- The patient and/or family members should be informed in detail about the circumstances. Allergy testing may also be recommended.

References

1. Rosero EB, Adesanya AO, Timaran CH, Joshi GP. Trends and outcomes of malignant hyperthermia in the United States, 2000 to 2005. *Anesthesiology* 2009;**110**:89–94.

2. Denborough MA, Forster JFA, Lovell RRH, Maplestone PA, Villiers JD. Anaesthetic deaths in a family. *Brit J Anaesth* 1962;**34**:395–96.

3. Malignant Hyperthermia Association of the United States. http://www.mhaus.org/

4. Larach MG, Dirksen SJH, Belani KG, *et al.* Creation of a guide for the transfer of care of the malignant hyperthermia patient from ambulatory surgery centers to receiving hospital facilities. *Anesth Analg* 2012;**114**(1):94–100.

5. Krause T, Gerbeshagen MU, Fiege M, *et al.* Dantrolene – A review of its pharmacology,

therapeutic use and new developments. *Anaesthesia* 2004;**59**(4):364–73.

6. Litman RS. Management of MH and MH-Susceptible Patients in the Ambulatory Setting, ASA refresher course lecture at 2010 ASA Annual Meeting.

7. Mulroy F. Systemic toxicity and cardiotoxicity from local anesthetics: Incidence and preventive measures. *Reg Anesth Pain Med* 2002;**27**(6):556–61.

8. Heavner JE. Cardiac toxicity of local anesthetics in the intact isolated heart model: A review. *Reg Anesth Pain Med* 2002;**27**(6):545–55.

9. American Society of Regional Anesthesia and Pain Medicine. Checklist for Treatment of Local Anesthetic Systemic Toxicity. http://www.asra.com/checklist-for-local-anesthetic-toxicity-treatment-1-18-12.pdf

10. Sampson HA, Munoz-Furlong A, Campbell RL, *et al.* Second symposium on the definition and management of anaphylaxis: Summary report – Second National Institute of Allergy and Infectious Disease/Food Allergy and Anaphylaxis Network symposium. *J Allergy Clin Immunol* 2006;**117**(2):391–97.

11. Dewachter P, Mouton-Faivre C, Emala CW. Anaphylaxis and anesthesia: Controversies and new insights. *Anesthesiology* 2009; **111**(5):1141–50.

Chapter 15

Office-based anesthesia

Johann Patlak, MD, Fred E. Shapiro, DO, and Richard D. Urman, MD

Introduction

The number of outpatient surgical procedures performed outside of hospital settings has increased dramatically over the past three decades. A significant portion of this growth has been in the office-based setting, with office-based surgical procedures making up an estimated 1/6th of all outpatient procedures in 2005.[1] This growth has been driven by economic and reimbursement factors along with patient and provider convenience and comfort. Ultimately, it has been the growing understanding and acceptance of office-based anesthesia (OBA) that has enabled surgeons to move increasing surgical volume to their offices.

With healthcare reform likely to change how services are paid for, the trend of hospital acquisition of ambulatory surgical centers and private physician practices seems poised to continue. Despite this, accountable care organizations or other hospital-based payment groups are likely to be interested in the same economic efficiencies as the private practitioner. Thus, it seems reasonable to expect that the number of office-based procedures will only increase.

Patient safety remains the paramount concern in the office-based setting, but definitive statements on the subject are difficult to make. The quality of data on the subject is limited by the relative youth and ongoing evolution of the subspecialty, lack of homogeneity across OBA practices and settings, and lack of consistent reporting of complications.[2] While drawing lessons from retrospective analysis of safety, an anesthesiologist entering the field of OBA must primarily look for approaches to maximize future patient outcomes. This chapter does not seek to discuss specific pharmacological approaches to OBA, which are essentially similar to those presented elsewhere in this book. Instead, it will focus on some of the unique concerns and pitfalls encountered by the anesthesiologist in the office-based setting.

Administrative issues

Prior to administering any anesthetic in an office-based setting, the anesthesiologist must ensure a safe and functional operating environment. This responsibility extends well beyond the anesthesia machine itself, and covers elements that might be taken for granted in a hospital setting.

Accreditation and classification

Perhaps the best starting point when evaluating a potential site for OBA is to inquire about the office's accreditation status. Accreditation requirements for office-based surgery (OBS) practices vary by state, with some states having no specific requirements. Other states, meanwhile, have extensive guidelines and regulations for OBS. The Federation of State Medical Boards currently maintains a state-by-state listing.[3,4] States without current regulations may create these in the future, so up-to-date information should be verified.

OBS practice accreditation can be obtained through one of three organizations: The Joint Commission (TJC), the Accreditation Association for Ambulatory Healthcare (AAAHC), and the American Association for Accreditation of Ambulatory Surgery Facilities (AAAASF). The basic requirements for each of these groups are similar. With the exception of the AAAHC, which has the ability to accredit OBA practices independently, the responsibility for obtaining accreditation lies with the owner of the OBS practice.

For the purposes of accreditation and state regulatory compliance, OBS practices are generally divided into three levels. Two classification schemes exist, one ranging from Level I to III and the other

Practical Ambulatory Anesthesia, ed. Johan Raeder and Richard D. Urman. Published by Cambridge University Press. © Cambridge University Press 2015.

Table 15.1 American Society of Anesthesiologists (ASA) Guidelines for Office-Based Anesthesia.[7]

For office-based anesthesia practices that are not accredited, several professional organizations have provided a basic set of guidelines that serve as a minimum benchmark for all providers. Examples from the American Society of Anesthesiologists (ASA) Guidelines for Office-Based Anesthesia include the following:

- The presence of a medical director responsible for verifying adequate training and credentialing of all anesthesia providers and staff.
- Ongoing quality improvement, continuing education, and risk management activities.
- Appropriate patient selection based on comorbidities and surgical complexity.
- Adherence to all basic anesthesia and ambulatory anesthesia guidelines as provided by the ASA, including for standard monitoring equipment.
- Appropriate space and staffing for post-anesthesia recovery evaluation.
- Facilities with adequate emergency equipment and backup power supply.
- Written plans for medical and non-medical emergencies including specific patient transport and transfer protocols.
- The immediate presence of the anesthesiologist during the entire intraoperative period.

from Class A to C. The Level system focuses somewhat more on surgical complexity, while the Class system is defined by level or technique of anesthesia. Ultimately, both systems are defined by the likelihood of unconsciousness and anesthetic complications.[5] Level I/Class A allows for local or distal nerve blocks with only mild oral anxiolysis. Level II/Class B allows for mild to moderate parenteral sedation and analgesia. Level III/Class C allows for deep sedation, general anesthesia, and regional or neuraxial blocks. Understanding the level at which a potential OBA site is accredited is important, as this determines which anesthetic techniques are allowed. Confusingly, some state boards deviate from these systems. Texas, for example, uses Levels I–IV, with only IV allowing general anesthesia.[6]

Facility evaluation and infrastructure

While OBS practice accreditation suggests compliance with basic standards, the ASA rightly cautions that the office setting may lack rigorous mechanisms and staff for maintaining adherence between accreditation

cycles.[5] Any anesthesiologist starting or joining an OBA practice should independently verify a number of factors at each OBA site. The following are examples of potential problem areas, but should not be taken as an exhaustive list of requirements. For the latter, the various accrediting bodies offer detailed handbooks or manuals available outside of the formal accreditation process. The ASA offers an OBA handbook with in depth discussion of these and other issues.

The anesthesia machine and monitors are likely owned by the surgeon who owns the OBS practice but may have little anesthesia experience. It is the responsibility of the OBA provider to verify that the equipment meets current standards and remains factory-supported. Maintenance and calibration need to be completed in accordance with manufacturer recommendations. The American Society of Anesthesiologists maintains guidelines for determining anesthesia machine obsolescence and recommends against obsolete machines being used in any setting.[8] Mobile anesthesia machines that travel with the anesthesiologist may make it easier to ensure equipment maintenance across OBS practices, but facility-specific equipment such as defibrillators should still be inspected.

Medical gas supply should be verified if coming from outside the immediate operating room (OR). Protocols for checking and replenishing gas supplies should be in place. A redundant backup system is a necessity. Waste gas scavenging is important for both patient and staff safety, and purpose-built office operating rooms may include adequate exterior venting of the scavenging system. This should be examined, however, especially in converted office space. While physician office space should meet minimum occupational health guidelines for ventilation and air exchange, these may be inadequate for an OR environment that includes electrocautery smoke and leaked anesthetic agents.

Fire safety must be considered in any OBS setting. OR fires can have devastating effects, and prevention requires awareness and participation on the part of all OR staff. Anesthetized patients or those under regional or neuraxial block present very different challenges from regular medical office patients in the event of an evacuation. All staff should be aware of OR-specific fire response plans, including evacuation of intubated patients, and these should be practiced in an organized fashion.

Electrical systems should be evaluated both for electroshock prevention and adequate backup power capability. Hospital construction regulations no longer require isolated circuits in ORs, and these would not be expected in an office setting. Ground fault circuit interrupter (GFCI)-type outlets offer the next best level of protection against accidental electroshock from short-circuited equipment and should be tested regularly. Backup power should be redundant and must be available in uninterrupted fashion to all life support, anesthesia machine, monitor, and suction pump outlets.

Anesthetic drugs, controlled or otherwise, must be securely stored in the absence of a central pharmacy. Whether controlled drugs are procured via the DEA license of the surgeon or of the anesthesiologist, it is the responsibility of the OBA provider to adequately document daily usage and waste. A protocol for reordering medication and monitoring usage rates to avoid medication expiration should be established.

Infection control remains an important concern in the OBS setting. In a cost-driven environment, there may be a temptation to find efficiency by splitting multi-dose vials between patients and minimizing the number of syringes and needles opened per case. Detailed guidelines are available for minimizing the risk of patient to patient transmission of infectious diseases, and the anesthesiologist should follow these carefully.[9] As medications may be administered by support staff in the pre-op or recovery room settings, a general infection control policy for all staff should be available and enforced.

Finally, emergency equipment, supplies, and medications should be easily available and fully functional. This includes a code cart, defibrillator, difficult airway supplies, and emergency medications. Required medications include ACLS drugs, the availability of dantrolene if any malignant hyperthermia-triggering agents are used or could potentially be used in the office, and the intralipid solution for local anesthetic toxicity management. Naloxone and flumazenil should also be available if opioids or benzodiazepines, respectively, are being administered. The ASA OBA manual includes in-depth tables of recommended emergency drugs.[5] Resuscitative equipment and medications will generally be provided by the surgical office, but the anesthesiologist's responsibilities include verifying their availability and functionality prior to any clinical care. Furthermore, a written plan for the emergency transfer of patients to a hospital setting must be verified. Easy access to ambulance and pre-hospital emergency care should be planned for and available. These plans should be present regardless of the surgeon's admitting privileges.

Providers and staff

In addition to a well-maintained facility, safe OBA requires an appropriately trained and effective perioperative team. This necessarily begins with the surgeon, who should be licensed to perform the desired procedures and should be in good standing with the state medical board. These inquiries must be made tactfully, but it should be understood that physicians will confirm each other's credentials before working in the potentially unregulated OBS setting. While unpleasant to consider, significant disparity in malpractice insurance coverage between surgeon and anesthesiologist could provide an incentive to include the better-insured provider in malpractice suits.[10] At a minimum, the anesthesiologist should have current ACLS certification and well-maintained airway management skills. Ideally, other OR staff will also have ACLS certification. All clinical staff need at least BLS certification.

Staff availability should be confirmed with the office manager or head nurse. While the goal of OBA is to minimize recovery times, lengthy cases ending in the late afternoon may still require recovery room staff to stay into the evening. A clear staffing plan for dealing with unexpected delayed recovery must be in place.

All providers and staff should participate in ongoing quality improvement and assurance activities. Unlike larger hospital- or ACS-based settings, the office-based anesthesiologist may not have the same level of informal and formal peer discussion about techniques and problems. The ASA recommends formal peer review for all anesthesiologists, even those in solo practice.[5] The OBS office as a whole should document and track surgical and anesthetic outcomes and adverse events. Complication rates should be quantifiable, reportable, and comparable to other similar practices. Submitting reports to large-scale databases such as the Anesthesia Quality Institute's National Anesthesia Clinical Outcomes Registry will help determine possible future safety concerns in OBA.[11]

Clinical care

Patient and procedure selection

The clinical care of the office-based surgical patient begins with careful patient and procedure selection. Not all surgical procedures are suitable for an OBS practice. In many ways, the OBA provider shares the same concerns as the anesthesiologist practicing in an ASC. While the ASC may have increased resources compared to an independent office, the goals of complication-free surgery and rapid recovery and discharge are the same.

Prior to scheduling a patient for a new type of procedure, the surgeon and anesthesiologist need to assess for possible complications that could be difficult to manage in a non-hospital setting. These include concerns about blood loss, postoperative pain control, postoperative nausea and vomiting, and the potential for excessive case length.[5]

Once acceptable procedure types have been agreed upon, the next important step is patient screening. Some patients may be at increased risk when having their procedure performed in the office rather than the hospital. This assessment should go beyond the basic ASA Physical Status Classification.[10] Patients with known or likely difficult airways based on physical exam are best avoided in the OBA setting, even if only sedation is planned. Similarly, patients with obstructive sleep apnea are at increased risk of intraoperative respiratory complication and of needing airway support in the recovery room. Postoperative pain control in chronic pain patients may provide a barrier to efficient discharge. Social issues also need to be taken into account, including the presence of a responsible person to bring the patient home. The OBS practice lacks the safety net of easy hospital admission to handle postoperative issues, and this fact should influence patient selection. Written guidelines can assist the surgeon in determining which patients require anesthesiologist consultation prior to booking and which can safely be seen immediately prior to surgery.

Perioperative care

On the day of surgery, all patients should be seen by the anesthesiologist prior to sedation. Separate consent forms for surgery and anesthesia should be reviewed and signed with the patient. NPO status and a ride home need to be confirmed. Surgical side and site marking should be performed prior to all procedures and should be confirmed prior to placement of any regional block. Time-outs and checklists have been shown to improve surgical safety in a number of settings.[12] ASCs are now required by CMS to use checklists.[13] Although this is not yet a reimbursement-driven requirement for OBS, a formal checklist can help ensure fulfillment of all perioperative requirements and may condition staff to notice and address potential problems early. The Institute for Safety in Office-Based Surgery (ISOBS) has created an OBS specific checklist and encourages OBA providers to introduce it to the surgical offices in which they practice.[14]

Intraoperatively, patients can be cared for with either general anesthesia or monitored anesthesia care as outlined elsewhere in this book. The same goals of balanced anesthesia and multimodal analgesia apply to OBA. Patients should be monitored at the same level that they would be in the hospital or ASC setting. Per the ASA Standards for Basic Anesthetic Monitoring, this includes end-tidal CO_2 ($ETCO_2$) monitoring for all patients undergoing moderate to deep sedation.[15] $ETCO_2$ monitors should be present in all settings where general anesthesia is performed, but may not be automatically present in sedation settings. Early recognition and treatment of respiratory depression or airway obstruction is critical for avoiding potentially severe complications and death.

The recovery phase is very important to a successful office-based anesthetic. Patients must be monitored by dedicated staff until they are ready for discharge. Ideally, recovery time should be short. The ASA OBA manual offers a post-anesthesia recovery scoring system, including criteria for fast-tracking patients directly to a waiting room setting, bypassing the need for a physical recovery space.[5] The ability to achieve this will depend very much on the procedure and anesthetic technique, but a plan and personnel for managing delayed discharge should be in place. The ISOBS checklist continues through this period.

Practice management

A detailed discussion of the financial implications of an OBA practice is beyond the scope of this chapter. The ASA OBA manual offers a brief discussion of the differences in surgeon reimbursement in the OBS versus ASC setting and how this may affect the anesthesiologist.[5] Furthermore, there are legal requirements regarding fair market value payment for anesthesiology services in order to avoid anti-kickback statutes.[10] In short, legal counsel with knowledge of the healthcare field should be involved in all contract negotiations.

Summary points

- Office-based surgery and anesthesia is likely a growing field, but is currently subject to a broad and evolving spectrum of state-by-state regulations.
- Accreditation by one of the three bodies providing this status to OBS practices is a good starting point, but the office-based anesthesiologist must be vigilant across a wide variety of issues to ensure ongoing quality and safety of care.
- Careful patient and procedure selection are the first line in the avoidance of complications.
- Clinical care need not vary dramatically from other ambulatory settings, but the anesthesiologist may need to take additional steps to ensure consistent, high-quality perioperative care throughout the practice.

References

1. TrendWatch Chartbook 2009: Trends Affecting Hospitals and Health Systems. Chapter 2. [Internet]. Washington DC: American Hospital Association (AHA); 2009 [cited 2014 Jul 2]. Available from: http://www.aha.org/research/reports/tw/chartbook/2009/chapter2.pdf

2. Urman R, Punwani N, Shapiro F. Patient safety and office-based anesthesia. *Current Opinion in Anesthesiology.* 2012;25(6):648653.

3. Federation of State Medical Boards. Office Based Surgery, States A-M [Internet]. 2014 [2 July 2014]. Available from: http://www.fsmb.org/Media/Default/PDF/FSMB/Advocacy/GRPOL_Office_Based_Surgery_A-M.pdf

4. Federation of State Medical Boards. Office Based Surgery, States N-Z [Internet]. 2014 [4 July 2014]. Available from: http://www.fsmb.org/Media/Default/PDF/FSMB/Advocacy/GRPOL_Office_Based_Surgery_N-Z.pdf

5. Office-Based Anesthesia [Internet]. 2nd ed. Park Ridge, IL: American Society of Anesthesiologists; 2008 [31 February 2014]. Available from: https://ecommerce.asahq.org/p-319-office-based-anesthesia-considerations-in-setting-up-and-maintaining-a-safe-office-anesthesia-environment.aspx

6. Texas Medical Board. Office Based Anesthesia [Internet]. 2014 [2 July 2014]. Available from: http://www.tmb.state.tx.us/page/renewal-office-based-anesthesia

7. American Society of Anesthesiologists. Guidelines for Office-Based Anesthesia [Internet]. 2009 [2 July 2014]. Available from: https://www.ahttps://www.asahq.org/For-Members/~/media/For%20Members/documents/Standards%20Guidelines%20Stmts/OfficeBased%20Anesthesia

8. American Society of Anesthesiologists. Guidelines for determining anesthesia machine obsolescence [Internet]. 2012 [2 July 2014]. Available from: https://www.asahq.org/~/media/For%20Members/About%20ASA/ASA%20Committees/ASA%20Publications%20Anesthesia%20Machine%20Obsolescence%202041.pdf#search=%22machine obsolescence%22

9. Centers for Disease Control. Safe Injection Practices to Prevent Transmission of Infections to Patients [Internet]. 2011 [4 July 2014]. Available from: http://www.cdc.gov/injectionsafety/IP07_standardPrecaution.html

10. Kurrek M, Twersky R. Office-based anesthesia: how to start an office-based practice. *Anesthesiology Clinics.* 2010;28(2):353–367.

11. Anesthesia Quality Institute. AQI – Introduction to NACOR [Internet]. [2 July 2014]. Available from: https://www.aqihq.org/introduction-to-nacor.aspx

12. Rosenberg N, Urman R, Gallagher S, Stenglein J, Liu X, Shapiro F. Effect of an office-based surgical safety system on patient outcomes. *Eplasty.* 2012;12:e59.

13. Ambulatory Surgery Center Association. Safe Surgery Checklist Information [Internet]. [2 July 2014]. Available from: http://www.ascassociation.org/federalregulations/qualityreporting/safesurgerychecklistinformation/

14. Institute for Safety in Office-Based Surgery. Safety Checklist for Office Surgery Development [Internet]. [2 July 2014]. Available from: http://isobsurgery.org/?page_id=330

15. American Society for Anesthesiologists. Standards for Basic Anesthetic Monitoring [Internet]. 2011 [2 July 2014]. Available from: https://www.asahq.org/For-Members/~/media/For%20Members/documents/Standards%20Guidelines%20Stmts/Basic%20Anesthetic%20Monitoring%202011.ashx

Controversies in ambulatory anesthesia

Steven Butz, MD

Preoperative screening

Gone are the days that every patient got a complete blood count and urinalysis prior to surgery. In 2002, the American Society of Anesthesiologists put out a practice advisory that routine preoperative testing was not a valuable part of preoperative screening. Instead, indicated testing may be of benefit in assessing patients prior to surgery.[1] Now it appears that even these reflexive tests are not appropriate.

Frances Chung, MD, and her group in Toronto, Canada, have done extensive research in this area. She has determined that for many ambulatory procedures, there is little association between test findings and the outcome of the anesthetic. A 2000 study by Schein *et al.* demonstrated that all testing can be eliminated for patients undergoing cataract surgery despite these patients usually having significant coexisting disease.[2] Chung proposed that testing may be dropped for all ambulatory surgeries.[3] She randomized 1061 patients to either have no testing or complete blood count, electrolytes, blood glucose, creatinine, electrocardiogram, and chest x-ray. The procedures and patients were similar between the two groups. The outcomes were the rate of perioperative adverse events and the rates of adverse events at postoperative days 7 and 30. She demonstrated that there was no increase in adverse event rates.

Cardiac testing can be very tempting when dealing with a geriatric patient or someone with known cardiac issues. Routine ECG testing is not indicated, especially in a patient without cardiac disease. As mentioned previously, there is no evidence that preoperative ECGs improve patient outcomes. In fact, they may lead to further testing and expense. There are indications for echocardiography to be performed preoperatively that have been published in *Circulation*. Generally speaking,

the indications are grade C and include non-innocent murmurs, heart failure, symptoms of endocarditis, syncope, ischemia, or known structural defects.[4]

Testing that should be done is blood glucose testing in diabetic patients. The reason is that glucose levels fluctuate greatly and are likely more abnormal in diabetic patients on the day of surgery. This is because they have to be fasted and likely have to alter their medication therapies. Although there is no glucose number that absolutely would preclude a successful anesthetic, it will definitely change the immediate management of the patient. A hypoglycemic patient would need glucose and a hyperglycemic patient would likely require hydration. Furthermore, glucose monitoring is on track to become part of the Surgical Care Improvement Project that is supported by the Centers for Medicare and Medicaid Services (CMS). Documentation that testing is done may soon become a required report to maintain full CMS billing.

Routine pregnancy testing remains very controversial. The issues on either side of the coin are the benefits of doing a test with low yield versus protection of an unborn fetus from the neurodevelopment issues with general anesthesia. Studies give a range of unexpected positive results from 0.3% to 1.2%.[5,6] A critical piece of data, though, is that a positive test influenced the management of the anesthetic 100% of the time. The other issues to consider are if the test is being done with or without consent, who is notified of the results in the case of a minor, and how to collect the specimen. Specimens are usually from urine, but is the urine produced timely in a fasted patient or what is the alternative to urine and is it available in a free-standing center? If the specimen is brought from home, is the preoperative test result still valid? There are no clear answers to these questions, but a

Practical Ambulatory Anesthesia, ed. Johan Raeder and Richard D. Urman. Published by Cambridge University Press.
© Cambridge University Press 2015.

thoughtful and considerate discussion needs to be made at a management level.

General inhalation-based anesthesia versus total intravenous anesthesia

The clinical issues to focus on when choosing an anesthetic technique are: rapid induction, smooth maintenance, rapid emergence, and adequate pain control, so that after the procedure the patients are fully awake and not suffering side effects such as nausea, vomiting, and shivering. When general anesthesia is provided with intravenous agents alone, this is called total intravenous anesthesia (TIVA). The TIVA concept is simple. An intravenous line is the only prerequisite, and everything needed for general anesthesia is supplied through this line, obviating the need for sophisticated gas delivery systems and scavenger equipment. The TIVA drugs are generally less toxic than inhalational agents, have less risk of causing malignant hyperthermia, and do not pollute the environmental air or atmosphere. TIVA usually necessitates component therapy, with different drugs dedicated to achieving different effects; typically one drug for the hypnotic effect (propofol, ketamine, methohexital, midazolam), and another for analgesia and antinociception (remifentanil, other opioids, ketamine).

Inhalational anesthesia usually implies inhalational maintenance, with or without opioid supplementation, after an intravenous induction in adults. In a study of septorhinoplasty, Gokce et al.[7] did not find any significant differences between desflurane + remifentanil maintenance versus propofol + remifentanil. In a more detailed study of micro-surgical vertebral disk resection, Gozdemir et al. found shorter emergence and less nausea, but more shivering and postoperative pain in the propofol + remifentanil group, when compared with the desflurane + nitrous oxide group.[8] Increased incidence of postoperative shivering was also found after remifentanil + propofol in Röhm et al.'s comparison with desflurane + fentanyl.[9] Moore et al. confirmed the well-known benefit of reduced postoperative nausea and vomiting (PONV) after TIVA with propofol in mixed-case day surgery.[10] Similarly, reduced PONV was found by Hong et al. after breast biopsy with propofol + remifentanil anesthesia.[11] However, their result may be biased by the use of a longer-acting opioid, fentanyl, in the control group. Inhalational induction with

sevoflurane + nitrous oxide was slower, but smoother (i.e., less bradycardia and apnea) and associated with slower emergence and less postoperative pain compared to the TIVA technique in this study.[11] In a large study of 1158 adults in ambulatory mixed surgery, Moore et al. compared different methods of sevoflurane with/without nitrous oxide induction and/or maintenance versus propofol TIVA.[10] They found more injection pain and hiccups with propofol and more breath-holding and recalled discomfort with sevoflurane induction. Sevoflurane was associated with more PONV, but the major outcome results, such as time to discharge and unplanned hospital admissions, were similar in both groups.[10]

In 2004, Gupta, et al. performed a meta-analysis with 58 articles comparing aspects of recovery of adults between different inhalational agents and propofol. They found that comparing desflurane with propofol showed that patients were awake sooner with desflurane, but had more PONV. There was no difference in time to discharge. With sevoflurane, propofol showed earlier arousal, less PONV, and earlier discharge home. Home-readiness was earlier with sevoflurane, but was very heterogeneous. As expected when comparing the effect of sevoflurane and desflurane on postoperative recovery, patients who received desflurane had earlier awakening and earlier ability to follow verbal instructions. However, sevoflurane showed early transfer from immediate recovery to second phase of recovery. Propofol versus all inhalational anesthetics demonstrated superior protection against PONV.[12]

General anesthesia versus regional or local anesthesia

Regional anesthesia can have significant benefits over general anesthesia. For procedures that are amenable to being performed under local or regional anesthesia, it becomes possible to avoid the complications associated with general anesthesia such as nausea and vomiting or postoperative sedation. The cost of avoiding general anesthesia is paid in terms of set up and the time it takes for the local or regional anesthesia to work. There also need to be allowances in case the regional anesthetic either does not work or wears off before the procedure ends. Postoperative pain needs to be included and addressed so that the patient is not left in pain without relief.

The majority of cases that can have regional anesthesia are orthopedic. Sedation and local anesthesia can be commonly applied to superficial cases or those common in plastic surgery. Although some plastic surgeons can accomplish bigger procedures under local anesthesia, patients need to be prepared that unlike a general anesthetic, some discomfort may be expected.

In a 2013 review of regional anesthesia in ambulatory surgery, Moore, Ross, and Williams evaluated different regional techniques and evaluated them in regard to quality of recovery. Part of what they evaluated patients with was the WAKE Score to bypass first stage of recovery.[13] Williams suggests that other scoring systems, such as the modified Aldrete Score, do not account for the effects of regional anesthesia. The WAKE Score does not require movement of all extremities to get a full score on that part of the evaluation.

Regional anesthesia can impact the WAKE scores in the following ways. Blood pressure may be strongly affected by a spinal anesthetic, but regional to an extremity is likely to have a small effect. Drugs such as propofol may be vasodilating, but the effects dissipate quickly. Wakefulness is more affected by heavy sedation or general anesthesia that can be avoided with regional anesthesia. Likewise, respiratory effort is more strongly affected by opioids and sedation. An exception is possible diaphragmatic paralysis related to a supraclavicular block or chest wall paresis due to paravertebral blocks. Oxygen saturation is affected similarly to respiratory effort. Pain scores tend to be lower with regional anesthesia because the hyperalgesia of opioids is avoided. Both forms of anesthesia benefit from multimodal anesthesia. PONV is less likely with a regional or local anesthetic as stated before.[14]

Prior to the proliferation of ultrasound use in regional anesthesia, many techniques were technically difficult and had a lower success rate. The use of ultrasound allows for smaller volumes of local anesthetic to be used and significantly reduces the risk of vascular puncture. Theoretically, this will also reduce the risk of local anesthetic toxicity, as most reports of cardiovascular collapse occur due to intravascular injection. Ultrasound guidance has also demonstrated a shorter procedure time to place the block, a faster onset time, and longer duration of the block.[15]

Airway management: supraglottic airway versus endotracheal tube

Compared with the facial mask, a supraglottic airway offers the option of spontaneous breathing and leaves the anesthetist's hands free for other tasks. With a good, tight fit the free airway is stable; there is minimal leakage of inhalational agents into the surroundings and good control of the gas mixture going into and out of the airways rather than anywhere else (i.e., pollution, patient's stomach). If there is no need for high-pressure ventilation, the laryngeal mask airway (LMA) has quite similar characteristics of use as an endotracheal tube (ETT), but the protection afforded against aspiration from a full stomach may be less. The LMA is always potentially more prone to being dislodged, with subsequent problems. This may be a particular problem if surgery is in the mouth or pharynx area, such as adenoidectomy and tonsillectomy. The LMA is also somewhat larger than an ETT, and cannot be so readily repositioned for surgical access. Although the LMA stimulates the pharyngeal structures and may traumatize the mucous membranes, there is less need for deep analgesia (or muscle relaxation) and fewer reports of postoperative sore throat and airway problems (i.e., spasm, coughing) than with the ETT. Whereas the only concern for fit for an ETT is the diameter of the tube, in some patients the LMA may be difficult to fit. If the seal pressure has to be very high (i.e., more than 45 cmH$_2$O) it may be a sign of improper fit and the high pressure may then cause mucous membrane trauma in those places where the fit is tight. If the fit remains poor after optimal cuff inflation, a different size of LMA should be attempted or another brand of LMA may be successful. Because each brand is designed slightly differently, there is a different success rate in individual patients. Although the LMA does not provide a 100% seal of the trachea, it is still argued that it protects the airway very well against modest amounts of mucus or blood from the pharynx area, as the whole entrance of the larynx is covered and protected. However, if the pharynx for some reason (marked bleeding, regurgitation from a full stomach) is "flooded" with fluid, the LMA will not protect fully against airway aspiration, whereas an ETT with a properly inflated cuff will.

The benefits of a properly placed ETT with inflated cuff are: close to 100% control of all inspiration and expiration in the patient; robustness against the need for high airway pressures; minimal danger of dislocation or aspiration. Classical dogma has been to add muscle relaxants during anesthesia induction to relax the vocal cords and facilitate the ETT placement; however, this practice has been challenged by the availability of modern anesthetic agents. With deep levels of anesthesia the vocal cords will be fairly well relaxed and other airway reflexes (coughing) will be abolished, thus the ETT can be placed without the need for specific muscle relaxation. However, there are reports of airway damage with this approach, claiming that the use of relaxants makes the intubation more gentle.[16] A more common problem with intubation without relaxants is that the timing of the short intubation trauma may not quite match the peak of the strong analgesic effect, thus a period of severe hypotension may occur before or after the intubation procedure with this approach.

A meta-analysis was performed on randomized prospective trials comparing the LMA with other forms of airway management to determine if the LMA possessed any advantages over ETT or face-mask. Advantages of LMA over the ETT included: increased speed and ease of placement by both inexperienced and experienced personnel; improved hemodynamic stability at induction and during emergence; minimal increase in intraocular pressure following insertion; reduced anesthetic requirements for airway tolerance; lower frequency of cough during emergence; improved oxygen saturation during emergence; and lower incidence of sore throat in adults. Disadvantages over the ETT were lower seal pressures and a higher frequency of gastric insufflations.[17]

In 2002, the ProSeal model of the LMA was released. It addresses some of the shortcomings of the standard or classic LMA. It has a channel built into it that allowed access to the esophagus via a separate port and has a built-in bite block. A better seal means the ProSeal can be used to ventilate at higher airway pressures without creating as much gastric distension as the classic model.[18] Because the airway conduit is flexible, it has a designed airway inserter. However, papers abound using other stylets such as oro-gastric tubing, Eschmann stylets, and FlexiSlip stylet.[19–21] The ProSeal is a reusable model; the single-use model also by Teleflex is called the LMA Supreme. It has a similar gastric channel, but the airway conduit is more rigid. Papers comparing the two models demonstrate a slightly faster insertion time and slightly lower leak pressures with the Supreme.[22–25] The literature describes using these two devices ranging for cases that are gynecologic, laparoscopic, or prone-positioned and patients that are pediatric or obese.[23,24,26–28] One contraindication for this type of airway is a known or suspected

full stomach.[29] Otherwise, the only time an ETT would be indicated in the ambulatory setting would be if the supraglottic device itself interfered with the surgical site or surgical access.

The difficult airway can create anxiety in the ambulatory setting. Rather than the mental image that the words "difficult airway" draw, policy and judgment should be focused on concrete issues. The medical staff needs to make a multidisciplinary decision regarding the type of known difficult airways allowed. The unexpected difficult airway can always occur and a facility always needs to be prepared for this. In assessing a patient with a known difficult airway, what makes the airway difficult needs to be defined. Is the patient easily ventilated, but unable to have a successful laryngoscopy? Or has the patient had a failure of a supraglottic airway device? The most significant is the patient that cannot be successfully ventilated, as this is the most likely to cause life-threatening hypoxia. In the ambulatory surgery setting, the bony structures of the mandible and cervical spine are not likely to change with surgery. Still, there may be significant problems in a few patients; for example, patients with rheumatoid arthritis or Bechterew and a totally stiff neck, or patients with jaw problems. The soft tissue of the pharynx may change as a result of the surgery (i.e., tonsillectomy, excision of lingual lesion) or positioning (i.e., prolonged, prone procedure). By defining the source of the difficulty and the procedure, it may be acceptable for the known difficult airway to undergo a procedure. However, a patient with a known, more minor issue may become inappropriate if bony issues are combined with the risk of significant soft-tissue swelling. For example, a patient with a known history of difficult intubation can have a successful blepharoplasty under local anesthesia. A patient for a prolonged, posterior liposuction may need to be further evaluated for the presence of a beard or bull neck. In the end, the facility needs to have the ability to serve the patient safely.[30]

The difficult airway cart is a necessity for the unknown, difficult airway patient. There are no requirements for specific instrumentation, but it needs to be usable by the anesthesia staff at the facility. There is a significant risk of anesthesia providers losing their airway skills if they are not exposed to difficult airway scenarios frequently.[31] Therefore, providers need to keep their skills up by using the specialized equipment on hand and maintaining continuing education on the topic. The equipment should not be useful only to a certain provider, but appeal to most and be in good repair. The difficult airway cart itself needs to be well-organized. There should be uniformity between it and other places that providers frequent. Batteries, drugs, expiration dates, and equipment need to be checked regularly and documented. An annual or biannual assessment should be done to see if the equipment is still appropriate for the setting. Lastly, the staff (nursing and anesthesia provider) needs to have regular drills for airway emergencies.

Intravenous fluid management in ambulatory surgery

Most practitioners probably handle intravenous fluid (IVF) management as they did during their residency. We were taught the 4-2-1 principle of dehydration during times of fasting and that insensible losses need to be replaced in the operating room. That is, the amount of fluid a patient loses during fasting is equal to 4 cc/kg/h for the first 10 kg of weight plus 2 cc/kg/h for the next 10 kg of weight, then 1 cc/kg/h for additional kg of weight greater than 20 kg. This means a 70 kg person fasting for 8 h would have a fluid deficit of (10 kg × 4 cc/kg/h × 8 h) + (10 kg × 2 cc/kg/h × 8 h) + (50 kg × 1 cc/kg/h × 8 h) = (320 cc + 160 cc + 400 cc) = 880 cc. Blood loss is supposed to be replaced at a 3 to 1 ratio with IVF. Newer data may signal that it is time for a change in thinking. The issues to consider are: the best choice for fluid replacement, how much fluid replacement, and does colloid therapy belong in ambulatory surgery. Additionally, the goals of IVF therapy need to be considered in terms of prevention of dehydration and, perhaps, PONV.

Much of the literature comparing "restrictive" and "liberal" fluid management is based on inpatient, colorectal surgery. The first problem in comparing the studies is that there is not a consistent definition of either term. The second is that it is not ambulatory data. However, the main themes can be applicable. According to a review by Bamboat et al., focused on inpatient bowel surgery, the restrictive approach increases hemodynamic instability and postoperative nausea while decreasing end-organ perfusion and tissue oxygenation. Liberal fluids may promote poor wound healing, heart failure, and interstitial edema as well as delay gastric emptying and return of normal bowel function.[32] For patients that are more comparable to ambulatory patients, Holte et al. looked at amounts of fluid being given to knee arthroplasty patients. Interestingly, their group gave a combination of crystalloid and colloid fluid in each group. Each group was equally fasted and received 0.7 cc/kg of colloid solution. The liberal group also received a 10 cc/kg bolus of lactated Ringer's with 30 cc/kg/h intraoperatively. The restricted group received 10 cc/kg/h of lactated Ringer's intraoperatively. The groups were compared for pulmonary function, exercise capacity, coagulation, postoperative hypoxia, postoperative ileus, and subjective recovery score. The group with the "liberal" IVF administration showed significantly less PONV, improved pulmonary function, and increased hypercoagulability.[33]

The constituent components of the fluids used in surgery is currently popular in the literature. Very recently, McClusky et al. demonstrated that increased hyperchloremia in non-cardiac surgery increased morbidity and mortality. His group reviewed over 22,000 patients that underwent inpatient surgery at his facility. The patients that used normal saline instead of lactated Ringers had elevated chloride levels and higher 30-day postoperative mortality.[34] A commentary in the same journal noted that although there is not enough power in the literature, and the McClusky et al. study was retrospective and not conclusive, the best recommendation based on available studies is to use a balanced salt solution such as Normosol, Plasmalyte, or lactated Ringers "for intravascular volume resuscitation in surgical patients."[35] This obviously involved cases and patients not typical for ambulatory surgery. The addition of dextrose to IVF may be moving out of the pediatric realm and into the adult world for its effects on PONV. There have been many small studies and posters presented at recent meetings. One recent study by Dabu-Bondoc et al. looked at 62 patients undergoing gynecologic surgery. The two groups were equal for amounts of IVF, prophylactic anti-emetics, and opioids administered. The difference was one group received 1 liter of lactated Ringer's and the other received 1 liter of lactated Ringer's with 5% dextrose in the recovery room after surgery. It was found that the group receiving dextrose had less-frequent treatment for nausea in recovery and a shorter length of stay in recovery.[36]

In the debate between crystalloid and colloid, a review of basic fluid homeostasis is revealing. The extracellular volume (ECV) of total body fluid is about 15 liters in the adult, 3 liters in plasma, and the remaining in the interstitium. The osmotic gradients keep the balance of the free water as described above. The ability of small solutes to easily cross cellular barriers allows cellular metabolism to occur freely. Trauma during surgery and the resulting inflammation decreases the ability of the lymphatic system to return fluid to the circulation and increases "third-spacing" or interstitial fluid (controversial term). Ideal replacement of blood lost would be drop for drop with whole blood. As this is not a reasonable approach for many reasons (expense, infection, etc.), crystalloid is typical. At this rate, only 20% stays intravascular with 80% gradually going to the interstitium. Transfusion only occurs at levels that are individually based on patient risk factors. The hemodilution is actually beneficial as it improves the rheology of the blood to maximize perfusion and oxygenation. Current fasting of patients preoperatively actually results in very little intravascular dehydration. The body can accommodate this easily when there is no associated bowel preparation. Loading volume to "correct" the dehydration results in increases in interstitial volume and increases vascular volume at the end of surgery when the vasodilating anesthetic wears off. The kidneys cannot function well to clear the extra volume and the patient has resulting weight gain, swelling, and possible pulmonary edema.[37]

There is an endothelial glycocalyx that acts to modify the permeability of the vascular endothelium. It also has a role in preventing platelet aggregation. The glycocalyx accounts for the difference between measured oncotic pressure between intra- and extracellular compartments by making the oncotic pressure relevant only between the plasma and a minelayer of fluid just deep to the glycocalyx. The glycocalyx acts as a filter for proteins and large colloids so they cannot pass as freely. Disruption of the glycocalyx occurs from trauma, and inflammatory mediators such as tumor necrosis factor (TNF), and antinatriatic peptide (ANP). The effect of disruption is local tissue swelling in the area of the disruption. Recall that ANP is released in response to fluid expansion of the vascular compartment. Hence, the findings of tissue swelling and hypercoagulability in studies where the patients have received liberal IVF management.[34,35] The glycocalyx is also damaged by ischemia, proteases, and oxidized, low-density lipoproteins.[37]

Chappell *et al.* recommends using crystalloid or colloid solutions as drugs with indications. Crystalloids should be used to replace insensible losses and urine output. This replaces the losses that come from a primary interstitial location as crystalloid ends up 80% in the interstitium. He also warns that measured insensible losses are far below the classic training of 5–20 cc/kg/h of exposed abdomen. Colloid should be used to replace intravascular volume that occurs due to disruption of the glycocalyx. This would be from blood loss or pathologic shifting due to capillary leak from a damaged endothelium. To avoid giving colloid, anesthesia should be aimed at reducing the "stresses" that degrade the glycocalyx. One is to avoid overhydration. Another is to utilize regional analgesia techniques that decrease surgical stress and TNF release.[37] This would represent a shift in thought for most ambulatory anesthesiologists and it has not been studied. However, it may represent a logical approach to take with less-healthy patients or larger, ambulatory procedures.

Obesity and obstructive sleep apnea

The Society for Ambulatory Anesthesia (SAMBA) has released a consensus statement on the treatment of patients with obstructive sleep apnea (OSA) in the ambulatory setting in 2012. There was also a recent review of current literature that was applicable to treatment of obese patients in ambulatory anesthesia in 2013. In the absence of research, expert opinion was used.

The American Society of Anesthesiology released a consensus statement on management of patients with OSA in 2006. It was based on inpatient data and was very restrictive in recommendations that virtually eliminated outpatient surgery.[38] SAMBA looked to update the recommendations based on literature since 2005. Much of the work came from Chung's group in Toronto and her work to develop a screening tool. The STOP-Bang questionnaire was the product of her labor. It is a simple tool that has a high sensitivity. Its specificity can be raised by increasing the number of positive responses from > 2 to > 5.[39] The questions involved are:

1. Do you Snore?
2. Do you feel Tired, fatigued or sleepy during the day?
3. Has anyone Observed you stop breathing in your sleep?

4. Do you have high blood **Pressure**?
5. Is your **BMI** > 35?
6. Is your **Age** > 50?
7. Is your **Neck** size > 15.7 inches or 40 cm?
8. Are you male **Gender**?

The SAMBA statement makes many recommendations. The significant comorbidities associated with OSA need to be optimized prior to surgery. Those with poorly controlled heart disease or diabetes may not be ideal ambulatory candidates. Painful procedures associated with opioid use may be avoided in the ambulatory setting because opioid use exacerbates OSA. In contrast to the ASA statement, upper abdominal, laparoscopic surgery showed no increased risk, but airway surgery could not be evaluated on an ambulatory basis. Patients using a continuous positive airway pressure (CPAP) device should bring it to the ambulatory facility if the facility does not have one of their own. The patients should also use the CPAP device whenever they are sleeping for several days as the risk for apnea is highest on the third postoperative day in patients with moderate to severe OSA.[40] As opioids do negatively impact OSA, efforts should be made to avoid or minimize an OSA patient's exposure to them.[41]

The advice from SAMBA is that complications arise from the interplay of OSA and coexisting diseases. As with any ambulatory procedure, the medical condition of the patient should be optimized. A discussion should be had with the surgeon preoperatively regarding pain management strategy. The use of acetaminophen and non-steroidal drugs should be maximized. The opioid-sparing effect of steroids is also recommended. CPAP and BiPAP should be continued postoperatively. If a patient is not medically optimized, refuses to use CPAP or BiPAP, or pain can only be treated with opioids, then the patient with OSA (or presumed OSA) is not a good ambulatory candidate.[41]

The review of obesity in the literature was not robust enough to create a consensus statement. It did provide a current look at relevant literature. What the authors found was that obesity (BMI) does not seem to be a risk factor for transfer to a hospital from a free-standing facility. It did increase the risk of respiratory complications such as need for oxygen, bronchospasm, and airway obstruction. Morbid obesity (BMI 40–49) does not increase the 30-day mortality as reported to American College of Surgeons National Quality Improvement Program. The super-obese (BMI > 50) did have longer operative times and more comorbidities. The super-obese did also have more superficial and deep postoperative wound infections, sepsis, septic shock, and mortality. Readmission rates have been associated with male gender, symptomatic asthma, gastro-esophageal reflux disease, and history of deep vein thrombosis or pulmonary embolism. Another study added employment status of disabled or retired as a risk factor.[42]

The recommendations of the authors are that the only limit to how large a patient can be is perhaps that a BMI greater than 50 presents an independent risk factor. Otherwise, each patient needs to be considered independently and have an assessment based on how well coexisting diseases are managed and what the proposed procedure is.[42] Recovery factors may also come into play and the level of care the patient will require postoperatively.

Depth of anesthesia monitoring

The idea of "depth-of-anesthesia-monitoring" (DAM) is to provide an evaluation of the pharmacologic effect of anesthetic drugs that is more accurate and precise than end-tidal monitoring of gases or simulation of IV plasma levels. DAM should also be more sensitive and specific than the clinical monitoring of effects, such as sympathomimetic output, hemodynamics, and movements. As it is potentially harmful to have a level of anesthesia that is either too light or too deep, it is a good idea to provide some "warning" of clinical changes in either direction. The two indications for DAM are prevention of awareness (i.e., underdosing) and more precise titration of the correct drug dose (i.e., over- or underdosing).

There are numerous commercial methods and devices for DAM.[43] Many use the recorded EEG, whereas others use the EEG response to a stimulus. These methods are depth-of-sleep monitors, but there are other devices that attempt to measure the nociception-induced stress level, by using the R-R interval in ECG, muscle tension, pulse amplitude, or sweating.[44] The most-used and best-documented device is the BIS monitor, which transforms a passive, sampled frontal EEG and compares it using an algorithm with a data bank of empirical EEG patterns.[45] The BIS is calibrated to give a signal of 0–100, where values below 60 indicate unconsciousness or sleep in most patients. Keeping the BIS value in the 40–60 range (or even better the 50–60 range) during general anesthesia ensures rapid emergence and less risk of overdosing in individual patients. Shortcomings with

BIS include the inability to account for the influence of opioid or nitrous oxide supplements, and a paradoxical increase in the BIS value when ketamine is given to a sleeping patient.

Awareness is quite rare, about 1 per 500 in newer studies without DAM.[46] Unpleasant awareness only occurs in fully curarized patients, because noncurarized patients will move if they are uncomfortable and are becoming aware. In order to be aware it seems that a period of at least 4 min of BIS above 60 is needed.[46] It has been shown in two studies, one in high-risk procedures (mostly emergency)[47] and the other in inhalational-based inpatient anesthesia,[46] that awareness is significantly reduced by 80% if BIS monitoring is used. The cost–benefit relevance of these studies for ambulatory cases is disputed, as muscle relaxation in ambulatory surgery is infrequent and the costs of BIS electrodes range from 10 to 15 dollars per unit. It has also been claimed that, with inhalational anesthesia, keeping the end-tidal gas level at appropriate values (1 MAC or more) may be as sensitive and as specific as BIS monitoring for avoiding reaction and awareness.[48] BIS values above 60 for more than 4 min happens in about 20% of cases, and only 1 out of 500 of these will be aware.[46] Where the BIS is observed to be above 60 drugs may be dosed more generously; therefore, overall the costs of implementing procedures to avoid just one case of awareness are quite high. Nevertheless, if economy permits, it may be a good choice in terms of the patient's quality of experience to provide BIS or other DAM monitoring for those patients who are fully paralyzed in ambulatory practice as well as in the inpatient setting. Depth of anesthesia monitoring becomes particularly useful in patients with an unpredictable need for drugs, such as the obese, the elderly, drug addicts, patients with hypermetabolism, and patients on liver-enzyme-inducing drugs.

Cases of special patient populations may require special consideration in BIS monitoring. Geriatric patients were found to have decreased emergence times after undergoing major orthopedic, inpatient procedures when guided by BIS values.[49] However, White's group found that faster emergence and recovery were not present with minor procedures requiring general anesthesia in the ambulatory setting.[50] Pediatric patients do have lower total doses of inhalational agents and faster recovery when a bispectral index or related technology is used. What was not realized was a difference in emergence delirium.[51] As a matter of fact,

delirium was not found to be correlated to the amount of time spent in "deep anesthesia" with bispectral indices less than 45, either.[52] Obese patients have similar BIS values at similar depths of anesthesia. As a matter of fact, most studies comparing the pharmacokinetics of anesthetic agents in obese patients use the BIS value to create an accepted equivalent level of anesthesia.[53,54]

Patients with brain injuries have altered bispectral indices when compared to their non-injured counterparts. Pediatric patients with cerebral palsy have typical responses to inhalational anesthesia according to their bispectral index; however, the numerical value runs lower when compared to children without cerebral palsy.[55] Stroke patients will have an altered bispectral index, but this is greatly dependent on the size and age of the infarction. Patients with mental retardation have no differences in bispectral index compared to their normal peers.[56] White's group found an interesting correlation in patients undergoing electro-convulsive therapy. The pre-ECT BIS value correlated with the duration of both the motor and EEG seizure activity. The peak post-ECT BIS value correlated with the duration of the EEG seizure activity. A positive correlation was also found between the EEG seizure duration and the time to eye opening. However, the BIS value at time of emergence was highly variable.[57]

When DAM is used in non-paralyzed patients, then the focus is different. These patients will move when anesthesia becomes too light, so DAM should focus on highlighting when patients become anesthetized too deeply following standard dosing. By giving these individual patients less anesthetic and thus speeding their emergence, the average drug consumption and emergence for the whole group of patients will be reduced.[43] Again, this may be especially useful in patients with unpredictable drug requirements (see above) and also during procedures of unpredictable duration and sudden end. In such cases it is hard to titrate the drugs carefully down during the planned end of the procedure, and maintaining an appropriate (not too deep) level at all times is very useful.

Target-controlled infusions and computer-assisted patient sedation

Target-controlled infusion (TCI) anesthesia involves giving an IV-based anesthetic that is controlled by a computer algorithm to a goal effect. The effect is generally a sedation score necessary to accomplish a surgical or endoscopic procedure or a depth of anesthesia score such as BiS. However, more complex systems may use plasma concentration or calculated concentration. The technology has been around for over a decade and the IV agents of choice are propofol and remifentanil.

In 2008, a Cochrane database review was done to compare TCI versus manually controlled infusions by anesthetists. It demonstrated higher drug use by TCI, but less airway interventions. There was no difference in quality of anesthesia or adverse events. The studies were very heterogeneous and, therefore, no firm recommendations could be made.[58] The comparison of costs between TCI and human management is extremely variable depending on insurance or employment contracts and acquisition cost for the computer system. Even though a TCI may be free of the use of an anesthetist, many regulatory agencies still require someone present whose sole responsibility is the monitoring of the patient and sedation. The final costs are very dependent on the local market where the services are being provided.

The next evolution of TCI is computer-assisted patient sedation (CAPS). In the approved version, only the provider is allowed to increase the level of sedation to be more sedated. It is not TCI because it does not seek to manage the end-effect of propofol infusion. It will reduce the infusion rate of propofol when signs of over-sedation are detected. The system approved in the United States is Sedasys by Ethicon. It will monitor oxygen saturation, blood pressure, and heart rate on its bedside unit. On its procedure room unit, it adds capnography and automated responsiveness monitoring. The functions for propofol and oxygen administration are on the procedure room unit, too. Another feature is a PRN function that allows additional propofol given for times of increased patient discomfort. It becomes controversial that this function can be used to bypass the safety shut-offs meant to prevent over-sedation. The system is set to treat low oxygen saturations by decreasing propofol infusion rate and giving oxygen to meet a saturation goal. The propofol rate is also dropped when the patients do not respond quickly to auditory stimulus by pushing a hand-held button when directed.

The goal of Sedasys is to create minimal to moderate conscious sedation. To that end, it appears to be successful. From the literature, patients use less propofol and recover more quickly. They are also less

sedated and required no airway support. There was desaturation under < 90% for > 15 seconds in 6% and apnea > 30 seconds in 38%.[59] On the pro-anesthetist side, the machine takes longer to get to desired effect as there are limits to how quickly the propofol infusion rates can be started. It also treats possible airway obstruction with oxygen therapy. The providers using the device should be trained to rescue deeper-than-intended sedation and be able to successfully assess a patient for risks of sedation. Furthermore, the system is still using a drug with a narrow therapeutic window. It is only approved for ASA class I and II patients 18-years-old or greater undergoing colonoscopy or esophagogastroduodenoscopy. An anesthesia professional must also be immediately available.[60]

References

1. Practice advisory for preanesthesia evaluation: a report by the American Society of Anesthesiologists Task Force on Preanesthesia Evaluation. *Anesthesiology* 2002;**96**:485–96.

2. Schein OD, Katz J, Bass EB, *et al*. The value of routine preoperative medical testing before cataract surgery. Study of Medical Testing for Cataract Surgery. *N Engl J Med* 2000;**342**:168–75.

3. Chung F, Yuan H, Yin L, Vairavanathabn S, Wong D. Elimation of preoperative testing in ambulatory surgery. *Anesth Analg* 2009;**108**:467–75.

4. Roberts JD, Sweitzer BJ. Perioperative evaluation and management of cardiac disease in the ambulatory surgery setting. *Anesthesiol Clin* 2014;**32**:309–20.

5. Azzam FJ, Gurpreet SP, DeBoard JW, Krock JL, Kolterman SM. Preoperative pregnancy testing in adolescents. *Anesth Analg* 1996; **82**:4–7.

6. Manley S, de Kelaita G, Joseph NJ, Salem R, Heyman HJ. Preoperative pregnancy testing in ambulatory surgery. *Anesthesiology* 1995; **83**:690–93.

7. Gokce BM, Ozkose Z, Tuncer B, *et al*. Hemodynamic effects, recovery profiles, and costs of remifentanil-based anesthesia with propofol or desflurane for septorhinoplasty. *Saudi Med J* 2007;**28**:358–63.

8. Gozdemir M, Sert H, Yilmaz N, *et al*. Remifentanil–propofol in vertebral disk operations: hemodynamics and recovery versus desflurane-N(2)O inhalation anesthesia. *Adv Ther* 2007;**24**:622–31.

9. Röhm KD, Riechmann J, Boldt J, *et al*. Total intravenous anesthesia with propofol and remifentanil is associated with a nearly twofold higher incidence in postanesthetic shivering than desflurane–fentanyl anesthesia. *Med Sci Monit* 2006;**12**: CR452–CR456.

10. Moore JK, Elliott RA, Payne K, *et al*. The effect of anaesthetic agents on induction, recovery and patient preferences in adult day case surgery: a 7-day follow-up randomized controlled trial. *Eur J Anaesthesiol* 2008;**25**:876–83.

11. Hong JY, Kang YS, Kil HK. Anesthesia for day case excisional breast biopsy: propofol–remifentanil compared with sevoflurane–nitrous oxide. *Eur J Anaesthesiol* 2008;**25**:460–67.

12. Gupta A, Stierer T, Zuckermann R, Sakima N, Parker S, Fleisher L. Comparison of recovery profile after ambulatory anesthesia with propofol, isoflurane, sevoflurane and desflurane: a systematic review. *Anesth Analg* 2004;**98**:632–41.

13. Williams BA, Kentor ML. The WAKE score: patient-centered ambulatory anesthesia and fast-tracking outcomes criteria. *Int Anesthesiol Clin* 2011;**49**:33–43.

14. Moore J, Ross S, Williams B. Regional anesthesia in ambulatory surgery. *Current Opin Anesthesiol* 2013;**26**:652–60.

15. Gray A, Laur J. Regional anesthesia for ambulatory surgery: where ultrasound has made a difference. *Int Anesthesiol Clin* 2011;**49**:13–21.

16. Combes X, Andriamifidy L, Dufresne, *et al*. Comparison of two induction regimes using or not using muscle relaxant: impact on postoperative upper airway discomfort. *Br J Anaesth* 2007;**99**:276–81.

17. Peirovifar A, Eydi M, Mirinejhad M, Mahmoodpoor A, Mohammadi A, Golzari S. Comparison of postoperative complication between Laryngeal Mask Airway and endotracheal tube during low-flow anesthesia with controlled ventilation. *Pak J Med Sci* 2013;**29**(2):601–05.

18. Brimacombe J, Keller C. The ProSeal laryngeal mask airway. *Anesthesiol Clin N Am* 2002;**20**(4):871–91.

19. Nagata T, Kishi Y, Tanigami H, *et al*. Oral gastric tube-guided insertion of the ProSealTM laryngeal mask is an easy and noninvasive method for less experienced users. *J Anesth* 2012;**26**:531–35.

20. El Beheiry H, Wong J, Nair G, *et al*. Improved esophageal patency when inserting the ProSeal laryngeal mask airway with an EschmannTM tracheal tube introducer. *Can J Anesth/J Can Anesth* 2009;**56**:725–32.

21. Chen HS, Yang SC, Chang Chien CF, Spielberger J, Hung KC, Chung KC. Insertion of the ProSeal laryngeal mask airway is more successful with the Flexi-Slip stylet than with the introducer. *Can J Anesth/J Can Anesth* 2011;**58**:617–23.

22. Hosten T, Gurkan Y, Ozdamar D, Telin M, Toker K Solak M. A new supraglottic airway device: LMA-Supreme comparison with LMA-Proseal. *Acta Anaesthesiol Scand* 2009;**53**:852–57.

23. Lee AKY, Tey JBL, Lim Y, Sia ATH. Comparison of the single-use LMA Supreme with the reusable ProSeal LMA for anaesthesia in gynaecological aparoscopic surgery. *Anaesth Intens Care* 2009;**37**:815–19.

24. Belena JM, Nunez M, Anta D, *et al*. Comparison of Laryngeal Mask Airway Supreme and Laryngeal Mask Airway Proseal with respect to oropharyngeal leak pressure during laparoscopic cholecystectomy: a randomised controlled trial. *Eur J Anaesthesiol* 2013;**30**(3):119–23.

25. Hosten T, Gurkan Y, Kus A, *et al*. Comparison of ProSeal LMA with Supreme LMA in paediatric patients. *Acta Anaesthesiol Scand* 2013;**57**:996–1001.

26. Lopez AM, Valero R, Hurtado P, Gambus P, Pons M, Anglada T. Comparison of the LMA SupremeTM with the LMA Proseal for airway management in patients anaesthetized in prone position. *Br J Anaesth* 2011;**107**(2):265–71.

27. Nicholson A, Cook TM, Smith AF, Lewis SR, Reed SS. Supraglottic airway devices versus tracheal intubation for airway management during general anaesthesia in obese patients (Review) Copyright © 2014 The Cochrane Collaboration. Published by JohnWiley & Sons, Ltd.

28. Lim B, Pawar D, Ng O. Pressure support ventilation vs spontaneous ventilation via ProSealTM laryngeal mask airway in pediatric patients undergoing ambulatory surgery: a randomized controlled trial. *Pediatr Anesth* 2012;**22**:360–64.

29. ProSeal LMA Instructions for use. Copyright © 2013 Teleflex Incorporated.

30. Greenland K. Difficult airway management in an ambulatory surgery center? *Curr Opin Anesthesiol* 2012;**25**:659–64.

31. Greenland KB, Acott C, Segal R, *et al*. Emergency surgical airway in life-threatening acute airway emergencies: why are we so reluctant to do it? *Anaesth Intens Care* 2011;**39**:578–84.

32. Bamboat Z, Bordeianou L. Perioperative fluid management. *Clin Colon Rectal Surg* 2009; **22**:28–33.

33. Holte K, Kristensen B, Valentiner L, Nicolai BF, Husted H, Kehlet H. Liberal versus restrictive fluid management in knee arthroplasty: a randomized, double-blind study. *Anesth Analg* 2007;**105**:465–74.

34. McCluskey S, Karkouti K, Wijeysundera D, Minkovich L, Tait G, Beattie WS. Hyperchloremia after noncardiac surgery is independently associated with increased morbidity and mortality: a propensity-matched cohort study. *Anesth Analg* 2013;**117**:412–21.

35. Butterworth J, Mythen M. Should "normal" saline be our usual choice in normal surgical patients? *Anesth Analg* 2013;**117**:290–91.

36. Dabu-Bondoc S, Vadivelu N, Shimono C, *et al.* Postoperative antiemetic rescue treatment requirements and postanesthesia care unit length of stay. *Anesth Analg* 2012;**117**:591–96.

37. Chappell D, Jacob M, Hofmann-Kieferr K, Conzen P, Rehm M. A rational approach to perioperative fluid management. *Anesthesiology* 2008;**109**:723–40.

38. Practice guidelines for the perioperative management of patients with obstructive sleep apnea. *Anesthesiology* 2006;**104**:1081–93.

39. Chung F, Yang Y, Liao P. Predictive performance of the STOP-Bang score for identifying obstructive sleep apnea in obese patients. *Obes Surg* 2013;**23**(12):2050–57.

40. Chung F, Liao P, Fazel H, *et al.* What are the factors predicting the postoperative apnea–hypopnea Index. *Chest* 2010;**138**:703A.

41. Joshi G, Ankichetty SP, Gan TJ, Chung F. Society for Ambulatory Anesthesia consensus statement on preoperative selection of adult patients with obstructive sleep apnea scheduled for ambulatory surgery. *Anesth Analg* 2012;**115**:1060–68.

42. Joshi G, Ahmad S, Riad W, Eckert S, Chung F. Selection of obese patients undergoing ambulatory surgery: a systematic review of the literature. *Anesth Analg* 2013;**117**:1082–91.

43. White PF. Use of cerebral monitoring during anesthesia: effect on recovery profile. *Best Pract Res Clin Anaesthesiol* 2006;**20**:181–89.

44. Gjerstad AC, Storm H, Hagen R, *et al.* Skin conductance or entropy for detection of non-noxious stimulation during different clinical levels of sedation. *Acta Anaesthesiol Scand* 2007;**51**:1–7.

45. Hoymork SC, Hval K, Jensen EW, Raeder J. Can the cerebral state monitor replace the bispectral index in monitoring hypnotic effect during propofol/ remifentanil anesthesia? *Acta Anaesthesiol Scand* 2007;**51**:210–16.

46. Ekman A, Lindholm ML, Lennmarken C, Sandin R. Reduction in the incidence of awareness using BIS monitoring. *Acta Anaesthesiol Scand* 2004;**48**:20–26.

47. Myles PS, Leslie K, McNeil J, *et al.* Bispectral index monitoring to prevent awareness during anesthesia: the B-Aware randomised controlled trial. *Lancet* 2004;**363**:1757–63.

48. Alpiger S, Helbo-Hansen HS, Vach W, Ording H. Efficacy of the A-line AEP monitor as a tool for predicting successful insertion of a laryngeal mask during sevoflurane anesthesia. *Acta Anaesthesiol Scand* 2004;**48**:888–93.

49. Wong J, Song D, Blanshard H, Grady D, Chung F. Titration of isoflurane using BIS index improves early recovery of elderly patients undergoing orthopedic surgeries. *Can J Anesth* 2002;**49**:13–18.

50. White PF, Tang J, Wender RH, *et al.* Desflurane versus sevoflurane for maintenance of outpatient anesthesia: the effect on early versus late recovery and perioperative coughing. *Anesth Analg* 2009;**109**(2):387–93. doi:10.1213/ ane.0b013e3181adc21a.

51. Zohar E, Luban I, White P, Ramati E, Shabat S, Fredman B. Bispectral index monitoring does not improve early recovery of geriatric outpatients undergoing brief surgical procedures. *Can J Anesth* 2006;**53**(1):20–25.

52. Liao WW, Wang JJ, Wu GJ, Kuo CD. The effect of cerebral monitoring on recovery after sevoflurane anesthesia in ambulatory setting in children: a comparison among bispectral index, A-line autoregressive index, and standard practice. *J Chin Med Assoc* 2011;**74**:28–36.

53. Faulk D, Twite M, Zuk J, Pan Z, Wallen B, Friesen RH. Hypnotic depth and the incidence of emergence agitation and negative postoperative behavioral changes. *Pediatr Anesth* 2010;**20**:72–81.

54. Zeidan A, Mazoit JX. Minimal alveolar concentration of sevoflurane for maintaining bispectral index below 50 in morbidly obese patients. *Acta Anaesthesiol Scand* 2013;**57**:474–79.

55. Choudhry DK, Brenn BR. Bispectral index monitoring: a comparison between normal children and children with quadriplegic cerebral palsy. *Anesth Analg* 2002;**95**:1582–85.

56. Ponnudurai RN, Clark-Moore A, Ekulide I, *et al.* A prospective study of bispectral index scoring in mentally retarded patients receiving general anesthesia. *J Clin Anesth* 2010;**22**:432–36.

57. White PF, Rawal S, Recart A, Thornton L, Litle M, Stool L. Can the bispectral index be used to predict seizure time and awakening after electroconvulsive therapy? *Anesth Analg* 2003;**96**:1636–39.

58. Leslie K, Clavisi O, Hargrove J. Target-controlled infusion versus manually-controlled infusion of propofol for general anaesthesia or sedation in adults. *Cochrane Database of Systematic Reviews* 2008;Issue 3: CD006059.

59. Pambianco DJ, Whitten CJ, Moerman A, Struys MM, Martin JF. An assessment of computer-assisted personalized sedation: a sedation delivery system to administer propofol for gastrointestinal endoscopy. *Gastrointest Endosc* 2008;**68**:542–47.

60. Ethicon Endo-Surgery, Inc. (2013). Taking sedation to a new place: Sedasys sedation redefined. [brochure].

Chapter 1

Current and future trends in ambulatory anesthesia

Steven Butz, MD

A short historical perspective

Ambulatory surgery continues to grow in terms of number of cases, types of cases, and locations that the cases are performed. As we advance in technical skill and creativity to approach surgical pathology, there are more and more opportunities to practice advanced cases in patients expecting to go home. The settings for these cases are expanding away from the hospital operating suite and ambulatory surgery centers, too. Office-based anesthesia is expanding rapidly and the "office" may now be a radiology suite, a gastroenterology suite, dental or surgeon's office.

Office-based cases moved from the early, tentative steps of excisions of small, skin lesions to now a wide spectrum of plastic and reconstructive surgery. Orthopedics and urology joined in along with dental, gynecology, and general surgery. Typical cases may now include breast augmentations and facelifts, dental rehabilitation, cystoscopy and prostate surgery, egg harvests and uteroscopy, upper and lower endoscopies. The cases are now only limited by expectations for patients to go home and amount of time for case to be performed and recovery due to staffing. The American Society of Plastic Surgeons recommends that the cases be completed in 6 hours and before 3 pm. This was not based on known safety data, but more a common sense to have staff and resources available in a setting not flush in redundancy as in a hospital.

Initially, cases were performed using only conscious sedation. Now, general anesthesia is very common. Part of the move was driven by better anesthesia drugs. Primary among that was propofol. Its rapid recovery and beneficial recovery profile make it perfect for the ambulatory setting. Furthermore, it requires no special handling such as waste gas scavenging and has no potential to trigger malignant hyperthermia. Accrediting bodies including the Centers for Medicare and Medicaid Services dictate that the use of succinylcholine and potent inhalational agents requires providing dantrolene for a crisis. Dantrolene at this time carries about a $2000 price for 36 vials. The synthetic opioids are favored and the use of remifentanil has made total intravenous anesthesia a more feasible possibility. It is very often combined with propofol to create a complete anesthetic. Ketamine has found more widespread uses and has been found to reduce opioid requirement when used in very small doses. The expansion of anti-emetics beyond droperidol and promethazine (and their black box warnings) to create effective drugs with less side effects was also very important.

New and up-coming anesthetic agents

Very new agents and those with promise to ambulatory anesthesia are becoming fewer. However, a few that are already available deserve attention. One is an old drug with a new carrier, Exparel®. This is bupivacaine dissolved in a liposomal emulsion. It was released in October 2011. The emulsion gives it the same white appearance as propofol, so syringe labeling is critical. The benefit is that the bupiviacaine is now a slow-release drug that decreases opioid use for days instead of hours. The emulsion has been used for drugs for infiltration or infusion, but it is the infiltration that seems the best use in this instance. It has not been approved for central nervous system use. A small, prospective study by Marcet *et al.* demonstrated significant opioid reduction and decreased cost and length of stay when used as part of a multimodal approach to pain control in patients undergoing ileostomy reversal. The opioids administered via patient-controlled analgesia were, 20 mg in the Exparel® group versus 112 mg. The

Practical Ambulatory Anesthesia, ed. Johan Raeder and Richard D. Urman. Published by Cambridge University Press. © Cambridge University Press 2015.

hospital cost was $6482 versus $9282 with a 2.1 decrease in stay from 5.1 days.[1] A limitation with this drug is the limited amount of bupivacaine released per hour, which may not be comparable to a wound catheter infusion in terms of analgesic efficacy, but is definitely more versatile.

Another drug class of benefit is the NK-1 antagonists. With non-sedating side effects, these drugs will add a new modality to the multimodal approach of nausea prophylaxis without the increase in postoperative length of stay. Aprepitant is the primary example of this drug. Previously, it was only available as an oral, but now has an intravenous form. The advantage of the drug is its long half-life; in the IV form, it is 9–13 hours. This drug has an indication for postoperative nausea and vomiting, but so far much of the marketing and research is targeted on chemotherapy-induced nausea and vomiting.[2]

There are now intravenous forms of old friends available and new recommendations for others, too. Intravenous acetaminophen finally made it to US shores and has been used successfully in many practices. IV ibuprofen has been available for a couple years more. The benefit touted is reduction in opioid use that should translate into less postoperative nausea and vomiting and shorter recovery times.[3,4] Both have the additional benefit of indications for fever reduction according to their package inserts. However, IV acetaminophen does not reduce opioid usage in all studies, but at least improved the quality of pain relief.[5] A few studies have shown that acetaminophen works centrally in the serotonergic system and the analgesic effects of acetaminophen may be blocked by the co-administration of a 5-HT$_3$ antagonist.[6] It is unknown if the effects of whole 5-HT$_3$ class anti-emetics are negatively affected by acetaminophen; neither is it known if the sequence of giving ondansetron before or after acetaminophen has any impact. There are also cautions from the Federal Drug Agency (FDA) about limiting the dosages of acetaminophen. If an IV form is given, care must be taken that excessive doses are not given through home management of postoperative pain. The newer federal recommendations are reflected in lower acetaminophen doses available in oral opioid combinations with oxycodone and hydrocodone. Lastly, in a related pain topic, the FDA released a statement in February 2013 warning about the use of codeine in postoperative tonsil patients.[7] Codeine has to be metabolized into an active form of morphine in order to be an effective analgesic. The problem lies in genetic range of metabolism. Some people cannot metabolize the codeine at all, leaving them with inadequate analgesia. On the other hand, the very rare patients that are ultra-fast metabolizers are at risk of death. What happens in these patients is the entire dose of oral codeine is converted into morphine quickly and acts like a large bolus. If the patient has a diagnosis of sleep-disordered breathing or sleep apnea, they may suffer a respiratory arrest. The same may be for children receiving breast milk from a mother with ultra-fast metabolism.

Sugammadex shows promise for its ability to completely reverse the non-competitive neuromuscular blocking agents, vecuronium and rocuronium. It was hoped that this would allow succinylcholine to be replaced. It would also theoretically prevent residual neuromuscular blockade with the associated respiratory risks and feelings of malaise. Furthermore, a complete reversal of blockade would make rocuronium and vecuronium safe for use in patients with neuromuscular disorders.[8] Sugammadex is expensive and has not yet been approved by the FDA in the US, but has been approved in 50 countries including several countries in Europe, Australia, and Japan.

Examples of drugs coming to a TIVA recipe near you are remimazolam and methoxycarbonyl etomidate. Remimazolam is a benzodiazapine that is metabolized by non-specific plasma esterases into a carboxylic acid form that is 400-times less potent. Only a prolonged infusion should create a level of metabolite high enough to cause behavioral effects. Phase 1 trials demonstrate the context-sensitive half-life has a maximum of 7–8 minutes after infusions of 2 hours or more. It also appears to have a recovery time independent from length of time of infusion. A significant advantage over propofol is that the effects of remimazolam can be antagonized or reversed by flumazanil.[9] This has implications for the training required to use remimazolam for sedation, that has limited propofol use to anesthesia-trained providers only.

Methoxycarbonyl etomidate (MOC-etomidate) is similarly quickly metabolized by esterases such as remifentanil and remimazolam. The therapeutic effects of hypnosis and hemodynamic stability are still present, but the sedation and adrenal suppression both quickly dissipate with the discontinuation of an infusion. The carboxylic acid metabolite from MOC-etomidate is 300–400-times less potent at the GABA$_A$ receptor than MOC-etomidate. The metabolite does accumulate rapidly to levels that cause a clinical effect. New efforts are being made to create a drug that is more potent and more resistant to hydrolysis so that the more potent drug will overwhelm the weaker metabolite by lasting longer. Less active drug would be given with subsequent less metabolite created.[9]

Another promising drug is being investigated by a Japanese manufacturer. JM-1232 (–) acts on the $GABA_A$ receptor and is inhibited by flumazanil. However, it is not structurally a benzodiazepine. It can be dissolved in an aqueous solution and has hypnotic effects with hemodynamic stability at clinically relevant doses. It also has anti-nociceptive properties. The most important feature is that it has a therapeutic index of >38.5, which is greater than propofol, midazolam, or etomidate.[9]

New horizons in procedures

Some of the greatest growth for ambulatory surgery will be evolution of surgical procedures and surgical techniques. The gastroenterologists may be on the verge of displacing general surgeons in much the same way interventional cardiologists have encroached on areas once only belonging to cardiac surgeons. NOTES and POEM are two examples. NOTES is Natural Orifice Transluminal Endoscopic Surgery. It is essentially gaining access to intra-abdominal or intra-pelvic organs with an endoscope that passes through the mouth and esophagus into the stomach. From the stomach, the other organs are accessed via an incision made in the stomach. After the procedure, the stomach is closed with endoscopic clips. Other orifices tried include the vagina and the rectum. Most of the work was experimental in the late 2000s and in animals. It is progressing and in 2007 at least one person in India underwent a NOTES excision of an appendix because the abdomen was extensively scarred from a burn. One of the benefits of NOTES is a lack of abdominal incision with less scar and pain. Hernia formation, infection, and adhesions are also reduced. A more difficult question to answer may be who should be doing the surgery? Endoscopists certainly have more dexterity with an endoscope, but they are less familiar with intra-abdominal anatomy than surgeons. It is unknown where the cases are best placed: a GI suite or an operating room. Also unknown is where and who best to do the training. The surgeons and endoscopists have become proactive and created a joint society to address these issues.[10]

POEM is Per Oral Endoscopic Myotomy. It is performed in patients that are usually too ill to otherwise undergo a myotomy for the relief of achalasia.[11]

This procedure involves an endoscope through the mouth and creating an incision in the esophageal lining. A dissection plane is created to the muscle layer and inflated with carbon dioxide. The muscle layers are divided to relieve the obstruction into the stomach and food is allowed to pass. Initial papers came from Japan, and Johns Hopkins is a main center performing this in the United States. It is quickly spreading to other centers, though.

Other surgeries are becoming less invasive as distal structures are being accessed via lumens and structures not previously possible. There are biopsies via the bronchial tree for peripheral lung lesions. Abscesses and pseudocysts of the pancreas can be drained via the stomach. Not all of these may be in ambulatory patients, but the work is being done and as it spreads, it will move more procedures out of the inpatient operating rooms.

Orthopedics is not wanting to be left out and can do joint replacement surgery on an ambulatory basis. The approach for knees is to leave the posterior compartment intact so the surgery is less painful and the new joint more stable. Anesthesia is often a general with a regional nerve catheter placed for postoperative pain management.[12] For hip surgery, the surgeons do a hemi-arthroplasty and, again, regional for pain relief is critical although the regional may be an epidural.[13] Also, mini-invasive techniques are being developed where small pieces are introduced through a minor incision, and then assembled into a complete prosthesis inside the joint area. To be successful, the patients should be done early in the morning as they need to participate in physical therapy in the afternoon. Discharge criteria beyond anesthesia are that they can ambulate, get into and out of bed and a chair, as well as walk down steps. This is aggressive surgery and requires careful patient selection. At the time of this writing, such knee surgery is becoming more common but hip surgery is still being studied for feasibility.[12,13]

Vascular surgeons are now able to do aortic repairs endovascularly. The procedures involve an approach through the femoral artery and deployment of a device to prevent or treat an aneurysm. In the United States, a feasibility study in 2014 looked at 79 patients having AAA repair. The authors allowed home discharge after an uneventful repair and 6-hour recovery. Of the 79 patients, 23 were able to be discharged home and only one was readmitted on postoperative day 3. There was a tendency for fewer

ASA class 4 patients and a higher percentage of general anesthesia in the group that went home. The patients participating had to have a good functional capacity and supportive home life. The cost studies may prove prohibitive if readmission rates become too high.[14] Another group was able to perform and publish on 96 outpatient endovascular aneurysm repairs. This group found high patient satisfaction, good cost comparison, and a low readmission rate (4%). Again, the patients were all carefully screened and had to meet discharge criteria including consent of the surgeon and anesthesiologist. All patients had an office visit for postoperative days 1 and 5.[15] In both cases, it seems the possibilities are only limited by advancing techniques and good patient selection.

Patient selection

In the United States, the average of the population is getting older as the Baby Boomer generation continues to age. Along with age come the inevitable debilities. In the previous chapter, we have already discussed the effective use of preoperative testing. Testing should only be driven by history and with a specific reason for the evaluation. By corollary, it is possible to perform anesthesia on patients who get classified as an ASA 3 or 4 in the ambulatory setting. The paper by Fleischer *et al.* described evaluation for cardiac risk factors for non-cardiac surgery in 2007, and was recently updated in 2014. The taskforce he was a member of determined that as the surgery itself becomes more "low-risk", sicker patients can be considered.[16] Rating a patient as an ASA class 3 or 4 means that the disease they have is either poorly controlled or places them at a constant threat of death. In order to do these cases, it means that the surgery itself becomes less of a physiologic assault and that the anesthetic can be performed in a way that homeostasis can be maintained during and after. Cataract surgery demonstrates this perfectly. Lens replacement started out as a multiple-hour procedure that required patients to lie very still the entire time. The only way to accomplish this was through general anesthesia. As the surgeons and techniques progressed, the level of anesthesia lessened. Now, an implant can be placed in minutes and with a topical eye drop. It would be naïve to think that as we continue to evolve surgical and anesthesia care, that we do not need to widen who may be considered.

Creating a patient alliance

The Internet has been a boon for the information society. It is now very easy to use a symptom or physical complaint in an Internet search engine and come up with a number of diagnoses and advertisements for medical providers to treat it all on the same webpage! Medicine was once a mystery that was only known to those who went to medical school. Now, anyone can search a term, read a blog, and read reviews of treatments and providers. We always seek to have informed consent from our patients, but it is now possible that patients get too much information without the appropriate filters to distinguish what is relevant. Marketers also reach out to patients with print and broadcast advertising to offer solutions to medical problems that they need to request from their providers. It is important to realize that patients are not likely searching terms just because they want to treat themselves. If that were true, they would never appear in your facility. Instead, they are likely trying to alleviate anxiety about an issue cognitively by learning as much as they can and projecting a path they need to travel in order to heal. Without the temper of medical training to guide them, their expectations may not reflect reality.

The answer to successfully manage patients like these is one magic word: because. Patients cannot perform their own anesthetics and need services from a provider in order to have surgery. Often the anesthesia provider is a stranger whom they meet on the day of surgery. Dismissing a patient's questions that they found on the Internet is not a good way to form a therapeutic relationship. Instead, try listening earnestly. When you have formulated a plan, tell them why. For example, someone may say he does not want a general anesthetic because he fears being paralyzed and awake. He read about it online and demands that you use one of those "awareness monitors" on him. You may reply, "For this procedure I feel confident it is not necessary *because* paralytic agents are not routinely used and every breath is monitored for how much anesthesia gas you are receiving. It is very well documented what levels of anesthesia are needed for unawareness and patients have movement before recall. However, I will use the extra monitor if you wish *because* I want you to feel at ease." These statements demonstrate that you are considering an important issue the patient has. It also gives you the opportunity to be a consultant of anesthesia the way you were trained.

Pay for performance and outcome measurement

The epiphany by the federal government was that they wanted measurable quality healthcare that they could pay less for. In order to achieve this, a group of quality measures were developed for all types of medical practices by the Centers for Medicare and Medicaid Services (CMS). Four of them apply to anesthesia and they are all process measures and not outcomes. They are:

- Measure #30 Perioperative Care: Timely Administration of Prophylactic Parenteral Antibiotics
- Measure #44 Coronary Artery Bypass Graft: Preoperative Beta-Blocker in patients with Isolated CABG surgery
- Measure #76 Prevention of Catheter-Related Bloodstream Infections
- Measure #193 Perioperative Temperature Management

The measures are fairly straightforward. Number 30 requires that an appropriate antibiotic is started within an hour of skin incision or procedure start if no incision is made. A two-hour window is allowed for quinolones and vancomycin. The preferred antibiotics are first- or second-generation cephalosporins. Measure #44 requires a dose of beta-blocker be given within 24 hours of incision for coronary bypass operations. Measure #76 requires use of a bundle for insertion of central lines. Measure #193 requires patients that have an anesthesia billed time of 60 minutes or greater have a temperature of at least 36.0°C between the time of 15 minutes prior to arrival in recovery and 30 minutes after arrival. If a forced-air warming device was used, the goal is met regardless of temperature.

These measures are part of a Physician Quality Reporting System (PQRS) approved by CMS to ensure quality. The program is initially geared to reward simple reporting. As it matures, it will reward achieving threshold goals by increasing CMS payments by 1% or 2%. That will be followed by penalizing payments by 2% for non-reporting or not meeting thresholds. Decreases in CMS payments can also be avoided if practices or providers are involved in other approved CMS quality projects such as developing or participating in an Accountable Care Organization (ACO). The information given here is relatively general and dates and measures remain in flux. In order to see what is most current, the CMS website would be the best resource, and the information is available at www.CMS.gov. The information currently resides under the Medicare tab, then under the Physician Quality Reporting System in the Quality section.

Choices exist in where to report practice data. It can be directly to PQRS via billing data. It can also be reported via an approved database. The American Society of Anesthesiologists support a database managed by the Anesthesia Quality Institute (AQI). Its database can report the data and membership in AQI is included in ASA member's dues. The AQI also works with sub-specialty databases to include them in PQRS reporting, too. The Society for Ambulatory Anesthesia currently is one of the sub-specialty societies that manages a database with an AQI relationship.

Whereas much attention is being paid to the CMS mandates, other payers of medical care are joining in. Some private insurers such as Anthem and Aetna are negotiating payment rates that have a pay-for-performance aspect to them. Examples are use of preferred generic medications, documenting compliance with an asthma plan, or providing aspirin administration to patients in the emergency department with complaints of chest pain. There are no anesthesia requirements now, but it is presumed they will be developed. Whereas they may be completely reward-based, they, too, may evolve to be more of a stick and less of a carrot to influence providers. It would probably be best to be proactive in creating meaningful measures in anesthesia practices so that the measures are relevant and not just useless mandates.

Politics of anesthesia practice: present and future

Medical practice in the United States is in a state of dramatic flux. Not only are payments to providers shifting from fee-for-service toward quality-based parameters, but patients are evolving, too. As mentioned before, the Internet is a ready source of unfiltered medical information. Patients are also becoming more responsible for paying for healthcare. As cost of coverage rises, plans with greater deductibles are becoming a less-expensive option. This means that patients need to be careful how they spend their money and may choose what procedures they are willing to have done. Transparency of cost will be a strong benefit to those practicing in the ambulatory setting. Whereas predicting a hospital bill from a procedure can be very difficult, the flat fees charged by ambulatory centers are very predictable. To maintain a patient base, groups may have to place their costs at a more competitive level to maintain insurance contracts. All the while, quality indicators have to be maintained and made available for patients to see and evaluate.

Organized anesthesia will be very critical in creating agreed standards and measurements. It can also be a communication source for the specialty of anesthesia. Government controls CMS reimbursement and gives money for resident and fellowship training. Having a strong voice when these issues are discussed will be critical for the future of anesthesiology. The development of ACOs means that a given dollar for a procedure will have to be divided among all of the providers. Strong leadership will help ensure a fair anesthesia share. As national databases are managed and researched, finer points of anesthesia care may emerge. In order to see that these be properly translated into standards, a strong society needs to lead it. Much of anesthesia care and the high level of safety afforded to patients is in part due to the propagation of standards of care by our society.

Individually, anesthesia providers can make themselves more visible to hospital leadership and community providers. Becoming involved with management of the operating rooms is critical. We have a unique view that sees how many of the equipment and personnel pieces fit together. Managing a daily schedule efficiently will be even more valued as the pot of healthcare dollars shrinks. Involvement in hospital or facility committees is very important so our voices are heard and expertise can be appreciated. Participation in local and national anesthesia societies will also carry our voice and give us control over our future.

Like medical practice in general, board certification is evolving. Maintenance of Certification in Anethesiology (MOCA) has been around for more than a decade. For anesthesiologists young in their practice, it is a reality. For the more senior members, lifetime certification may not be good enough. Hospitals and groups may require MOCA for ongoing privileging. CMS has joined in by increasing payments by 0.5% to providers enrolled in the ABA MOCA program. Certification in a sub-specialty

area by the American Board of Anesthesiology (ABA) requires MOCA participation, too. MOCA went from a simple exam to a four-part requirement. There is: professional standing, evidence of lifelong learning, cognitive evaluation, and practice performance assessment and improvement. Professional standing requires the diplomat to hold an unrestricted medical license. It is required to have 250 continuing medical education (CME) credits, limited by year. Ninety CME credits need to be from approved self-assessment and 20 CME credits need to be about patient safety. The examination is a 200-question test that takes place in years 7 through 10 of the 10-year cycle. The practice assessment and improvement require performing a quality project to demonstrate improvement in a measure of the anesthesiologist's practice. It also requires an assessment via a simulation exercise. Either one may be performed in the first 5 years, and the other in the next 4. There is an attestation that must be made in year 9. The most current certification information can be found on the ABA website: www.theABA.org.

References

1. Marcet JE, Nfonsam VN, Sergio Larach S. An extended pain relief trial utilizing the infiltration of a long-acting multivesicular liposome formulation of bupivacaine, EXPAREL (IMPROVE): a Phase IV health economic trial in adult patients undergoing ileostomy reversal. *J Pain Res* 2013;**6**:549–55.

2. Highlights for prescribing information [for Emend]. Copyright © 2008, 2009 Merck Sharp & Dohme Corp., a subsidiary of Merck & Co., Inc.

3. Singla N, Rock A, Pavliv L. A multi-center, randomized, double-blind placebo-controlled trial of intravenous-ibuprofen (IV-ibuprofen) for treatment of pain in postoperative orthopedic adult patients. *Pain Med* 2010;**11**:1284–93.

4. Sinatra RS, Jahr JS, Reynolds LW, Viscusi ER, Groudine SB, Payen-Champenois C. Efficacy and safety of single and repeated administration of 1 gram intravenous acetaminophen injection (paracetamol) for pain management after major orthopedic surgery. *Anesthesiology* 2005 Apr;**102**(4):822–31.

5. Cakan T, Inan N, Culhaoglu S, Bakkal K, Başar H. Intravenous paracetamol improves the quality of postoperative analgesia but does not decrease narcotic requirements. *J Neurosurg Anesthesiol* 2008 Jul;**20**(3):169–73.

6. Pickering G, Loriot MA, Libert F, Eschalier A, Beaune P, Dubray C. Analgesic effect of acetaminophen in

humans: first evidence of a central serotonergic mechanism. *Clin Pharmacol Ther* 2006;**79**:371–78.

7. FDA Drug Safety Communication 02-20-2013.

8. Schaller SJ, Fink H. Sugammadex as a reversal agent for neuromuscular block: an evidence-based review. *Core Evidence* 2013;**8**:57–67.

9. Chitilian HV, Eckenhoff RG, Raines DE. Anesthetic drug development: novel drugs and new approaches. *Surg Neurol Int* 2013 Mar 19;**4**(Suppl 1):S2–S10.

10. Baron TH. Natural orifice transluminal endoscopic surgery. *Br J Surg* 2007;**94**:1–2.

11. Inoue H, Minami H, Kobayashi Y, *et al.* Peroral endoscopic myotomy (POEM) for esophageal achalasia. *Endoscopy* 2010;**42**:265–71.

12. Berger RA, Kusuma SK, Sanders SA, Thill ES, Sporer SM. The feasibility and perioperative complications of outpatient knee arthroplasty. *Clin Orthop Rel Res* 2009;**467**:1443–49.

13. Berger RA, Sanders SA, Thill ES, Sporer SM, Della Valle C. Newer anesthesia and rehabilitation protocols enable outpatient hip replacement in selected patients. *Clin Orthop Rel Res* 2009;**467**:1424–30.

14. Dosluoglu HH, Lall P, Blochle R, Harris LM, Dryjski ML. Ambulatory percutaneous endovascular abdominal aortic aneurysm repair. *J Vasc Surg* 2014;**59**:58–64.

15. Lachat ML, Pecoraro F, Mayer D, *et al.* Outpatient endovascular aortic aneurysm repair: experience in 100 consecutive patients. *Ann Surg* 2013;**258**:754–59.

16. Fleisher LA, Beckman JA, Brown KA, *et al.* ACC/AHA 2007 guidelines on perioperative cardiovascular evaluation and care for noncardiac surgery: a report of the American College of Cardiology/American Heart Association Task Force on practice guidelines (Writing Committee to revise the 2002 guidelines on perioperative cardiovascular evaluation and care for noncardiac surgery). *Circulation* 2007;**116**:e418–e500.

Index

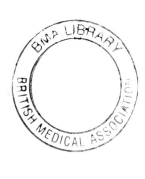